Cancer Treatment and Research

Volume 164

Series editor

Steven T. Rosen, Duarte, CA, USA

More information about this series at http://www.springer.com/series/5808

Karl Y. Bilimoria · Christina A. Minami
David M. Mahvi
Editors

Comparative Effectiveness in Surgical Oncology

Key Questions and How to Answer Them

Springer

Editors
Karl Y. Bilimoria
Department of Surgery
Northwestern University
Chicago, IL
USA

David M. Mahvi
Department of Surgery
Northwestern University
Chicago, IL
USA

Christina A. Minami
Northwestern University
Chicago, IL
USA

ISSN 0927-3042
Cancer Treatment and Research
ISBN 978-3-319-12552-7 ISBN 978-3-319-12553-4 (eBook)
DOI 10.1007/978-3-319-12553-4

Library of Congress Control Number: 2014959410

Springer Cham Heidelberg New York Dordrecht London

Printed on acid-free paper

Springer International Publishing AG Switzerland is part of Springer Science+Business Media (www.springer.com)

The opportunity to write a dedication gives me the unique chance to thank my parents and mentors for preparing me well to hopefully be successful in life, surgery, and research. I also appreciate beyond words the love and support from my wife and girls—I couldn't do it without you.

—Karl Y. Bilimoria

Preface

Most surgical oncology textbooks are distillations of the current literature that guide us in treatment decisions and clinical practice. They are reliable, practical, and comprehensive pictures of where our field stands. But how do we push forward? Major unresolved questions persist in the oncologic world despite tremendous strides in recent years. How do we address these and continue our advancement?

Comparative effectiveness research (CER) is a relatively new name for an old concept. By the Institute of Medicine's definition, it is the synthesis of evidence that compares the benefits and harms of alternative methods to prevent, diagnose, treat, and monitor a clinical condition or to improve the delivery of care. Though randomized controlled trials function as our gold standard, we must often, for a variety of reasons, look to alternative CER techniques for answers. These approaches may include well-conducted retrospective cohort studies from cancer registries and other data sources, decision and cost-effectiveness analyses, and other novel methodologies.

This book lays out the current critical questions for a variety of solid-organ malignancies, identifies the barriers to obtaining high-level evidence, and proposes potential approaches to the fundamental questions of each disease.

We would like to recognize the creativity and expertise demonstrated by all of the authors. While other textbooks require an intimate knowledge of a particular malignancy, this book also required the authors to imagine solutions to the most fundamental questions in their field. We believe that it is this type of progressive thinking and research that will spur the evolution of surgical oncology.

Karl Y. Bilimoria
Christina A. Minami
David M. Mahvi

Acknowledgments

The editors would like to acknowledge Ms. Remi Love for her dedication and attention to detail in helping us compile this book.

Contents

Contributors

Elliot A. Asare Department of Surgery, Medical College of Wisconsin, Milwaukee, WI, USA

Jim Belotte Division of Surgical Oncology, Department of Surgery, Northwestern University, Chicago, USA

David J. Bentrem Division of Surgical Oncology, Department of Surgery, Northwestern University, Chicago, USA; Robert H. Lurie Comprehensive Cancer Center of Northwestern University, Chicago, IL, USA; Jesse Brown VA Medical Center, Chicago, IL, USA

Karl Y. Bilimoria Department of Surgery, Feinberg School of Medicine, Surgical Outcomes and Quality Improvement Center, Northwestern University, Chicago, IL, USA

Jeanette W. Chung Department of Surgery, Feinberg School of Medicine, Northwestern University, Chicago, IL, USA

David Cosgrove Department of Medical Oncology, Johns Hopkins Hospital, Baltimore, MD, USA

Keith A. Delman Department of Surgery, Emory University, Atlanta, GA, USA

Lane L. Frasier Department of Surgery, University of Wisconsin Hospital and Clinics, Madison, WI, USA

Caprice C. Greenberg Department of Surgery, University of Wisconsin Hospital and Clinics, Madison, WI, USA

Katherine A. Hutcheson Department of Head and Neck Surgery, University of Texas MD Anderson Cancer Center, Houston, TX, US

Haejin In Departments of Surgery and Epidemiology, Albert Einstein College of Medicine, Bronx, NY, USA

Christine C. Jensen University of Minnesota, Minneapolis, MN, USA; Colon and Rectal Surgery Associates, Minneapolis, MN, USA

Christine V. Kinnier Department of Surgery, Massachusetts General Hospital, Boston, MA, USA

Lawrence M. Knab Division of Surgical Oncology, Department of Surgery, Northwestern University, Chicago, USA

Michael E. Kupferman Department of Head and Neck Surgery, University of Texas MD Anderson Cancer Center, Houston, TX, US

Carol M. Lewis Department of Head and Neck Surgery, University of Texas MD Anderson Cancer Center, Houston, TX, US

Robert D. Madoff University of Minnesota, Minneapolis, MN, USA

Hidayatullah G. Munshi Division of Hematology/Oncology, Department of Medicine, Feinberg School of Medicine, Northwestern University, Chicago, IL, USA; Robert H. Lurie Comprehensive Cancer Center of Northwestern University, Chicago, IL, USA; Jesse Brown VA Medical Center, Chicago, IL, USA

Heather B. Neuman Department of Surgery, University of Wisconsin Hospital and Clinics, Madison, WI, USA

Andrew J. Page Division of Surgical Oncology, John L. Cameron Professor of Alimentary Tract Surgery, Department of Surgery, Johns Hopkins Hospital, Baltimore, MD, USA

Sonali Patankar Department of Obstetrics and Gynecology, Columbia University College of Physicians and Surgeons, New York, US

Timothy M. Pawlik Division of Surgical Oncology, John L. Cameron Professor of Alimentary Tract Surgery, Department of Surgery, Johns Hopkins Hospital, Baltimore, MD, USA

Mitchell C. Posner Division of Surgical Oncology, Department of Surgery, University of Chicago, Chicago, IL, USA

Maria C. Russel Department of Surgery, Emory University, Atlanta, GA, USA

Seth A. Strope Division of Urologic Surgery, Washington University School of Medicine, St. Louis, MO, USA

Ana I. Tergas Department of Obstetrics and Gynecology, Columbia University College of Physicians and Surgeons, New York, US; Department of Epidemiology, Mailman School of Public Health, Columbia University, New York, US

Thomas K. Varghese Division of Thoracic Surgery, Department of Surgery, Harborview Medical Center, University of Washington, Seattle, WA, USA

Tracy S. Wang Department of Surgery, Medical College of Wisconsin, Milwaukee, WI, USA

Nabil Wasif Department of Surgery, Mayo Clinic Arizona, Phoenix, AZ, USA

Jason D. Wright Department of Obstetrics and Gynecology, Columbia University College of Physicians and Surgeons, New York, US; Herbert Irving Comprehensive Cancer Center, Columbia University College of Physicians and Surgeons, New York, US

Approaches to Answering Critical CER Questions

Christine V. Kinnier, Jeanette W. Chung and Karl Y. Bilimoria

Abstract

While randomized controlled trials (RCTs) are the gold standard for research, many research questions cannot be ethically and practically answered using an RCT. Comparative effectiveness research (CER) techniques are often better suited than RCTs to address the effects of an intervention under routine care conditions, an outcome otherwise known as effectiveness. CER research techniques covered in this section include: effectiveness-oriented experimental studies such as pragmatic trials and cluster randomized trials, treatment response heterogeneity, observational and database studies including adjustment techniques such as sensitivity analysis and propensity score analysis, systematic reviews and meta-analysis, decision analysis, and cost effectiveness analysis. Each section describes the technique and covers the strengths and weaknesses of the approach.

Keywords

Comparative effectiveness research · Surgical oncology · Observational and database studies · Pragmatic trials

C.V. Kinnier
Department of Surgery, Massachusetts General Hospital, Boston, MA, USA

J.W. Chung
Department of Surgery, Feinberg School of Medicine, Northwestern University, Chicago, IL, USA

K.Y. Bilimoria (✉)
Surgical Outcomes and Quality Improvement Center, Department of Surgery, Feinberg School of Medicine, Northwestern University, Chicago, IL, USA
e-mail: k-bilimoria@nmff.org

K.Y. Bilimoria et al. (eds.), *Comparative Effectiveness in Surgical Oncology*, Cancer Treatment and Research 164, DOI 10.1007/978-3-319-12553-4_1

Contents

1 Introduction

Significant advances in evidence-based medicine have occurred over the past two decades, but segments of medical care are still practiced without underlying scientific evidence. Many practice patterns are so firmly established as the standard of care that a randomized controlled trial (RCT) would be unethical. Where evidence from RCTs exist, the study population is narrow and not easily applicable to most patients. Finally, multiple treatments are firmly engrained in clinical practice and have never been rigorously questioned.

Answering most of these knowledge gaps with an RCT, however, would be unethical, impractical, or dissimilar to routine care. In the last case, this is because an RCT is concerned with measuring efficacy: the effect of an intervention as compared to placebo when all other variables are held constant. In other words, an RCT creates a study environment in which outcome differences are most attributable to the intervention. While RCTs accurately identify treatment effects under ideal conditions, patients do not receive their routine care under those conditions. When it comes to routine patient care, physicians are less interested in efficacy than effectiveness: the effect of an intervention under routine care conditions. In order to study effectiveness, health care investigators have developed a toolbox of alternative techniques, known collectively as comparative effectiveness research (CER).

Both researchers and policy agencies have recognized the power of studying effectiveness. The 2009 government stimulus package allocated $1.1 billion to CER [1]. The following year, the Affordable Care Act proposed multiple health care reforms to improve the value of the United States health care system. These reforms included the foundation of the Patient-Centered Outcomes Research Institute (PCORI), a publically funded, non-governmental institute charged with conducting and funding CER projects [2]. As a result, funding for CER has grown substantially in the past 5 years.

2 Randomized Controlled Trials: Limitations and Alternatives

RCTs are the gold standard of medical research because they measure treatment efficacy, but they remain dissimilar to routine care and are impractical under many circumstances. First, RCTs are often prohibitively expensive and time consuming. One study reported that Phase III, National Institutes of Health-funded RCTs cost an average of $12 million per trial [3]. RCTs also take years to organize, run, and publish. Consequently, results may be outdated by publication. Second, some events or complications are so infrequent that enrolling a sufficiently large study population would be impractical. Third, clinical experts working from high-volume hospitals follow RCT participants closely in order to improve study follow-up and treatment adherence. Following study conclusion, however, routine patients receiving routine care may not achieve the same level of treatment adherence. Therefore study outcomes and routine care outcomes for the same intervention may differ substantially. Fourth, and perhaps most importantly, RCTs are restricted to a narrow patient population and a limited number of study interventions and outcomes. These necessary restrictions also restrict the broad applicability of RCT results.

Clearly investigators cannot rely solely on RCTs to address the unanswered questions in surgical oncology. CER techniques offer multiple alternatives. We will introduce these approaches here and then describe each technique in more detail throughout the series.

3 Experimental Studies

The term "clinical trials" evokes images of blinded, randomized patients receiving treatment from blinded professionals in a highly specialized setting. These RCTs are highly sensitive to the efficacy of the intervention under investigation. In other words, an intervention is most likely to demonstrate benefit in a setting where patients have few confounding medical diagnoses, every dose or interaction is monitored, and patients are followed closely over the study period. Unfortunately, RCTs are often prohibitively expensive and require many years to plan and complete. Furthermore, a medication that is efficacious during a highly-monitored RCT may prove ineffective during routine care where patients more frequently self-discontinue treatment due to unpleasant side effects or inconvenience. Clinical trials performed with the comparative effectiveness mindset aim to address some of these limitations.

3.1 Pragmatic Trials

Due to the constraints of an RCT, results may not be valid outside the trial framework. Pragmatic trials attempt to address this limition in external validity by testing an intervention under routine conditions in a heterogeneous patient population. These routine conditions may include a broad range of adjustments. First, pragmatic trials may have broad inclusion criteria; ideally trial patients are only excluded if they are not intervention candidates outside of the study. Second, the intervention may be compared to routine practice, and clinicians and patients may not be blinded. This approach accepts that placebo effect may augment intervention outcomes when used in routine practice. Third, pragmatic trials may use routine clinic staff rather than topic experts, and staff may be encouraged to adjust the medication or intervention as they would in routine practice. Fourth, patient-reported outcomes may be measured in addition to—or instead of—traditional outcomes. Finally, patients are usually analyzed according to their assigned intervention arm; this is also known as intention-to-treat analysis. Pragmatic trials may range anywhere along this spectrum: on one end, an otherwise traditional RCT may use an intention-to-treat analysis; on the other, investigators may aim to conduct the study under completely routine circumstances with the exception of intervention randomization. The investigators must determine what level of pragmatism is appropriate for their particular research question.

Pragmatic trials help determine medication or intervention effectiveness in a more realistic clinical setting. The adjustments that make pragmatic trials more realistic, however, also create limitations. Pragmatic studies are conducted under routine clinical circumstances, so an intervention that is effective in a large, well-funded private clinic may not be equally effective in a safety-net clinic. Therefore, clinicians must consider the study setting before instituting similar changes in their own practice. In addition, pragmatic trials include a broad range of eligible patients and consequently contain significant patient heterogeneity. This heterogeneity may dilute the treatment effect and necessitate large sample sizes and extended follow-up periods to achieve adequate statistical power. This may then inflate study cost and counterbalance any money saved by conducting the trial in a routine clinic with routine staff.

3.2 Cluster Randomized Trials

Cluster randomized trials (CRTs) are defined by the randomization of patients by group or practice site rather than by individual. Beyond group randomization, CRTs may use either traditional RCT techniques or pragmatic trial techniques. Group level randomization has multiple effects. Group contamination is uncommon since participants are less likely to know study participants from other sites. This makes CRTs ideally suited for interventions that are organizational, policy-based, or provider-directed. With these education or resource-based interventions, well-intentioned participants or physicians may distribute information to control-arm participants without the investigator's knowledge. Risks of cross contamination are significantly lowered when participants from different study arms are separated by site and less likely to know one another. Group randomization also better simulates real-world practice since a single practice usually follows the same treatment protocol for most of its patients. Finally, physicians and clinic staff can be educated on the site-specific intervention and then care for patients under relatively routine circumstances. In some circumstances this may help to coordinate blinding, minimize paperwork, and reduce infrastructure and personnel demands.

Clustered patient randomization, however, introduces analytical barriers. Patients often choose clinics for a specific reason, so patient populations may differ more among clinics than within clinics. Furthermore, differences may not be easily measurable (e.g., patients may differ significantly in how much education they expect and receive prior to starting a new medication), so adjusting for these differences may be difficult during analysis. Consequently, cluster randomization requires hierarchical modeling to account for similarities within groups and differences between groups, but hierarchical modeling produces wider confidence intervals. As with pragmatic trials, this may require increases in subject number and follow-up time in order to detect clinically significant outcome differences. Unfortunately, individual participant enrollment is usually limited within each cluster, so increasing a trial's statistical power usually requires enrollment of additional clusters.

3.3 Adaptive Trials

Due to a history of unethical research, like the Tuskegee Syphilis Study, RCTs now undergo multiple interim analyses [4]. These routine evaluations check for interim results that may make trial continuation unethical, such as changes in routine care, early and robust outcome differences, or failure to see outcome differences where expected. Early termination prevents the inferior outcome group from suffering further harm.

Simply initiating an RCT, however, requires significant time, funding, and energy. Rather than terminating a trial, adaptive trials take advantage of interim analyses to adjust the trial conditions or outcomes and address further treatment questions. Changes to adaptive trials may include adjustments to eligibility criteria, randomization procedure, treatment dose or duration, or the number of interim analyses. They may also incorporate the addition of concomitant treatments or secondary endpoints. To prevent the introduction of bias, both the adjustments and the circumstances under which they are introduced must be clearly delineated prior to trial initiation.

Unblinding the data for interim analysis may introduce bias, so data and resulting analyses must be sequestered from clinicians and patients still participating in the trial. Changing a study's outcomes may also cloak long term results. A medication that provides significant benefit after one year may have dangerous long term side effects that will remain unknown if a study is adapted. The investigator must therefore remember that any planned adaptations may affect important secondary outcomes.

4 Treatment-Response Heterogeneity

RCTs study the efficacy of a drug at a specific dose and frequency, but patients may vary widely in their ability to metabolize a medication or their response to a standard serum level. Furthermore, patient comorbidities may variably affect their susceptibility to drug side effects. These variations in effectiveness are collectively known as treatment-response heterogeneity.

There are three major techniques for addressing treatment-response heterogeneity. If the affected population and heterogeneity are already known, then a new trial may stratify patients according to the groups that require investigation and evaluate for outcome differences. If the affected population and heterogeneity are unknown, then data from a previous trial may be divided into subgroups and reanalyzed. This raises a number of analytical issues of which the investigator must be aware. The original trial may be insufficiently powered to detect differences in subgroups, especially when those subgroups are small segments of the larger study population. If the study is sufficiently powered, the investigator must analyze the subgroups appropriately. Evaluating the treatment effect within a subgroup is not sufficient to draw conclusions about treatment-response heterogeneity within that subgroup. Treatment effects within the subgroup must also be compared to remaining subgroups in order to determine if treatment-response heterogeneity truly exists within the subgroup of interest as compared to the general population. If subgroups are too small for formal subgroup analysis, the investigator may simply check for correlation between the concerning subgroup variable and the treatment. High correlation between the two suggests treatment-response heterogeneity.

Health care studies have recently employed a fourth technique known as finate mixture models [5]. These models allow certain covariate coefficients to vary for patient variables containing treatment-response heterogeneity. While new, this technique has been used with increasing frequency in health care cost modeling and is likely to find other applications in coming years.

5 Observational and Database Studies

In contrast to the experimental studies described above, observational and database studies examine patients and outcomes in the setting of routine care. Observational studies—which include cohort studies, case-control studies, and cross-sectional studies—and database studies help generate hypotheses when insufficient evidence exists to justify a randomized trial or when a randomized trial would be unethical.

5.1 Commonly Used Datasets

Databases are an excellent data repository for large numbers of patients. Data may be collected retrospectively or prospectively. While many institutions maintain their own databases to facilitate single institution studies, we will focus here on some commonly used and readily available national databases that are relevant to surgical oncology.

The Nationwide Inpatient Sample (NIS) [6] is the largest all-payer, inpatient database in the United States and is sponsored by the Agency for Healthcare Research and Quality. Data elements are collected retrospectively from administrative billing data and include primary and secondary diagnosis codes, procedure codes, total charges, primary payer, and length of stay. Data collection does not extend beyond discharge, however, and patient data cannot be linked across inpatient episodes. This means that even short-term variables like readmission and 30-day mortality cannot be measured. Limited information on patient demographics and hospital characteristics may be obtained by linking to other databases where permitted, but additional clinical details are unavailable. Consequently, patient-level risk adjustment and investigation of clinical complications or intermediate outcomes are largely impossible. Even with these limitations, the NIS is an all-payer, inpatient database. This makes the NIS a valuable resource for investigators interested in care and hospital cost differences associated with insurance coverage or changes in procedure use over time. Furthermore, NIS data is relatively inexpensive and available to any investigator that completes the online training.

The American College of Surgeons National Surgical Quality Improvement Program (ACS NSQIP) [7] maintains a database of 30-day outcomes for all qualifying operations at ACS NSQIP hospitals. In contrast to the NIS, data elements in ACS NSQIP are collected prospectively by a trained nurse registrar. This significantly improves data quality by minimizing missing data elements and standardizing data entry. Data elements include patient demographics and comorbidities, operative and anesthesia details, preoperative laboratory values and 30-day postoperative morbidity and mortality. Hospital participation in NSQIP is voluntary, so unlike the NIS, ACS NSQIP data skews toward large, well-funded hospitals. Datasets from the ACS NSQIP are free but only available to ACS NSQIP participants.

The reach of ACS NSQIP is expanded significantly by linking to the National Cancer Data Base (NCDB) [8]. The NCDB, is a joint program of the Commission on Cancer (CoC) and the American Cancer Society. Like ACS NSQIP, the NCDB is a prospective database collected by trained registrars that provides high quality, reliable data. The NCDB collects data elements on about 70 % of cancer patients who receive treatment at a CoC-accredited cancer program. In addition to patient demographics and tumor characteristics, the database also contains data elements regarding chemotherapy, radiation, and tumor-specific surgical outcomes that are not available through the standard ACS NSQIP database. Perhaps most powerfully, registrars enter 5-year mortality data for all patients in the database. The NCDB is moderately priced but is publically available once an investigator has completed the mandatory training. Data linking to the ACS NSQIP database, however, is only available to investigators from ACS NSQIP hospitals.

The NCDB only collects data from cancer patients who receive care at CoC-accredited hospitals. Consequently, many minorities are underrepresented within the NCDB. In order to encourage high quality research on cancer epidemiology, the National Cancer Institute developed the Surveillance, Epidemiology, and End Results Program (SEER) [9]. SEER is a prospective database that over-represents minority cancer patients. For example, SEER samples all cancer patients in Connecticut but only collects data on Arizona cancer patients who are Native Americans. Like the NCDB, SEER data is also compiled by trained registrars thus making the data high quality and reliable. SEER elements include patient demographics, cancer stage, first treatment course, and survival. SEER is publically available following mandatory training but does have a modest data compilation fee. SEER may also be linked to cost and payer datapoints through the Medicare database for an additional price.

While research using each of these databases is associated with its own challenges, databases remain an excellent resource for large sample, retrospective research and offer a good starting point for many effectiveness research questions.

5.2 Sensitivity Analysis

Third-party, observational databases like those described above rarely contain the precise data elements with the precise coding desired by the investigator. Investigators may need to merge data elements to create a new study variable or define parameters to categorize a continuous data element. These decisions may unintentionally affect analytic results. Investigators can determine whether study results are robust using sensitivity analysis. An analysis is first run using parameters and specifications identified by the investigator, and the results are noted. Slight changes to variable definitions are then made and the analysis is rerun. Substantial changes in results suggest the results are largely dependent on investigator-selected parameters and specifications. Conversely, unchanged or similar results suggest the results are robust.

5.3 Propensity Score Analysis

Observational studies are primarily limited by the absence of randomization. In routine care, clinicians guide patients towards certain treatments based on the clinician's experience and the patient's primary condition and comorbidities. In order to control for these non-random choices in clinical care, propensity score analysis (PSA) attempts to match treatment subjects to control subjects with similar traits that may influence treatment choice and outcome. The investigator first identifies covariates that are likely to predict which patients received treatment, such as patient comorbidities or underlying disease severity. Using logistic regression, a propensity score is then calculated for each subject. Subjects who received treatment are matched to subjects with similar propensity scores who did not receive treatment, and outcomes for the two subject groups are then compared using multivariable analysis.

Matching methods vary widely amongst investigators. One-to-one subject matching, where each subject receiving treatment A is uniquely matched to a single subject receiving treatment B, is the most common, but multiple treatment B subjects may be used to improve statistical power. In addition, matching techniques may either optimize matching for the entire group and thereby minimize the total within-pair differences in propensity scores, or matching may be optimized for each patient as they are encountered in the dataset. In the latter case, the within-pair difference is minimized for the first subject but within-pair differences may increase as control subjects are progressively assigned to patients in the treatment group. In some cases, control subjects are replaced so that they can be used as the matched-pair for multiple treatment subjects, but this must be done uniformly throughout the matching process.

PSA is most limited by the covariates available in the dataset. For example, if tumor size is not recorded consistently then tumor size cannot be used to calculate the propensity score, and treatment differences will not be matched for tumor size. Conversely, including too many irrelevant covariates during propensity score calculation may minimize differences between groups and produce false negative results. The investigator must therefore optimize the number of covariates in the model so that patients are adequately matched but real group differences may be detected.

5.4 Subgroup Analysis

As mentioned above, PSA corrects for measured confounders in a dataset, but there is often reason to suspect that unmeasured confounders may be affecting the analysis. Subgroup analysis is one way to identify whether results have been biased by unmeasured covariates. There are multiple ways to use subgroup analysis to identify bias caused by unmeasured covariates; two are described here.

Observational studies most often compare treatment subjects to control subjects, but control subjects may include multiple subgroups. For example, if the treatment of interest is a medication, investigators typically assume that control subjects are patients who are not currently taking, and have never taken, the medication. But it is possible that control subjects used the medication in the past but stopped many years ago (remote users) or used the medication in the past but stopped recently (recent users). Control subjects may also be actively receiving a similar therapy using a different class of medications (alternative users). These subgroups can be leveraged to determine whether the study results are robust. In a typical observational study interested in complications from a medication, the investigator would compare the treatment subjects to all control subjects. With subgroup analysis, the investigator might compare treatment subjects to each control subgroup. Significantly different results in each subgroup analysis suggest that unmeasured variables have affected treatment choice and outcomes. In contrast, similar results in each subgroup analysis suggest that unmeasured confounders do not exist and the results are robust. The ability to use this technique largely depends on whether relevant subgroups exist and whether those subgroups are large enough to detect statistical differences.

5.5 Instrumental Variable Analysis

Subgroup analysis can detect unmeasured confounders, but in some cases, an analysis can actually correct for unmeasured confounders using instrumental variable analysis. Instrumental variable analysis essentially simulates randomization in observational data through the use of an instrument: an unbiased variable that differentially affects subject exposure or intervention but is uncorrelated with the measured outcome. Subjects are then grouped by treatment adjusted for the instrument, and outcomes are evaluated. If outcomes are similar regardless of instrument group, then treatment does not affect outcomes; if outcomes differ, then differences in outcomes between instrument groups can be attributed to natural bias in group assignment.

A well-known example of instrumental variable analysis is the Oregon Medicaid health experiment. In 2008, Oregon expanded its Medicaid program. Due to funding limitations, Oregon used a lottery to select the additional individuals who would receive Medicaid and those who would not. Investigators took advantage of this natural experiment and used differential access to Medicaid as an instrument. Investigators then evaluated the effects of Medicaid enrollment on health outcomes in low-income Oregon residents [10]. Sudden and random policy changes are rare events, but unbiased instruments can be identified through creative thinking. For example, distance to a hospital offering partial nephrectomy has been used as an instrumental variable when evaluating the effect of surgical technique on kidney cancer outcomes [11].

Given that instrumental variable analysis can mitigate the effects of unmeasured confounders, it can be a powerful tool in observational research. Unfortunately, use of the technique is highly dependent on having a reliable and unbiased instrumental variable.

6 Systematic Reviews and Meta-Analysis

Large RCTs that produce definitive results are uncommon due to significant funding and coordination barriers. Frequently, multiple small RCTs will address similar research questions but produce conflicting or non-significant results. In this case, the results of these RCTs can be aggregated to produce more definitive answers.

6.1 Systematic Reviews

Multiple RCTs may address the same research topic with results published in widely varying journals over many years. A systematic review disseminates these research results more concisely through the methodical and exhaustive evaluation of current literature on a specific research question. Investigators start with a research question, or collection of related questions, that are not easily answered by a single study or review. Medical databases are then searched using precise terms. High quality systematic reviews search multiple databases covering multiple disciplines and use redundant and related search terms. While the number of search terms must be brief enough to keep the number of results manageable, authors commonly use too few search terms and therefore miss critical articles on the topic of interest.

Once a list of articles is assembled, each article is carefully screened for eligibility and relevance based on predetermined inclusion and exclusion criteria. Results should summarize not only study results but also the quality of the study. In addition to a traditional results section, systematic reviews typically include a table of articles along with the study results and the level of evidence.

In the surgical community, the CHEST guidelines on venous thromboembolism prophylaxis are perhaps the most well-known systematic review [12]. In addition, the Cochrane collaboration is a not-for-profit, independent organization that produces and publishes systematic reviews on a wide range of healthcare topics, many relevant to surgery [13]. Unfortunately, systematic reviews are limited by the current data and they are unable to merge outcomes from multiple small RCTs. Systematic reviews also become outdated quickly since they do not create any new data. The quality of the conclusions is also highly dependent on the quality of the underlying database review. Despite these limitations, systematic reviews are an effective way to consolidate and disseminate information on a research topic and are often able to reveal trends in study results that are not visible when presented across multiple unique publications.

6.2 Meta-Analysis

Meta-analysis is a form of systematic review in which results from the relevant publications are combined and analyzed together in order to improve statistical power and draw new conclusions. To begin, investigators perform a systematic review, being careful to define the inclusion and exclusion so that study populations are similar. An effect size is calculated for each study and then an average of the effect sizes, weighted by sample size, is calculated. If multiple previous but small studies trended towards an outcome but were not statistically significant, a meta-analysis may produce clear and statistically significant results. If previous studies provided conflicting results, a meta-analysis may demonstrate a significant result in one direction or the other.

A meta-analysis, however, will not necessarily predict the results from a single, large RCT. This is because the results of the meta-analysis are largely dependent on the quality of studies. A few, high-quality RCTs will produce more robust results than multiple, small, low-quality RCTs. In addition, meta-analysis is highly subject to publication bias. Studies with strong, significant results are more likely to be published than studies with equivocal or negative outcomes. This can skew meta-analysis toward a false positive result.

7 Decision Analysis

The comparative effectiveness techniques discussed so far compare one or many treatment options to one another, but they are not equipped to address treatment consequences, including the need for additional evaluation and treatment. Decision analysis attempts to estimate the downstream costs and benefits of these treatment choices. First, a decision tree is developed that includes initial treatment options as well as potential outcomes and their impact on future evaluation and treatment needs. The root of the decision tree will center at either the disease or the sign or symptom requiring evaluation. The final branches of the decision tree should terminate with either treatment cessation or cure or with definitive diagnosis of the sign or symptom in question. The investigator then assigns probabilities to each of the branch points as well as costs and benefits associated with each step in the course of treatment or work up. Finally, the maximum expected utility for each possible pathway in the decision tree is calculated. Some have argued that decision analysis makes an intuitive process cumbersome and time consuming, but research repeatedly demonstrates that high quality decision analysis produces more effective decisions than intuition alone.

The investigator should optimize decision tree usefulness rather than maximize potential complexity. Keeping the target decision maker in mind helps to identify which decision points are necessary and which can be collapsed into existing branches. If the investigator is unsure whether a decision point is necessary, then extreme cost and benefit values can be substituted for a questioned decision point. If the optimal outcome is unaffected, then the decision point is superfluous.

Decision analysis highly depends on assignment of accurate probabilities as well as costs and benefits. This is most challenging with non-monetary, analog outcomes such as quality of life or emotional distress. Without realistic estimates, however, the entire decision analysis will be inaccurate. The burden falls on the analyst to thoroughly research each treatment branch and estimate costs and benefits based on the best available data. If sufficient information is not available to develop an accurate decision analysis, then preliminary studies may be needed before decision analysis is attempted.

8 Cost Effectiveness Analysis

As more attention is focused on the disproportionate costs of the United States healthcare system compared to other countries, researchers have attempted to identify treatments that have the most favorable cost-to-benefit ratio. Investigators first focus on the costs and health benefits associated with each treatment option for a particular condition. Costs, at minimum, include the direct costs of the healthcare for which the provider is reimbursed. They may also include measures of indirect costs to the provider or the patient such as time or lost work productivity, intangible costs such as pain or suffering, and future costs. Future costs may relate to additional disease treatment or may be unrelated to the disease and treatment. Health benefits are most often measured as a difference in the quality-adjusted life years attributable to the intervention as compared to an alternative treatment. This measure accounts for both the expected life years remaining following treatment as well as the quality of life of those years. The quality of remaining years is usually discounted over time. For each treatment option, the ratio of total cost to health benefit is calculated and treatments are compared. The lowest ratio is identified as the most cost effective treatment, requiring the lowest cost for each quality-adjusted life year of benefit.

Cost effectiveness analysis is a valuable tool in policy development or insurance policies that are implemented at the population level. It may also provide some benefit for an individual who pays for healthcare out of pocket, but clinicians are unlikely to find cost effectiveness analysis helpful when counseling individual patients.

9 Conclusion

This chapter provided an overview of common CER techniques. Subsequent chapters will describe these techniques in further detail and provide examples of potential applications in surgical oncology. We hope that these examples will stimulate research ideas and encourage surgical oncologists to embrace CER techniques and use them in their own research fields. Interest in effectiveness research will only increase as policy makers attempt to rein in exponential healthcare costs in the United States. If surgical oncologists begin using CER techniques now, they will be well prepared for the culture shift that is already mounting.

References

1. Pear R (2009) US to compare medical treatments. The New York Times, 16 Feb 2009
2. GovTrack HR (2009) Patient protection and affordable care act. In: 3590–111th congress. Accessed 25 Feb 2014. http://www.govtrack.us/congress/bills/111/hr3590
3. Johnston S, Rootenberg J, Katrak S, Smith W, Elkins J (2006) Effect of a US national institutes of health programme of clinical trials on public health and costs. Lancet 367 (9519):1319–1327
4. National Advisory Heart Council (1967) Organization, review and administration of cooperative studies (Greenberg Report)
5. Hunsberger S, Albert PS, London WB (2009) A finite mixture survival model to characterize risk groups of neuroblastoma. Stat Med 28(8):1301–1314
6. Overview of the Nationwide Inpatient Sample (NIS) (2014) http://www.hcup-us.ahrq.gov/nisoverview.jsp. Accessed 25 Feb 2014
7. Welcome to ACS NSQIP (2014) http://site.acsnsqip.org/. Accessed 25 Feb 2014
8. National Cancer Data Base (2014) http://www.facs.org/cancer/ncdb/. Accessed 25 Feb 2014
9. Data and Software for Researchers (2014) Surveillance, epidemiology, and end results program http://seer.cancer.gov/resources/. Accessed 25 Feb 2014
10. Taubman SL, Allen HL, Wright BJ, Baicker K, Finkelstein AN (2014) Medicaid increases emergency-department use: evidence from Oregon's Health Insurance Experiment. Science (New York, NY) 343(6168):263–268
11. Tan HJ, Norton EC, Ye Z, Hafez KS, Gore JL, Miller DC (2012) Long-term survival following partial versus radical nephrectomy among older patients with early-stage kidney cancer. JAMA J Am Med Assoc 307(15):1629–1635
12. Guyatt GH, Akl EA, Crowther M, Gutterman DD, Schuünemann HJ (2012) Executive summary: antithrombotic therapy and prevention of thrombosis, 9th ed: american college of chest physicians evidence-based clinical practice guidelines. CHEST J 141(2_suppl):7S–47S
13. The Cochrane Collaboration (2014) http://us.cochrane.org/cochrane-collaboration. Accessed 25 Feb 2014

Leveraging Comparative Effectiveness Research to Improve the Quality of Multidisciplinary Care for Breast Cancer Patients

Lane L. Frasier, Caprice C. Greenberg and Heather B. Neuman

Abstract

Breast cancer is the most commonly diagnosed cancer among women. To date, the use of efficacy randomized controlled trials (RCTs) in breast cancer have resulted in dramatic improvements in oncologic outcomes for this disease. However, not every question pertinent to breast cancer is amenable to such efficacy trials. This chapter will discuss some of the unique aspects of breast cancer that make efficacy RCTs challenging and/or impractical, how comparative effectiveness research can be used to address these issues, and identify several key questions which would benefit from ongoing comparative effectiveness research.

Keywords

Comparative effectiveness research · Breast cancer · Breast conserving therapy (BCT) · Mastectomy · Sentinel lymph node biopsy · Axillary lymph node dissection · Hormonal therapy · Hormone receptor status

Contents

L.L. Frasier (✉) · C.C. Greenberg · H.B. Neuman
Department of Surgery, University of Wisconsin Hospital and Clinics, Madison, WI, USA
e-mail: LFrasier@uwhealth.org

K.Y. Bilimoria et al. (eds.), *Comparative Effectiveness in Surgical Oncology*,
Cancer Treatment and Research 164, DOI 10.1007/978-3-319-12553-4_2

1 Introduction

Breast cancer is the most commonly diagnosed cancer and the second leading cause of cancer death for women in the United States. As a result of numerous randomized controlled trials (RCTs) addressing key breast cancer questions, great strides have been made in the detection, treatment, survival, and quality of life outcomes for this disease. However, not every question pertinent to breast cancer is amenable to such efficacy trials. There is also significant uncertainty in how the data generated in the highly-controlled clinical trial setting translates into "real world" practice. Comparative effectiveness studies are the optimal means of addressing both of these issues, and can generate critical evidence which complements the data generated through efficacy trials, potentially improving the quality of care we provide breast cancer patients. This chapter will begin with a brief representation of the critical role efficacy RCTs have played in breast cancer management, followed by a discussion of the unique characteristics of breast cancer which make some aspects of care difficult to assess with a RCT. We will next identify several important issues amenable to investigation with comparative effectiveness research (CER), and finally, discuss potential approaches which might lead to high-quality evidence for these issues.

2 The Roles and Limitations of Randomized Controlled Trials in Breast Cancer Research

Efficacy RCTs have played a critical role in advancing breast cancer care. With the enrollment of thousands of women across several decades, RCTs have been the driving force behind current best-practice guidelines for the multidisciplinary management of breast cancer. These studies were most commonly designed to compare oncologic endpoints (survival, recurrence, treatment adverse events) in selected patient populations receiving different therapies. The role of RCTs in defining the surgical management of breast cancer is especially noteworthy, with the evolution from the Halstead radical mastectomy to the current option of breast conserving therapy (BCT) with sentinel lymph node (SLN) biopsy (Fig. 1). The majority of these surgical trials have focused on overall survival and local recurrence. However, many surgical breast RCTs have increasingly incorporated alternative patient-centered outcomes, such as quality of life, [1] physical function, [2] and arm range of motion. [3].

However, even as we acknowledge the important role of RCTs in defining the management of modern breast cancer, it is important to recognize their limitations. RCTs are conducted within a tightly controlled environment with strict inclusion and exclusion criteria. Practically speaking, this may result in the exclusion of patients with unfavorable baseline characteristics, such as significant comorbidities or advanced age. As an example, in National Surgical Adjuvant Breast and Bowel

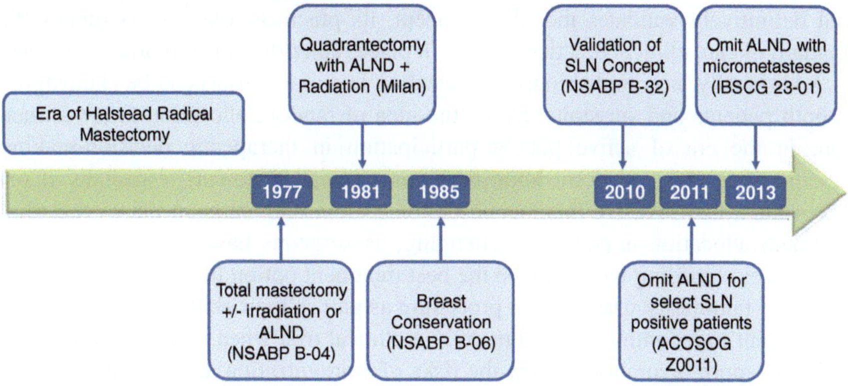

Fig. 1 Impact of efficacy randomized controlled trials on the surgical management of breast cancer (select trials represented)

Project (NSABP)-B06, the clinical trial which defined our current surgical management of breast cancer, women over the age of 70 were excluded. Given that ~40 % of current breast cancer diagnoses occur in women over the age of 70, [4] exclusion criteria such as these have the potential to limit clinicians' ability to apply trial findings to real-life patient populations. Similarly, RCTs require strict adherence to treatment protocols, and may include central auditing of pathology and imaging findings, surgical credentialing, and enhanced patient follow-up; however, many of these components may be altered or omitted as these treatments are implemented in clinical practice, potentially impacting outcomes observed. In contrast to the highly-controlled environment of efficacy trials, effectiveness research provides insight into treatment effects under 'real-world' conditions, which may differ substantially from the trial setting.

There are also a number of factors specific to surgery which make conducting RCTs challenging. In general, the field of surgery has traditionally depended less on RCTs to test new surgical interventions compared to other aspects of medicine, such as clinical drug trials. Consequently, many new surgical techniques (especially those that represent a less invasive or morbid approach) are disseminated into clinical practice prior to any RCT data supporting their efficacy or safety, making it challenging to then generate the supporting data. A pertinent example of this is the SLN biopsy for breast cancer. The SLN biopsy for breast cancer was first described in two small, single-institution studies [5, 6]. In 1999, a RCT began with the intent to validate the SLN biopsy concept [7]. Patients were randomized to SLN biopsy followed by either immediate axillary lymph node dissection (ALND) versus ALND only if the sentinel node was positive. Ultimately, this trial, reported in 2010, demonstrated equivalent overall and disease-free survival as well as regional control with a SLN biopsy [7]. However, in the intervening years between trial initiation and reporting of results, the practice of SLN biopsy became broadly incorporated into standard breast surgery practice, with 59 % of early stage breast cancer patients undergoing SLN biopsy rather than ALND by 2004 [8]. Although the NSABP-B32 trial definitively validates the SLN concept, its practical role was to support the standard of care clinical practice already in place rather than inform practice change.

Additionally, accomplishing randomization in surgical trials can be challenging, as both patients and surgeons dislike the idea of random allocation to a treatment arm. In the era of active patient participation in therapeutic decision-making, patients often resist randomization between surgical treatments, especially if one represents a less invasive therapeutic option. Addressing surgeon biases regarding treatment allocation is equally challenging, as surgeons have their own personal preferences regarding what may be the best treatment option for their patients and a particular familiarity with a given procedure as part of their skill set. Surgeons may be reluctant to recommend enrollment in a clinical trial when they view one of the trial arms more favorably or view the risks of randomization as unacceptably high. Several examples of patient and provider bias can be seen in the execution of prior RCTs in breast cancer. For example:

- American College of Surgeons Oncology Group (ACOSOG) Z0011: This study examined whether ALND is necessary after positive SLN biopsy in women undergoing BCT for invasive breast cancer. Women with positive SLNs were randomized to completion axillary dissection versus observation, and overall survival and local recurrence was determined to be similar between the two groups [9, 10]. Target enrollment was 1,900 patients; however, the study closed early due to lower than expected accrual (<50 % of target) and event rates. This trial began accrual in 1999, at a time when the SLN concept was still being disseminated into wide-spread clinical practice [8]. The timing of trial initiation is likely one factor that influenced the slow accrual, as it may reflect surgeons' reluctance to enroll patients on a trial that avoided an ALND for node positive patients when many were still performing an ALND for even clinically node negative patients. This concept of surgeon bias is further indirectly supported by the low volume axillary disease of patients enrolled in the trial (~40 % with micrometastases), supporting that surgeons selectively enrolled their very low risk patients in the trial [9, 10]. As a result of this clinical trial, women undergoing breast conservation with 1 or 2 positive SLN may be spared a completion ALND. However, the selective accrual of "low-risk" patients to this trial limits the patient populations these findings can be applied to.
- Cancer and Leukemia Group B C9343: This study evaluated patients >70 years of age undergoing BCT to determine whether whole-breast radiation along with tamoxifen improved outcomes compared to tamoxifen alone [11]. Outcomes (recurrence, overall survival) were similar between the groups, and omitting radiation from the adjuvant treatment of women over the age of 70 is now a standard of care option for appropriate women. It is noteworthy that at initiation of the trial, eligibility criteria included T1 or T2 (tumors up to 4 cm) with no restrictions on estrogen receptor (ER) status. However, "in an attempt to broaden participation by physicians concerned about the upper size limit", eligibility criteria was changed to limit tumor size to 2 cm and require ER status to be positive or unknown. Following this change, accrual was rapidly completed. Of note, at accrual completion, only 14 of 636 women had T2 tumors, and only ten

were ER negative [11]. As a result of this clinical trial, women over the age of 70 may consider omitting radiation from their breast conservation treatment plan, although the applicability of this study's findings is limited to a small subset of the older breast cancer patient population due to its strict inclusion criteria.

These examples highlight the challenges associated with randomization in surgical trials, as well as how surgeon bias can affect trial accrual and even lead to early trial closure. Ultimately, these issues will impact generalizability of the clinical trial to the real world setting.

3 Breast Cancer-Specific Limitations to Efficacy Trials

In addition to the general challenges associated with conducting RCTs, there are a number of unique characteristics associated with breast cancer which make some aspects of care difficult to assess with a RCT (Table 1). These largely reflect our

Table 1 Limitations of efficacy randomized controlled trials in breast cancer and possible solutions provided by comparative effectiveness research

	Challenges to performing RCT in breast cancer	Use of CER to overcome challenges
Improved outcomes (survival, recurrence)	Large number of patients required to identify small differences in oncologic outcomes	Retrospective evaluation of large data sets (i.e. administrative data, etc.)
	Extended follow-up period to assess delayed outcomes	Meta-analysis to evaluate pooled data
	Often prohibitively time and financially intensive, given favorable overall prognosis	Decision-modeling to evaluate theoretical outcomes associated with different options
	Discrepancy between outcomes in clinical trial and real life	Pragmatic clinical trials to evaluate real life outcomes with incorporation of patient-centered outcomes
	Improved outcomes may increase relative importance of other patient-centered outcomes (see below) as surrogate endpoints	
Patient preferences	Breast cancer management especially preference-sensitive	Retrospective evaluation of large data (avoids need for randomization but requires selection bias controls)
	Patients may resist randomization if not aligned with their values	Use of qualitative research to explore patient values
	Some questions not amenable to randomization	Development of validated decision aids
Patient-centered outcomes	Few validated tools for objective measurement of outcomes	Expanded research to develop tools assessing outcomes valued by stakeholders
	Subjective and objective measures may not correlate	Qualitative research methods to explore stakeholder values

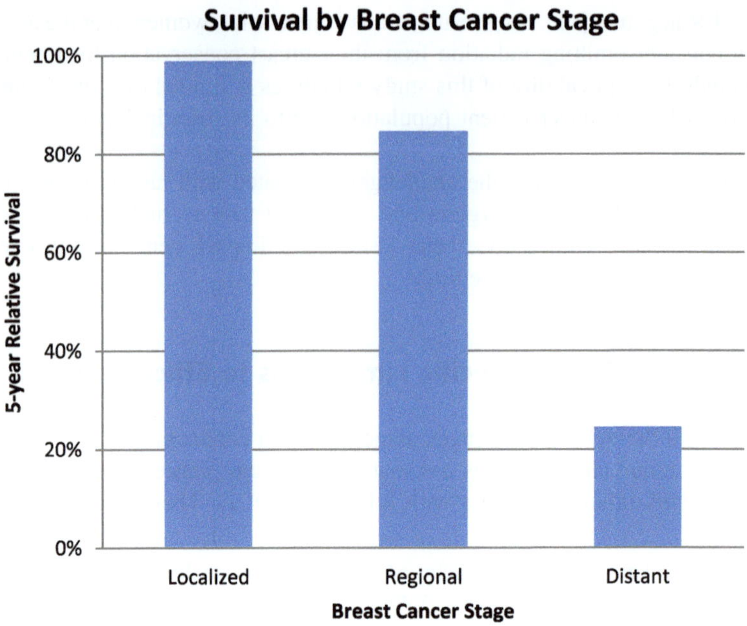

Fig. 2 5-Year Breast Cancer Survival by Cancer Stage [4]

success in treating breast cancer (with an associated improved survival) and the increasing role patients and their preferences play in treatment decision-making.

Implications of Prolonged Survival: With improvements in cancer detection and treatment, the prognosis for breast cancer patients has markedly improved in the past 20 years. The 3-year survival for the 3 million breast cancer survivors currently living in the United States exceeds 97 % for localized (node negative) and 84 % for regional (node positive) disease (Fig. 2) [4]. The increased overall survival and decreased local recurrence associated with modern breast cancer treatment represents a challenge in conducting efficacy RCTs, as predicted differences between treatment groups will be small and require an extended period of follow-up to identify. Conducting such trials would therefore require large patient cohorts to have adequate power which will be prohibitively expensive and time-intensive, and may not yield a meaningful clinical outcome.

One option to address this challenge is to limit inclusion criteria for clinical trials to select "higher-risk" sub-groups for whom differences may be more easily observed. However, such inclusion criteria may increase the difficulty in patient accrual, and would not represent a feasible method for studying processes with high cure rates like DCIS.

Patient Preference: When compared to other cancers, decision-making surrounding breast cancer management is especially preference-sensitive (decisions regarding mastectomy versus breast conservation, reconstruction choices, etc.). These preferences may also determine how patients perceive and ultimately decide to participate in, a clinic trial. Investigators must therefore address this in their trial design to ensure adequate trial accrual. For example, NSABP-06 randomized women between one of the three treatment arms: mastectomy, segmental mastectomy followed by breast irradiation, or segmental mastectomy alone. These treatment arms represent therapies with relevant differences in patient-centered outcomes including quality of life and body image. In recognition of the challenges to randomly assigning women to one of these very different arms, investigators designed the trial using a "pre-randomization" technique. After assessing women for eligibility this study, patients were pre-assigned to one of the treatment groups. Patients were then approached for participation and disclosure of their pre-randomization arm was included in the consent process. Only patients who accepted their pre-assigned therapy and provided informed consent were enrolled in the trial. A total of 2,024 women were randomized to the three treatment arms. Despite these measures, the assigned treatment was still refused by 175 patients, with 78 refusing mastectomy, 55 refusing segmental mastectomy plus breast irradiation, and 41 refusing segmental mastectomy alone [12]. Overall, however, this "pre-randomization" design allowed patients to consider their personal preferences for treatment when deciding whether to participate in the trial and allowed successful completion of the trial, which defines our current standard of care for breast cancer surgery.

In addition to representing a challenge to trial accrual, patient preference limits to some degree what types of questions can be answered in efficacy trials, as randomization for many questions may be either unethical or not feasible. One pertinent example is examining outcomes of risk-reducing surgery for women at elevated risk of developing breast cancer (i.e. *BRCA1* and *BRCA2* mutation carriers). To date, there is no level 1 evidence supporting a survival benefit to risk-reducing surgery, and the necessary study is unlikely to ever occur given the ethics associated with randomizing high-risk women in such a preference–laden scenario. Other examples of clinical questions unlikely to be answered through efficacy RCTs include consideration of the role of contralateral mastectomy for women with a new cancer diagnosis and outcomes after different types of post-mastectomy reconstructive procedures.

Studying Patient-Centered Outcomes: With the improvement in recurrence and survival observed in breast cancer, increasing emphasis has been placed on alternative patient-centered outcomes such as range of motion, quality of life, sexual function, cosmesis, and patient satisfaction. These outcomes can be negatively impacted by the breast cancer treatment administered, and are highly valued by breast cancer survivors. Unfortunately, it can be challenging to measure these outcomes as appropriate and sensitive tools are not always available. Additionally, the relative importance of many of these outcomes may vary based on the individual patient, and objective and subjective measures of the same outcome may not correlate. For example, in a prospective study of lymphedema in women who underwent SLN biopsy or an ALND, significant differences were observed in the rates of patient-reported (subjective) and objectively measured lymphedema [13]. Further, many survivors with objectively measured changes in limb volume did not report having clinical symptoms of lymphedema. This example highlights some of the challenges associated with evaluating patient-centered outcomes and even defining what outcomes should be measured.

Further, understanding patient satisfaction in relation to surgical decision-making, reconstruction, and cosmesis is in its infancy. Although reconstruction plays a key role in patient satisfaction for their surgical breast cancer treatment, it has no effect on cancer recurrence or survival and is therefore rarely reported in RCTs. Assessment of cosmetic outcome is extremely challenging and difficult to quantify, although robustly validated measurement tools are becoming more readily available [14]. Patients' assessment of their cosmetic outcome is heavily impacted by preoperative expectations and their overall satisfaction with their cancer care, resulting in possible discordance between objective and subjective measures. Finally, there are notably wide regional, socio-economic, and demographic variations in rates of breast reconstruction after mastectomy that are poorly understood. Although these variations are likely multi-factorial, patient preferences and values play an important role in patient decision-making for reconstruction and the differences in priorities between different populations represent an additional challenge in assessing these and similar outcomes.

4 Breast Cancer Clinical Questions Amenable to Comparative Effectiveness Research

In day-to-day practice, physicians routinely encounter clinical questions about breast cancer care which have not been satisfactorily addressed with RCT data and are unlikely to be ever addressed in this manner. However, many of these questions may be appropriate to examine using CER methodologies. Summarized below are several key clinical questions in breast cancer which do not currently have RCT-based evidence available to guide decision-making. We will discuss why these particular questions are important to address as we strive to improve the quality of care we provide breast cancer patients, examine why they are not amenable to study using typical efficacy trials, and explore how these questions may be approached from a CER perspective.

Breast Cancer Screening: Significant controversy surrounds the recent recommendation from the United States Preventive Services Task Force (USPSTF) that routine screening mammography for average-risk women begin at age 50 [15]. The rationale for this recommendation stems from the lower rate of breast cancer and the higher rate of false positive results in women under the age of 50. Significant controversy exists, however, because mammography represents a low-cost, non-invasive screening tool. In addition, recommendations represent those for the average woman, and specific guidance is not providing regarding how to adapt these guidelines for subgroups of women at increased risk of breast cancer (i.e. those with a strong family history). While several RCTs have been completed comparing mammography to no intervention [16] and found a statistically significant mortality benefit, these studies were not powered to evaluate the benefits of mammography for patients based on individual risk factors. Given our relatively limited ability to identify younger women at high risk of breast cancer who may benefit from initiation of earlier screening, critics of the new guidelines feel that screening of the entire population is warranted to minimize the incidence of missed cancers. Given the wide-spread acceptance by both clinicians and women of the importance of mammography in breast cancer screening, the question of whether or not to screen women under the age of 50 with mammography will never be addressed in a RCT, making it appropriate for a comparative effectiveness approach. This question could be addressed through a number of mechanisms. One option would be to perform observational or retrospectives studies using existing data sources, such as mammography registries. These often include more detailed information on individual risk factors than is available through cancer registry data (such as SEER) making these registries a rich data source. Systematic reviews represent one alternative approach. As an example, a recent meta-analysis of more than 60 studies sought to identify risk factors associated with increased risk of breast cancer in women ages 40–49 [15]. Although these systematic reviews are limited to data available in the studies included, this review was able to identify risk factors associated with 1.0–1.5, 1.5–2.0, or greater than 2.0- fold increased risk for invasive carcinoma which could then be used to guide screening decisions for younger women. Modeling techniques such as decision-analysis or cost-effectiveness analysis are another feasible approach. In a study by Schousboe et al. [17] mammography was found to be beneficial both in terms of quality-adjusted life years and cost-effectiveness for younger women who had either dense breasts or both a family history of breast cancer and personal history of breast biopsy. This study utilized data from the SEER program as well as the Breast Cancer Surveillance Consortium. These types of study design represent the most practical way to assess the impacts of discrete risk factors on breast cancer risk and subsequent potential benefit of screening mammography, and may guide the development of more individualized mammography screening recommendations.

Management of DCIS: With improved imaging techniques, diagnosis of DCIS has increased throughout the past two decades. While DCIS represents a pre-cancerous lesion, there is a range of histology and cell biology within this category and some risk of eventual conversion to invasive carcinoma. Unfortunately, data is scant on long-term outcomes for the various grades of DCIS and we are currently unable to predict which patients, if untreated, will progress to invasive cancer and which patients have a clinically insignificant lesion. Patients are therefore generally treated as a homogenous group with local surgical control, often combined with radiation and risk-reducing endocrine therapy. Given the excellent overall prognosis of patients with DCIS, the challenge lies in identifying not only statistically but also clinically significant differences in outcomes between various treatment approaches, applying these approaches to different subgroups of patients, and then incorporating patients' personal values into subsequent treatment decision-making. For example, although radiation after BCT decreases the risk of local recurrence, it has a limited impact on overall survival. Further, it may result in poorer cosmetic outcomes, increase the risk of lymphedema, limit future treatment options should cancer recur, and represents a significant time commitment on the part of the patient (with potential financial repercussions if radiation therapy appointments interfere with her ability to work). These patient-centered outcomes, although they factor into patient decision-making, are difficult to incorporate into traditional efficacy trial designs and make this question especially amenable to CER. The issue of management of DCIS has been addressed in a number of CER studies. A recent publication by Soeteman et al. [18] created a disease simulation model for six possible treatments of DCIS, utilizing outcome data from well-executed RCTs. Based on the grade of DCIS (low, intermediate, high) and simulated age at the time of diagnosis, the team identified the degree of benefit conferred by each therapeutic option in terms of breast preservation and disease-free, invasive disease-free and overall survival for a hypothetical patient. They found that overall, the survival benefits associated with different therapeutic approaches to management of DCIS were comparable, with the maximum difference in survival between therapeutic options estimated to be 12 months. Given that this could be perceived as a clinically "less significant" difference, the authors suggested therapy for DCIS could be tailored based on patient values, including preferences for breast preservation and/or their wish to avoid a recurrence.

A second example of CER and DCIS utilized SEER-Medicare data to evaluate outcomes for older women who underwent lumpectomy with or without radiation [19]. The team identified more than 3,400 women ≥65 years of age who underwent lumpectomy with or without radiation therapy for DCIS. Additional data were collected to evaluate high-risk features (age 66–69 years, tumor ≥2.5 cm, comedo- and/or high-grade histology). Patients were then followed to determine whether they experienced an ipsilateral recurrence and/or underwent ipsilateral mastectomy. Researchers determined that radiotherapy was associated with a significant reduction in ipsilateral recurrence and subsequent ipsilateral mastectomy, especially for those patients with high-risk features. This data has high utility in providing clinicians with information which can guide shared-decision-making conversations with older patients regarding the management of their DCIS.

Margin Status: BCT is a standard of care option for surgical management of breast cancer, and the importance of obtaining negative margins to minimize local recurrence is clear. However, controversy remains surrounding what constitutes an "adequate" surgical margin. Current NCCN guidelines indicate that margins of 1 cm are always adequate, while margins ≤1 mm (no ink on tumor) are not, [20] but there is no consensus on any margin between these values for either DCIS or invasive breast cancer. These variable definitions of what constitutes negative margins may place patients at increased risk of local recurrence or alternatively lead to unnecessary re-excisions. Although this question could be addressed through a standard efficacy trial, the number of patients required and the duration of follow-up necessary to assess local recurrence as an outcome makes such trials unfeasible.

A number of options exist, however, to address this question through CER using existing data. One option is a meta-analysis of published data. As an example, a recent study assessed patients with DCIS treated with lumpectomy and radiation found increased rates of ipsilateral recurrence with margins <2 mm compared to margins >2 mm; however, there were no significant differences in recurrence for patients with margins of 2–5 mm or >5 mm [21]. Retrospective analyses of prospectively collected data (i.e. data collected systematically for a different initial purpose such as a clinical trial) would be an alternative means of address this question and has the potential to have a significant impact on how breast cancer surgery is currently practiced.

Management of the Positive SLN: After establishment of SLN biopsy as standard of care for staging the axilla, thousands of women with node negative cancer have been spared ALND. With the publication of two recent RCTs, there is now data to support omitting ALND in some women even with positive axillary nodes. As discussed earlier, the ACOSOG Z0011 trial examined women undergoing breast conserving surgery and SLN biopsy for invasive breast cancer, and found the use of SLN biopsy alone to be non-inferior to ALND in terms of survival, for eligible women [9, 10]. Similarly, the recently reported European Organization for Research and treatment of Cancer After Mapping of the Axilla: Radiotherapy or Surgery? (AMAROS) trial evaluated outcomes for women with T1/T2 breast cancer and positive SLN's; women undergoing either mastectomy or BCT were included, although 82 % underwent BCT (making the study population very similar to that observed in ACOSOG Z0011) [22]. Women were randomized to either ALND or axillary radiotherapy to levels I-II, with optional radiotherapy to level III. Although the study was underpowered to evaluate its primary endpoint, axillary recurrence, no clinically meaningful difference between the groups was observed (0.54 % after ALND versus 1.03 % after axillary radiotherapy).

Although both of these studies were underpowered, they provide strong supporting evidence that not all women with a positive SLN biopsy require a completion ALND (Table 2). However, these findings are largely applicable only to women undergoing BCT, with AMAROS providing only limited data on women undergoing mastectomy. Given the challenges in completing both of these trials, it is unlikely that further RCT of SLN positive women undergoing mastectomy will be initiated in the near future. This represents a unique opportunity to examine this question using CER, likely through existing administrative and clinical databases (while acknowledging some of the selection biases reflected in these data sources).

Survivorship and Surveillance: Since the publication of the Institute of Medicine Report, "From Cancer Patient to Cancer Survivor: Lost in Transition," [23] the focus on the quality of survivorship for cancer patients has increased. One area of focus which has been increasingly recognized by stakeholders as a priority is follow-up surveillance, with the recognition that little data exists to support the follow-up recommendations that currently exist.

Given the high overall survival and uncertainty surrounding the true clinical efficacy of a clinical follow-up exam, it is unclear which breast cancer survivors truly need prolonged follow-up with an oncologist, and when, if ever, primary care providers should assume a primary role in surveillance. Reducing unnecessary clinic visits represents a potential benefit to patients as they transition from active treatment back to their activities of daily living, and a timely transition would alleviate the burden of routine surveillance on specialty providers. However, it is

Table 2 Review of two trials evaluating management of the axilla with a positive sentinel lymph node

Trial	Patient population	Trial arms	Patient accrual	Endpoints	Findings	Limitations to generalizability
ACOSOG Z0011	Adult women with T1/T2 tumors undergoing BCT, with 1–2 positive SLN	Completion ALND versus no further therapy	901 pts	Local and regional recurrence	Local recurrence: 1.8 % in SLN biopsy arm versus 3.6 % in ALND arm	Study closed early due to poor accrual (<50 % target) and was underpowered
					Regional recurrence: 0.9 % in SLN biopsy arm versus 0.5 % in ALND arm	Included patients had small tumors and low volume axillary disease
						Only included patients undergoing BCT
						All received whole breast radiation (no additional planned axillary tangents)
AMAROS	Adult women with T1/T2 tumors undergoing either mastectomy or BCT with a positive SLN	Axillary radiation versus ALND	1,425 pts	Axillary recurrence, overall- and disease-free survival, quality of life	Axillary recurrence: 0.54 % in ALND arm versus 1.03 % in axillary radiation	Study was underpowered
						Limited data on mastectomy pts (82 % underwent BCT)
						Included patients had small tumors and low volume axillary disease

also likely that different patient populations (based on age, tumor characteristics, and treatment received) may benefit differently from clinical follow-up, adding to the challenge of refining current follow-up. As a result of these factors, examining the impact of different surveillance regimens through traditional RCTs is difficult.

Further, the Institute of Medicine has recommended that all cancer patients receive at the completion of therapy a survivorship care plan [23]. This plan provides details about the patient's cancer history (diagnosis, surgery, and treatment), outlines details of ongoing surveillance (frequency of visits, labs, and imaging, and responsible health care provider), and provides information about support for possible side effects of therapy and general health promotion strategies. However, no data exist to date examining the true impact of care plans (positive or negative) on patients or providers.

CER represents a viable method of addressing these types of questions to improve the quality of comprehensive survivorship care. Administrative databases, such as SEER Medicare, with their available longitudinal data, allow current patterns of care studies to be performed, providing insight into how different patient factors may influence follow-up visits or receipt of imaging [24]. However, SEER-Medicare is limited by the composition of its population (patients over the age of 65), making generalizability of these findings to the greater breast cancer patient population difficult. Further, administrative data sources such as SEER-Medicare cannot provide insight into the decision-making underlying the patterns of care observed.

Other techniques, such as qualitative research methods (focus groups, interviews), may be necessary to understand the preferences of key stakeholders (patients, primary care physicians, medical, surgical, and radiation oncologists) for follow-up care and how these preferences influence follow-up care delivered and received. Findings from such mixed-methods studies will complement the quantitative data and will provide critical insight into how stakeholders perceive follow-up. Cost-effectiveness studies, with a focus on both the financial and "person" costs of follow-up, will also likely play a substantial role in refining current follow-up. These approaches are also the optimal means of evaluating the relative impact of current survivorship care plans on patient care.

Finally, comparison of various surveillance protocols will necessitate creative approaches to any future efficacy trials. Randomization of individual patients is impractical and would create significant hardship for participating centers. A clustered randomized controlled trial, in which groups of patients rather than individual patients are randomized, represents one possible approach that would simplify the study design but still allow some degree of randomization.

Disparities in Breast Cancer: Significant disparity exists in many aspects of breast cancer. When examined along racial or socio-economic lines, rates of breast cancer screening, diagnosis, treatment, reconstruction after mastectomy, and mortality vary widely. For example, in a recent literature review examining ethnic differences in breast cancer survival, Maskarinec et al. [25] found that compared to white women, African-American women had a hazard ratio of breast cancer-specific mortality of 1.2–1.3, while Latinas had a breast cancer mortality risk of 1.1. Asian-Americans as a whole have significant variability by sub-group, although women of Japanese descent have a survival advantage of about 20 % compared to Caucasians [25]. These authors also found that disparities were smaller but persistent in studies that controlled for confounding variables such as access to health care, obesity, and co-morbidities. They note that many of these confounders are closely tied to socio-economic status and may contribute to prognosis to multiple ways.

Given the under-representation of these populations in clinical trials, our efficacy RCTs can provide only limited insight into the factors underlying these disparities. In contrast, CER represents an opportunity to study these populations in "real world" settings, focusing on how geographic, socioeconomic, and cultural/social constructs impact treatment received and subsequent outcomes. Use of administrative databases combined with other research techniques such as qualitative interviews will be crucial in further investigative efforts.

5 Future Steps

CER for breast cancer represents a unique opportunity to address many of the pertinent questions that need to be answered to further improve the quality of care we provide to breast cancer survivors, while balancing the challenges associated with traditional efficacy trials. However, many of these questions remains difficult to address, and success will require the development of additional infrastructure to support CER efforts, creation of new data sources, and use of new research methodologies.

Fortunately, several new initiatives are in progress which will begin to address current deficits in data collection and coordination. One such initiative is the reorganization of the National Cancer Institute (NCI) trials network to include cancer care delivery research, which includes CER. Originally developed to facilitate efficacy RCTs, the NCI is interested in developing this infrastructure to support large research initiative. Cancer cooperative groups have accumulated data on patient demographics, treatment details, and longitudinal outcomes. Some of these outcomes of interest, including toxicity and cancer recurrence, are difficult to track from other currently available data sources (such as administrative data) and therefore represent a unique potential resource for cancer CER. This potential was recognized by the Alliance for Clinical Trials in Oncology, a merger of the former North Central Cancer Treatment Group, American College of Surgeons Oncology Group, and Cancer and Leukemia Group B. The American College of Surgeons Clinical Research Program (ACS-CRP), a joint initiative of the Alliance and The American College of Surgeons Cancer Program, was created with the goal of utilizing the Alliance's infrastructure to expand health services, patient-centered research, and CER. This will be executed through a partnership with the Commission on Cancer of the American College of Surgeons, which includes a national network of 1,500 hospitals involved in quality cancer care and research.

Another major initiative is the development of the Oncology NSQIP National Cancer Institute Center Consortium, composed of 51 hospitals accredited by the National Cancer Institute that are currently participating in NSQIP. Like the Alliance programs, this consortium was developed with the recognition of the importance of CER in addressing pertinent oncology questions and focus on sharing and comparison of oncology-specific data to improve outcomes; improvement and expansion of risk-adjustment, process measures, and short-term outcomes utilized by NSQIP; and providing infrastructure and resources for prospective and retrospective CER.

These coordinated efforts greatly expand the resources available to answer many important breast cancer-related questions. Additionally, the framework of CER, which encourages use of alternative research methodologies beyond traditional efficacy RCTs, is critical. These research methods and their potential contributions to clinical care are illustrated throughout this chapter. Methods such as cluster RCTs, decision modeling, meta-analyses, qualitative studies, and novel "big data" sources will allow us to understand key clinical problems when efficacy RCTs are impractical or impossible to conduct and, importantly, will allow the incorporation of patient-centered outcomes, an increasingly recognized focus. The clinician caring for breast cancer patients must be familiar with these approaches to stay current with the literature, and as we move into the twenty-first century, CER will play an expanded role in answering key clinical questions.

References

1. Fleissig A, Fallowfield LJ, Langridge CI et al (2006) Post-operative arm morbidity and quality of life. Results of the ALMANAC randomised trial comparing sentinel node biopsy with standard axillary treatment in the management of patients with early breast cancer. Breast Cancer Res Treat 95:279–293
2. Segal R, Evans W, Johnson D et al (2001) Structured exercise improves physical functioning in women with stages I and II breast cancer: results of a randomized controlled trial. J Clin Oncol 19(3):657–665
3. Ashikaga T, Krag DN, Land SR et al (2010) Morbidity results from the NSABP B-32 trial comparing sentinel lymph node dissection versus axillary dissection. J Surg Oncol 102:111–118
4. Howlader N, Noone AM, Krapcho M, Garshell J, Neyman N, Altekruse SF, Kosary CL, Yu M, Ruhl J, Tatalovich Z, Cho H, Mariotto A, Lewis DR, Chen HS, Feuer EJ, Cronin KA (eds) (2013) SEER Cancer Statistics Review, 1975–2010, National Cancer Institute. Bethesda MD, http://seer.cancer.gov/csr/1975_2010/, based on November 2012 SEER data submission, posted to the SEER web site, April 2013
5. Krag DN, Weaver DL, Alex JC et al (1993) Surgical resection and radiolocation of the sentinel lymph node in breast cancer using a gamma probe. Surg Oncol 2(6):335–339
6. Giuliano EA, Kirgan DM, Guenter JM et al (2010) Lymphatic mapping and sentinel lymphadenectomy for breast cancer. Ann Surg 252(3):426–432
7. Krag DN, Anderson SJ, Julian TB et al (2010) Sentinel-lymph-node resection compared with conventional axillary-lymph-node dissection in clinically node-negative patients with breast cancer: overall survival findings from the NSABP B-32 randomised phase 3 trial. Lancet 11:927–933
8. Rescigno J, Zampell JC, Axelrod D (2009) Patterns of axillary surgical care for breast cancer in the era of sentinel lymph node biopsy. Ann Surg Oncol 16(3):687–696

9. Giuliano AE, McCall L, Beitsch P et al (2010) Locoregional recurrence after sentinel lymph node dissection with or without axillary dissection in patients with sentinel lymph node metastases. The american college of surgeons oncology group Z0011 randomized trial. Ann Surg 252(3):426–432; discussion 432–433
10. Giuliano AE, Hunt KK, Ballman K et al (2011) Axillary dissection vs no axillary dissection in women with invasive breast cancer and sentinel node metastasis. A randomized clinical trial. J Am Med Assoc 305(6):569–575
11. Hughes KS, Schnaper LA, Berry D (2004) Lumpectomy plus tamoxifen with or without irradiation in women 70 years of age or older with early breast cancer. N Engl J Med 351 (10):971–977
12. Fisher B, Anderson S, Bryant J et al (2002) Twenty-year follow-up of a randomized trial comparing total mastectomy, lumpectomy, and lumpectomy plus irradiation for the treatment of invasive breast cancer. N Engl J Med 357:1233–1241
13. McLaughlin SA, Wright MJ, Morris KT et al (2008) Prevalence of lymphedema in women with breast cancer 5 years after sentinel lymph node biopsy or axillary dissection: patient perceptions and precautionary behaviors. J Clin Oncol 26(32):5220–5226
14. Pusic AL, Klassen AF, Scott AM et al (2009) Development of a new patient-reported outcome measure for breast surgery: the BREAST-Q. Plast Reconstr Surg 124:345–353
15. Nelson HD, Tyne K, Nalk A et al (2009) Screening for breast cancer: an update for the U.S. preventive services task force. Ann Intern Med 151:727–737
16. Kerlikowske K (1997) Efficacy of screening mammography among women aged 40 to 49 years and 50 to 69 years: comparison of relative and absolute benefit. J Natl Cancer Inst Monogr 22:79–86
17. Schousboe JT, Kerlikowske K, Loh A et al (2011) Personalizing mammography by breast density and other risk factors for breast cancer: analysis of health benefits and cost-effectiveness. Ann Intern Med 155:10–20
18. Soeteman DI, Stout NK, Ozanne EM et al (2013) Modeling the effectiveness of initial management strategies for ductal carcinoma in situ. J Natl Cancer Inst 105(11):774–781
19. Smith BD, Haffty BG, Buchholz TA et al (2006) Effectiveness of radiation therapy in older women with ductal carcinoma in situ. J Natl Cancer Inst 98(18):1302–1310
20. Network NCC (2013) NCCN Clinical practice guidelines in oncology breast cancer version 3.2013. http://www.nccn.org/professionals/physician_gls/pdf/breast.pdf. Accessed 1 Dec 2013
21. Dunne C, Burke JP, Morrow M et al (2009) Effect of margin status on local recurrence after breast conservation and radiation therapy for ductal carcinoma in situ. J Clin Oncol 27 (10):1615–1620
22. Rutgers EJ, Donker M, Straver ME et al (2013) Radiotherapy or surgery of the axilla after a positive sentinel node in breast cancer patients: final analysis of the EORTC AMAROS trial (10981/22023). ASCO meeting abstracts
23. From cancer patient to cancer survivor: lost in transition (2005) N. R. Council (ed). Institute of Medicine, Washington DC
24. Neuman HB, Weiss JM, Schrag D et al (2013) Patient demographic and tumor characteristics influencing oncologist follow-up frequency in older breast cancer survivors. Ann Surg Oncol 20(13):4128–4136
25. Maskarinec G, Sen C, Koga K et al (2011) Ethnic differences in breast cancer survival: status and determinants. Women's Health 7(6):677–687

Comparative Effectiveness in Melanoma

Maria C. Russel and Keith A. Delman

Abstract

The worldwide incidence of melanoma continues to rise. It is a leading cause of cancer death and the second leading cause of loss of productive years of life. Although the diagnosis of melanoma is straightforward, there remain many controversies regarding treatment and surveillance. This chapter addresses important questions in melanoma treatment such as sentinel lymph node biopsy, what to do with a positive sentinel lymph node, margins of resection for melanoma, radiation for primary, nodal and metastatic melanoma, and routine use imaging. Through this chapter, the evidence for these controversial subjects and the barriers to resolution will be elucidated.

Keywords

Melanoma · Sentinel lymph node · Completion lymphadenectomy · Melanoma margins · Melanoma radiation · Imaging for melanoma

Contents

M.C. Russel (✉) · K.A. Delman
Department of Surgery, Emory University, Atlanta, GA, USA
e-mail: Maria.c.russell@emory.edu

K.A. Delman
e-mail: kdelman@emory.edu

K.Y. Bilimoria et al. (eds.), *Comparative Effectiveness in Surgical Oncology*, Cancer Treatment and Research 164, DOI 10.1007/978-3-319-12553-4_3

1 Introduction

Melanoma remains one of the most confounding of solid tumors. Essentially refractory to cytotoxic chemotherapy, with a variable sensitivity to radiation, surgery remains the most effective tool in the armamentarium against this disease. While it may be one of the most well studied of malignancies from a surgical standpoint, with five radomized prospective clinical trials evaluating margin of excision, questions continue to abound about the appropriate application of therapies.

Though evidence-based medicine and cost are of paramount concerns for the clinician and the patient, many well-tested therapeutic interventions have never been proven to impact patients in a definitive manner. In addition, some of the newest therapies are so costly that their benefit has to be evaluated in the context of the patient's value system (i.e., what exactly is the cost of quantity and quality of life?). Perhaps more significantly, many interventions that have regularly been performed by clinicians, such as routine staging in asymptomatic patients, have *never* been shown to improve outcomes or quality of life in almost *any* malignancy. The driver of these procedures, however, continues to be the patient, and the false perception that these studies may offer early detection and improved outcomes.

The debate surrounding many of these questions may never truly be answered. Some argue that this is because the question will cost more to answer than just proceeding in a semi-blind dogmatic manner or that clinical judgment is sufficient to determine whether 1 or 2 cm margin would be optimal in a given location. It is incumbent upon us, however, to do our best to address these questions. At the very least it is imperative that we recognize the uncertainty around them, so that we can counsel our patients wisely, and preferably proceed thoughtfully and deliberately to answer them.

2 Sentinel Lymph Node

Lymphoscintigraphy was successfully used to identify regional draining nodal basins in melanoma patients in 1977 [1]. It would take another 15 years until results demonstrating the reliability and reproducibility of sentinel lymph node biopsy for melanoma were documented and led to the initiation of a prospective, randomized clinical trial [2]. In 2006, the initial results of the Multicenter Selective Lymphadenectomy Trial-1 (MSLT-1) were published and sentinel lymph node biopsy became the standard of care for patients with intermediate-thickness melanoma or in patients with thin melanoma and high-risk features. It is regarded as a safe and accurate procedure that allows for the evaluation of draining lymph nodes without exposing the patient to the morbidity of elective lymphadenectomy.

Sentinel lymph node status is the strongest prognostic factor in patients with melanoma and is used to stage patients in the American Joint Committee on Cancer (AJCC) guidelines. The introduction of this procedure has corresponded with a shift in survival curves for stage III patients that are likely a direct result of the routine use of the technique [3, 4]. Despite these changes, controversy continues to surround the routine use of sentinel node biopsy in patients with either thin (<1 mm) or thick (>4 mm) melanomas. The risk of a positive node in patients with thin melanomas is low enough that the risk-benefit consideration may not support routine use and the likelihood of systemic failure regardless of sentinel node status is so high in patients with thick melanomas that the benefit of the procedure is less definitive in this subpopulation of patients as well [3, 5].

3 Thin Melanomas and Sentinel Lymph Node

Thin melanomas account for nearly 70 % of all melanoma. In general, this population has excellent outcomes with a 90 % survival at 10 years [3, 6, 7]. Despite this success, 3–7 % of patients will develop regional disease. Performing sentinel lymph node biopsies on *all* patients with thin melanoma is not cost effective and would subject patients to the risks, albeit small, associated with the procedure. Ideally, a trial could address the optimal selection of patients in this population who would benefit from undergoing the procedure. Unfortunately, the number of patients required to discern a difference and the number of variables which would have to be accounted for makes such a study impossible. Factors that have been variably shown to increase the risk of nodal metastases in patients with thin melanomas include Breslow thickness ≥0.75 mm, Clark's level IV, ulceration, mitotic rate of one or more, vertical growth phase, lymphovascular invasion, and tumor regression [8–15] (Table 1).

Studies have reported an increased risk of nodal metastases in thin melanomas ≥0.75 mm when compared to <0.75 mm [8–10]. Han et al. [14] recently reported 6.3 % of melanomas ≥0.75 mm had positive lymph nodes, while only 2.5 % of melanomas <0.75 had positive lymph nodes. Other studies have reported rates of 5–15 % positive nodes for melanomas ≥0.75 mm, but 0–5 % for melanomas <0.75 mm [8–10, 12, 16–20] (Table 2). Positive nodes in melanomas <0.5 mm are even more unusual.

Table 1 Potential indications for sentinel lymph node biopsy in melanomas <1 mm

Biology	Depth	Patient
Ulceration	Positive deep margin	Excessive anxiety
Lymphovascular invasion	Regression	Age (younger)
Mitotic rate	Clark level IV or V	
Vertical growth phase	>0.75 mm	

Table 2 Rates of SLN positivity in thin melanomas and correlating characteristics

Study	Breslow thickness	Rate of SLN positivity (%)	Comments/other factors correlating with + SLN
Han et al. [8]	T1a < 0.76	0	Mitotic rate > 1/mm^2 ($p < 0.05$) Ulceration ($p < 0.05$)
	T1a ≥ 0.76	4.8	
	T1b < 0.76	18.2	
	T1b ≥ 0.76	12.5	
	T1 < 0.76	6	
	T1 ≥ 0.76	8.1	
Murali et al. [10]	0.51–0.74 mm	3.8	Lymphovascular invasion ($p = 0.018$)
	0.76–0.90 mm	5.3	
	0.91–1.00 mm	10.3	
Wright et al. [16]	<0.25 mm	8	Age < 50 ($p = 0.04$)
	0.25–0.50 mm	4	
	0.51–0.75 mm	4	
	0.76–1.00 mm	6	
Ranieri et al. [17]	<0.75 mm	2.3	Mitotic index > 6/mm^2 ($p = 0.006$) Clark level ($p = 0.01$)
	0.75–1.00 mm	10.2	
Wong et al. [18]	<0.75 mm	0	No other significant factors
	≤1 mm	3.6	
Hinz et al. [19]	<0.90 mm	0	No other significant factors
	0.90–1.00 mm	4.1	

SLN sentinel lymph node

Clark level has also been advocated by some as a predictor of nodal involvement in thin melanomas; however, the subjectivity of this classification has limited its utility. Ranges of SLN metastases in Clark level < IV are reported as 3.5–4.5 %, but this increases to 7.4–12.3 % in Clark level ≥ IV [14, 15, 17]. Additional studies have reported that Clark level is a predictor of disease when stratified by Breslow thickness to <0.75 and ≥0.75 mm [14]. Given this information, many continue to advocate for SLN biopsy with Clark IV tumors.

Although uncommon in thin melanomas, ulceration is a risk factor for more aggressive disease and secondarily, positive SLN. Yonick et al. [9] recently reported a five times increased risk in positive SLN in the presence of ulceration. Likewise, Han et al. [8, 14] reported ulceration increased the risk of a positive SLN. When stratified to Breslow thickness ≥0.75 mm, there was a 14.7% rate of nodal positivity in patients with ulceration, whereas only 6 % of patients without ulceration had a positive SLN [8].

Mitotic rate was included in the most recent iteration of the AJCC staging system, being used to discriminate stage IB patients from stage IA [3]. Although correlative for metastatic potential and an independent predictor of survival, the overall contribution of mitotic figures to lymph node positivity is yet to be clearly defined [15, 21–23]. Other studies have found a slight but nonstatistically significant increases in SLN positivity or a significance only among patients with lymph node positive disease [8, 10]. This is an area where further research is necessary.

Tumor regression refers to the tumor loss associated with inflammatory stromal changes around a melanoma [12]. The prognostic significance of this phenomenon is not entirely clear and conflicting data abounds, but it remains another factor that may be considered when deciding if a SLN biopsy is necessary. While some studies have advocated for a more aggressive approach to sentinel lymph node biopsy in the setting of thin melanoma and mitotic figures, others have found this unwarranted [14, 24–26]. Although currently used at some sites to promote SLN biopsy, regression is not currently a criteria according to the National Comprehensive Cancer Network guidelines nor was it suggested by the consensus guidelines published jointly by the SSO and ASCO in 2012 [27, 28].

Despite a litany of histologic features which make a thin melanoma "high risk" the risk of nodal involvement, even in patients with these features, is low. Importantly, the risk of the procedure and the cost remain modest, at worst, and the impact of identifying disease early is significant on outcomes. The cost of delaying intervention in patients with nodal metastases is likely considerable, as well [29]. Given these considerations, the comparative effectiveness of sentinel node biopsy in thin melanoma patients is a question with an ambiguous answer and unfortunately, preconceived biases and limited alternative approaches deter additional studies attempting to review this question.

4 Thick Melanomas and Sentinel Lymph Node

Thick melanomas are described as Breslow thickness ≥4 mm. These patients have a significant risk of regional metastases (60–70 %) but an equally high risk of systemic disease (70 %). The high risk of systemic disease in this population has therefore led many authors to question the utility of sentinel lymph node biopsy in patients with melanomas greater than 4 mm in depth rationalizing that their prognosis is more strongly linked to progression to stage IV illness than to lymph node status [30, 31]. Because the survival of these patients is poor overall, Balch et al. [32, 33] initially hypothesized that locoregional management via nodal dissection was unlikely to confer survival benefit. However, two recent studies advocated that sentinel lymph node status—even in patients with thick melanoma—was found to be an independent predictor of survival [30, 31]. Gershenwald et al. [31] looked at 116 patients with melanoma >4 mm thick and found that sentinel lymph node status was still the most powerful predictor of overall survival by univariate and multivariate analyses.

Ferrone et al. [34] likewise looked at 126 patients with thick melanoma and found comparable rates of positive SLN (30 % vs. 39 %) and 3-year recurrence-free survival (76 % vs. 72 %). In the presence of conflicting data, many institutions routinely perform SLN biopsy even in those with thick primary tumors. With the advent of more robust therapeutic options for visceral disease and investigations demonstrating promising early results for genetic profiling of tumors, the role of surgical staging via sentinel lymph node biopsy becomes more ambiguous, generating a greater series of questions. The opportunity for early intervention in high-risk patients without the potential morbidity of surgical lymphadenectomy may pose a better alternative than the current paradigm in a subset of patients.

5 Overall Benefit of Sentinel Lymph Node Biopsy

The MSLT-1 trial has proven that early detection of regional metastases improves survival (Fig. 1); however, because the ability to select patients to undergo sentinel lymph node biopsy is impeded by the limitations of using histologic characteristics to determine biology, the procedure itself does not afford an overall survival benefit for all comers (intervention can only impact survival in the 17 % of patients who actually have nodal disease). This is compounded by the significant heterogeneity observed in the node positive group, which–with increasing recognition of microscopic and immunohistochemically detected disease, is likely to become more diverse. Survival in this group can range from 64 to 91 % depending on the population [35]. The resulting limitation of the sentinel lymph node procedure therefore, is that even in patients who are at the highest risk for having nodal metastases, nearly two-thirds will be undergoing a procedure that they do not need and, therefore, can derive no benefit. Within this context, the optimal improvement in this procedure will not be a technical one, but rather an intervention which aids in improving selection. Unfortunately, the ability to make this improvement will likely rely upon techniques other than histology such as genetic analyses or similar. Likewise, improvments in selection will be dependent on an ability to accrue large numbers of patients in order to discern even small differences in study groups. There is still much work to be done to define the group most likely to benefit from sentinel node biopsy.

To work this direction, we could use large database studies, using propensity scoring to match those undergoing sentinel- lymph node biopsy with similar controls. While pooling of clinical data from multiple institutions has been done by the American Joint Committee on Cancer (AJCC), using a larger data set and standardizing the pathology variables (in which there was previously wide variability), could help us find an answer. Decision analyses could also assist in this process, and could effectively summarize the costs, benefits, and probabilities of each branch point. Though it may be difficult to assign accurate probabilities to some of the more qualitative outcomes, such as quality of life and patient satisfaction, application of the decision sciences could be very productive in defining the proper use of sentinel lymph node biopsies.

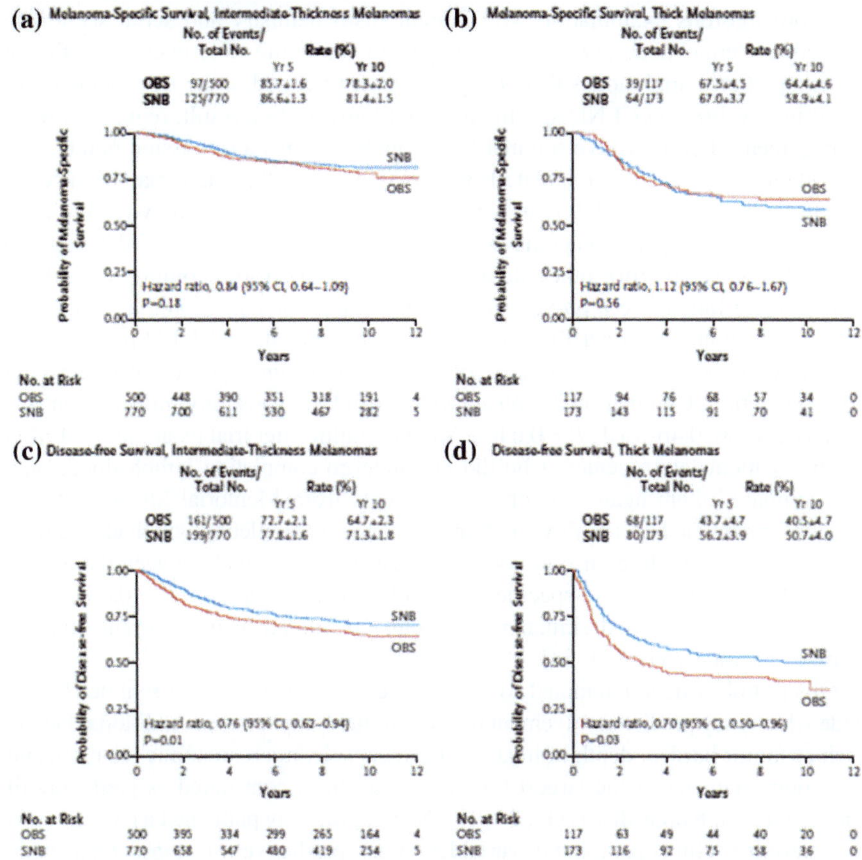

Fig. 1 Melanoma selective lymphadenectomy trial I (MSLT-1) results demonstrating both improved melanoma-specific survival and disease-free survival [29]. **a** Melanoma-specific survival, intermediate-thickness melanomas. **b** Melanoma-specific survival, thick melanomas. **c** Disease-free survival, intermediate-thickness melanomas. **d** Disease-free survival, thick melanomas

6 Completion Lymphadenectomy

The advent of sentinel node biopsy has made the management of nodal metastases even more controversial than the detection of nodal metastases. It is well recognized that in many diseases, management of regional disease is controversial (breast cancer, gastric cancer) and melanoma is similarly challenged. Using conventional histologic evaluation, only 20 % of patients undergoing CLND will have additional nodal disease, implying that as many as 80 % of SLN positive patients may be exposed to the risks of a second, more morbid procedure with potential long-term effects, without benefit. There are differences in the detection of metastatic deposits in sentinel nodes versus nodes in a completion lymphadenectomy specimen given the more rigorous examination with immunohistochemistry and serial sectioning applied to sentinel nodes. One could argue, that without the more intense scrutiny of the completion lymph nodes that is applied to sentinel nodes, the true incidence of nodal involvement in CLND specimens is not known. As a result, regional disease management after a positive sentinel lymph node remains a discussion point.

Although one might extrapolate from the MSLT trial that there may be survival benefit to clearing the nodal basin with completion lymphadenectomy (early detection of disease impacts outcome which would imply some potential benefit to regional disease control), other studies have not been so forthcoming. Outside of MSLT, there fails to be a proven survival advantage for undergoing a completion lymphadenectomy. Van der Ploeg et al. [36] recently evaluated 1,174 patients with sentinel node positive melanoma, 61 of whom did not undergo completion lymph node dissection. Completion lymphadenectomy did not show any influence on survival (HR 0.86, 0.46–1.61; $P = 0.640$). Another multicenter trial examined 134 SLN positive patients at 16 centers who did not undergo completion lymphadenectomy and compared them against a cohort of patients from Memorial Sloan Kettering Cancer Center who had a positive SLN and underwent completion lymphadenectomy [37]. There was no difference in nodal recurrence-free survival between the groups ($P = 0.07$) or in the disease-specific survival between the groups ($P = 0.65$). Other studies have documented similar results with no difference in recurrence-free or disease-specific survival [4, 38].

Other studies have attempted to delineate characteristics of the sentinel lymph node which may predict involvement of nonsentinel lymph nodes. Additional factors such as tumor burden, depth of invasion from capsule, microanatomic location, and maximum diameter of the largest tumor have all been considered as predictors of additional lymph node disease [4, 39–41]. Nagaraj recently published a metaanalysis to determine clinicopathologic variables most predictive of nonsentinel node metastases in the setting of a positive sentinel node [42]. There were nine factors including ulceration, satellitosis, neurotropism, >1 positive SLN, angiolymphatic invasion, extensive locations, macrometasases >2 mm, extranodal extension, and capsular involvement which predicted additional positive nodes beyond the sentinel lymph node. Unfortunately, this makes for a complex set of prognosticators when attempting to decide on completion lymphadenectomy and may not be as useful practically. Van der Ploeg et al. published a more straightforward study demonstrating that the burden of disease and allocation of tumor within the sentinel lymph node influences melanoma-specific survival. Patients with metastases <0.1 mm and found in the subcapsular area had a 5-year overall survival of 91 %. Nonsentinel lymph node rates for these patients was 2 %. The study concluded that completion lymph node dissection in these patients may be overtreating patients who have a survival that is equivalent to SLN negative patients [43].

The current guidelines of the 2008 National Comprehensive Cancer Network recommend either CLND or participation in a clinical trial for a positive sentinel lymph node. Despite these recommendations, only 50 % of patients in the National Cancer Data Base with a positive sentinel lymph node actually undergo CLND, clearly indicating some disconnect between recommendations and practice [44].

Reasons for lack of CLND in SLN positive patients are variable. Kingham et al. looked at over 2,000 patients who had undergone SLN biopsy, where 317 patients had positive SLN followed by lymphadenectomy and 42 patients with positive SLN did not. The patients not undergoing CLND were older (median age 70 vs. 56 years, $p < 0.01$) and had a trend toward thicker melanoma (Breslow 3.5 vs. 2.8 mm, $p < 0.06$). Additionally, as expected, there were a higher percentage of lower extremity melanomas in the group that did not undergo CLND (40 % vs. 13 %; <0.01) since many surgeons avoid groin dissections secondary to their high risk of complications and lymphedema. Bilimoria et al. and Cormier et al. [44, 45] found similar reasons for lower than expected rates of CLND such as older age, lower extremity melanoma, thin melanomas, and African-American race.

Perhaps most importantly, these studies, when analyzed in the context of the others, provide an ambiguity to the overall benefit to the patient undergoing completion lymphadenectomy. A survival benefit has not been proven, morbidity from many lymphadenectomies is high, and few patients in the sentinel node era actually recur in the nodal basin making palliative interventions a low priority. It is a challenge to demonstrate an overall comparative effectiveness to completion lymphadenectomy and it will be a long time before any data is available to provide any insight. Obstacles to our understanding this in greater detail include inherent bias toward the MSLT-2 trial (patients are only referred for possible observation if they are perceived as "lower risk"), low incidence of events in this population necessitating a large patient population with extended follow up, and finally a long "tail" in which events can occur before data is conclusively determined to represent a comprehensive review. With these obstacles, there will be a considerable delay before the questions surrounding lymphadenectomy can be answered.

Similar to the issues regarding the optimal use of sentinel lymph node biopsy, the uncertainty around completion lymph node dissections need to be explored using alternative research methods. Studies that make use of large databases and pooled multi-institutional clinical data will help us avoid the bias inherent in MSLT-2 and the long follow-up time required for meaningful results. Decision analyses can also help us examine how we should guide our patient through the process of choosing a completion lymphadenectomy or not.

7 Margins of Resection

7.1 1 versus 2 cm Margins

Until the 1970s, wide excision of all melanoma with 3–5 cm margins was the standard [46]. In the 1970s, there was recognition that different Breslow's thickness and Clark's levels may guide the need for a wider excision. In 1980s, the World Health Organization (WHO) melanoma group organized a randomized prospective clinical trial to determine optimal margin resection (1 cm vs. 3 cm) for thin melanoma <2 mm thick [47, 48]. There was no statistically significant local recurrence

Table 3 Randomized trials in primary melanoma excision margins

Trial	Melanoma thickness (mm)	Margins of resection	Local recurrence	Overall survival
WHO [46–48]	<2	1 cm versus 3 cm	12 year	12 year
			1 cm—2.6 %	1 cm—85.1 %
			3 cm—0.1 %	3 cm—87.2 %
				$p = 0.77$
Intergroup trial [49, 50]	1–4	2 cm versus 4 cm	10 year	10 year
			2 cm—2.1 %	2 cm—79 %
			5 cm—1 %	5 cm—7.6 %
				$p = 0.07$
Swedish melanoma study group [53]	0.8–2	2 cm versus 5 cm	10 year	10 year
			2 cm—0.6 %	2 cm—79 %
			5 cm—1.0 %	5 cm—76 %
French cooperative group [52]	<2.1	2 cm versus 5 cm	10 year	10 year
			2 cm—0.62 %	2 cm—87 %
			5 cm—2.4 %	5 cm—86 %
				$p = 0.56$
United Kingdom melanoma study group [51]	>2	1 cm versus 3 cm	5 year	5 year
			1 cm—3.3 %	1 cm—68.2 %
			3 cm—2.8 %	3 cm—70 %
				$p = 0.60$

between the two margins. A follow-up study from 1998 confirmed an insignificantly higher (2.6 % vs. 0.98 %) risk of local recurrence in the narrow margin group with no difference in overall survival [46]. Meanwhile the Intergroup Melanoma Surgical Trial randomized 1–4 mm melanomas to 2 cm versus 4 cm excisions [49]. Neither the local recurrence (0.8 % vs. 1.7 %) nor the 5-year survival (79.5 % vs. 83.7 %) were statistically significant. A follow-up study in 2001 confirmed that neither 10-year local recurrence (2.1 % vs. 2.6 %) nor overall survival (70 % vs. 76 %) was statistically significant in the narrow excision or wide excision groups [50]. Finally, the United Kingdom Melanoma Study Group Trial found no difference in local recurrence (3.3 % vs. 2.8 %) or overall 5-year survival (68.2 % vs. 70 %) in 1 cm versus 3 cm resection margins in melanomas >2 mm [51]. When combining local and regional disease recurrence, however, there was a significant difference (37.1 % vs. 31 %; $p = 0.05$) between the groups. In overlapping these trials, the recommendations of a 1–2 cm wide local excision for a 1–2 mm melanoma were created, allowing clinicians the liberty of taking a 1 cm margin in cosmetically sensitive locations (Table 3).

Two additional trials looked at even wider margins (Table 3). The French cooperative group randomized patients with thin or intermediate melanomas to 2 cm versus 5 cm local excision and found there was no difference in tumor recurrence, disease-free survival or overall survival for lesions <2 mm [52]. This was again confirmed in the Swedish Melanoma Study Group which looked at 2 cm

Table 4 Current recommendations for margins of excision

Breslow thickness	Margin of excision
In situ	5 mm
<1 mm	1 cm
1–2 mm	1 or 2 cm
2–4 mm	2 cm
>4 mm	2 cm

versus 5 cm margins in melanoma ≤2.1 mm thick [53]. There was no difference in overall survival or disease-specific survival at 10 years.

No randomized trials have ever examined 1 cm versus 2 cm margins and, while an international trial has been written and proposed, accrual to this trial is considered to be an obstacle. This concern is largely based on the fact that most clinicians have a predisposition to use a 1 cm margin where anatomically or physically constrained. A single institution study recently validated these data [54]. Hudson et al. reviewed 2,118 patients with T2 melanoma who underwent 1 cm versus 2 cm wide local excision. With a median follow-up of 38 months, the local recurrence was 3.6 months in the 1 cm group and 0.9 % in the 2 cm margin group ($p = 0.044$); however, on multivariate analysis, this difference was no longer significant ($p = 0.368$). Overall 5-year survival, likewise, was not statistically significant (29.1 months vs. 43.7 months). This validated the current NCCN recommendations; however, given the biases and uncertainty of retrospective analyses, a randomized controlled trial is required to put this question to rest.

For lesions greater than 2 mm, there remained controversy over margins of excision. Thomas et al. [51] published the results of a multi-institutional randomized trial of 1 versus 3 cm surgical margins in melanoma >2 mm. In the 900 patient trial, a 1 cm margin was associated with a statistically significant risk of recurrence but no difference in overall survival. Unfortunately, this trial did not use sentinel lymph node biopsy, had a poor definition for what constituted "local recurrence," and greater than 60 % of the recurrences were actually nodal in nature, which makes its modern applicability questionable. Still dissatisfied with the question of a 2 versus 4 cm resection margin for lesions >2 mm, Gillian et al. [55] published a trial specifically looking at these margins to determine overall survival. They found no difference in overall survival or in the risk of recurrence or death due to melanoma when using a 2 cm resection margin versus a 4 cm resection margin.

Thus, while the studies have compared different margins of excision based on Breslow depth of tumor, it has been globally accepted that a 2 cm margin is acceptable for melanomas >2 mm (Table 4). There appears to be no change in survival or recurrence with this margin. Importantly, the rate of primary closure with these resection margins is much higher than a 4 cm margin, which is associated with increased rates of skin grafts and their associated complications.

Despite the consensus regarding these approaches, there is increased morbidity with larger excisions, greater cost to the patient, and more days off from work. The goal of an excision is to perform complete removal of the tumor, and as has been noted with other malignancies, we have frequently overshot that mark. There is a considerable amount of data available on melanoma, but we are yet to find the smallest safe margin—which may even be less than 1 cm. At present, it will be extremely difficult to answer this question as biases have been set and although risks are definitely higher with larger excisions, the perceived morbidity is well tolerated.

However, if we could overcome these pre-conceptions, we could design a clinical trial similar to previous studies of wide local excisions, targeting cosmetically sensitive areas and patient populations that may be more willing to compromise in order to avoid wound healing issues or large grafts or flaps. There should also be efforts to design a trial that will tell us how deep a margin we truly need for a melanoma excision. In certain patients, on certain areas of the body (e.g., an obese patient with a thigh melanoma), it may not be necessary to excise all subcutaneous tissue down to the fascial level.

8 Radiation

8.1 Primary Cutaneous Melanoma

While the primary treatment of melanoma is surgical resection, radiation is often considered in both the primary and adjuvant setting. As the population ages, there are some elderly patients who are not candidates for surgical resection. In this scenario, there can be consideration for primary radiation therapy (RT) in patients with lentigo maligna and lentigo maligna melanoma. Small studies have shown that while the 5-year local recurrence rates are higher in patients treated with RT in head and neck melanoma, the difference may not be statistically significant (13.2 % vs. 6.8 %) [56]. This treatment is more often considered in Europe than in the United States.

Rates of local recurrence for cutaneous melanoma after appropriate wide local excision are approximately 5 %. However, there are certain conditions in which adjuvant radiation is considered including desmoplasia, neurotropism, microsatellites, positive resection margin not amenable to additional resection and recurrence after previous excision. Radiation is especially considered in cases of head and neck melanoma where further resection may simply not be feasible. Additionally, local control of lentigo maligna melanoma may be augmented with hypofractionated radiation [57]. Rao et al. [58] report that they are more likely to use radiation in patients with satellitosis because of the high risk of recurrence.

8.2 Radiation to Regional Nodal Basin

Studies have demonstrated benefit to adjuvant radiotherapy to regional nodal basins. Accepted criteria for this therapy include multiple positive nodes, large nodes, extracapsular extension, and recurrent disease. Recurrence rates of 60–80 % are reported for multiple nodes or nodes 6 cm or larger [59]. Likewise, extranodal extension is associated with an approximate 60 % recurrence rate [59, 60]. Finally, there are higher rates of relapses in the neck (35–45 %), whereas rates in the axilla

(25–35 %) and the groin (10–20 %) tend to be lower [59]. There are recent trials demonstrating decreased recurrence in high-risk nodal beds (multiple positive nodes, extracapsular extension, large nodes, or recurrent disease) [61, 62]. Burmeister et al. demonstrated a significant difference in reduced risk of lymph node field relapse to 16.3 % from 26.8 % (Hazard Ratio 0.56, 95 % confidence interval 0.32–0.98; $p = 0.41$), but no difference in relapse-free survival or overall survival in their randomized controlled trial.

Radiation is not without complications. Although cervical radiation is fairly well tolerated, complications are not infrequent in other sites. Complications following axillary radiation can be as high as 30 % at 5 years [58, 63]. In a study from the Melanoma Institute of Australia, arm lymphedema rates after axillary dissection with radiation were 53 % [64]. A similar study from MD Anderson demonstrated a 20 % incidence of lymphedema that necessitated medical treatment [65]. Complications in the groin after radiation and groin dissection can similarly be substantial, especially in those with a body mass index greater than 30 kg/m^2 [63]. Ballo et al. [66] demonstrated a 23 % incidence of clinically significant lymphedema after inguinal lymph node dissection and RT and a 40 % rate of clinically significant treatment-related complications of wound breakdown and healing complications. In the TROG study, Burmeister et al. [67] reported a 9 % incidence of lymphedema in patients with axillary disease undergoing lymphadenectomy and radiation. This number increases to a 19 % incidence of grade 3 lymphedema after ilioinguinal dissection and radiation. Although significant reductions in local recurrence are demonstrated, given these high complication rates, appropriate consideration should be given prior to instituting RT following lymphadenectomy. To balance the possible morbidity of this treatment against its benefits, more trial data would be helpful. Randomizing patients at a high risk of nodal disease (e.g., advanced Stage II) may help to delineate the limits of utility of this treatment in the clinical setting.

8.3 Brain Metastases

Up to half of patients with metastatic melanoma develop brain metastases [68]. Once brain metastases develop, the 1-year survival is less than 15 % [69]. Options for therapy include surgery, systemic therapy, whole brain radiation (WBR), and stereotactic radiosurgery. Although there are many studies on treatment of brain metastases, these often include multiple primary sites so applicability to metastatic melanoma in particular, may be limited.

8.4 Whole Brain

WBR has been described for many years in the treatment of metastatic lesions to the brain. When used alone, WBR does not have an appreciable survival benefit, but it can help with reducing symptoms and halting progression to allow for salvage therapy. Median survival after WBR is 3–5 months [70–72]. The addition of temozolomide may afford a slightly higher median survival of 6 months with an approximate 10 % response rate [73]. Finally, a recent phase 2 study evaluated temozolomide, thalidomide, and WBR to patients with brain metastases from melanoma and found only a 7.6 response rate with a median time to progression of 7 weeks and a median overall survival of 4 months [74]. Complications from WBR include neurocognitive toxicity and progressive dementia [58, 75].

8.5 Stereotactic Radiosurgery

Both gamma knife and linear accelerator-based radiosurgery have been used for cerebral melanoma metastases. TROG 9508 was a randomized trial of patients with one to three brain metastases (5 % melanoma primary) to WBR with or without the addition of SBRT and found an improvement in performance status at 6 months for those that received both therapies, but no survival advantage with the addition of SBRT. In patients with a single lesion, there was a benefit to adding SBRT to WBR [76]. Other studies have shown an improvement in relapse-free survival with the combination of WBR and SBRT [77, 78]. Finally, several studies have retrospectively evaluated melanoma-specific brain metastases and found SBRT to be beneficial for local control of melanoma, especially in those with a good performance status and a limited number of lesions, as well as control of extracranial metastases [79].

In summary, radiation is rarely used as the primary treatment of melanoma. Its use in control of high-risk lesions, as well as high-risk nodal basins after surgical resection remains in evolution, but has not shown definitive survival benefit. RT for central nervous system metastases could become more standard of care as newer techniques such as intensity modulated RT and image-guided RT enable more precise delivery to tumor with avoidance of normal tissue.

9 Staging and Follow up

Perhaps one of the least controversial yet equally minimally evidence-based aspects of the care of melanoma patients is routine imaging and patient follow up. Several studies have demonstrated little utility to routine exams and there is no evidence that radiographic imaging benefits patients in any manner [80–83]. Of all endeavors in the care of patients with a history of malignancy, radiographic imaging may be the most costly and the least proven. It is important to note that the timing of imaging rarely impacts therapeutic decision-making and the majority of scans performed in asymptomatic patients are negative. Furthermore, there is growing concern regarding the side effects from the radiation associated with repeated thin-cut CT scans.

In melanoma, as with many malignancies, the routine physical exam in follow up rarely yields a significant finding. Patients are instructed to contact providers to let them know of changes in between routine appointments. It is most often these interval evaluations that prompt further examination and investigation. Consider the scenario: in order for a routine visit to be the mechanism by which a patient identifies a recurrence or new lesion, the timing has to be that the lesion was first noticed within close proximity of the scheduled visit. Therefore, it is often the interval visits scheduled at the request of the patient that prompt additional testing for new concerns.

Perhaps most striking is that even with published NCCN guidelines many clinicians still routinely perform staging evaluations inclusive of aggressive radiographic imaging modalities in asymptomatic patients [83]. Even the most educated physicians who are aware of the evidence against routine scans will often acquiesce to radiographic studies "just to be sure." The solution to this is dependent on the education of the public—the public will need to understand that the routine scan has little benefit in the absence of symptoms—before the clamor for scans will begin to quiet. Despite these arguments against scanning, one cannot apply a value to the reassurance (false or real) provided by cross-sectional imaging. The ability to take a sigh of relief is an intangible, immeasurable quality that benefits patients and their families, despite the evidence against routine scans.

To determine the clinical utility of this practice, however, we need to perform rigorous cost-effective analyses and decision analyses. If findings of these speak against routine physical exam and imaging follow-up, the clinical conversation between surgical oncologist and patient will have to be accordingly tailored. Assessments of outcomes should then be performed; a recent Patient-Centered Outcomes Research Institute (PCORI) grant was giving to a project looking at patient self-management of distressing symptoms in centers treating breast, lung, prostate, and colon cancer. More projects in this vein could help to ease the anxiety that accompanies any cancer diagnosis.

10 Conclusion

As oncologists, we are faced with the challenges of decision-making in a less than informed environment. Charged with the task of applying evidence-based medicine in a field with a paucity of evidence and an enormous burden of bias, the challenge of making the right choices for our patients is overwhelming. It is unlikely that many of the questions in melanoma can be answered due to the complexity of the variables and the marginal differences expected. There are, however, opportunities for improving our understanding, enhancing our decision-making, and for the application of known data in a more effective manner. Importantly, these decisions cannot be made in the lay press and in the court of public opinion. It is imperative that knowledge be shared and choices be driven by data and not impression. Opportunities abound for investigation and the development of a better understanding of this disease and those must be pursued if we endeavor to provide the best care possible for patients.

References

1. Holmes EC, Moseley HS, Morton DL et al (1977) A rational approach to the surgical management of melanoma. Ann Surg 186:481–490
2. Morton DL, Wen DR, Wong JH et al (1992) Technical details of intraoperative lymphatic mapping for early stage melanoma. Arch Surg 127:392–399
3. Balch CM, Gershenwald JE, Soong SJ et al (2009) Final version of 2009 AJCC melanoma staging and classification. J Clin Oncol 27:6199–6206
4. Morton DL, Thompson JF, Cochran AJ et al (2006) Sentinel-node biopsy or nodal observation in melanoma. N Engl J Med 355:1307–1317
5. Wong SL, Kattan MW, McMasters KM et al (2005) A nomogram that predicts the presence of sentinel node metastasis in melanoma with better discrimination than the American joint committee on cancer staging system. Ann Surg Oncol 12:282–288
6. Gimotty PA, Guerry D, Ming ME et al (2004) Thin primary cutaneous malignant melanoma: a prognostic tree for 10-year metastasis is more accurate than American joint committee on cancer staging. J Clin Oncol 22:3668–3676
7. McKinnon JG, Yu XQ, McCarthy WH et al (2003) Prognosis for patients with thin cutaneous melanoma: long-term survival data from New South Wales Central Cancer Registry and the Sydney melanoma unit. Cancer 98:1223–1231
8. Han D, Yu D, Zhao X et al (2012) Sentinel node biopsy is indicated for thin melanomas ≥0.76 mm. Ann Surg Oncol 19:3335–3342
9. Yonick DV, Ballo RM, Kahn E et al (2011) Predictors of positive sentinel lymph node in thin melanoma. Am J Surg 201:324–327 (discussion 327–328)
10. Murali R, Haydu LE, Quinn MJ et al (2012) Sentinel lymph node biopsy in patients with thin primary cutaneous melanoma. Ann Surg 255:128–133
11. Koskivuo I, Suominen E, Niinikoski J et al (2005) Sentinel node metastasectomy in thin < or = 1-mm melanoma. Langenbecks Arch Surg 390:403–407
12. Morris KT, Busam KJ, Bero S et al (2008) Primary cutaneous melanoma with regression does not require a lower threshold for sentinel lymph node biopsy. Ann Surg Oncol 15:316–322
13. Olah J, Dobozy A (2003) The new TNM classification of malignant melanoma. Magy Onkol 47:59–61
14. Han D, Zager JS, Shyr Y et al (2013) Clinicopathologic predictors of sentinel lymph node metastasis in thin melanoma. J Clin Oncol 31:4387–4393
15. Kesmodel SB, Karakousis GC, Botbyl JD et al (2005) Mitotic rate as a predictor of sentinel lymph node positivity in patients with thin melanomas. Ann Surg Oncol 12:449–458
16. Wright BE, Scheri RP, Ye X et al (2008) Importance of sentinel lymph node biopsy in patients with thin melanoma. Arch Surg 143:892–899 (discussion 899–900)
17. Ranieri JM, Wagner JD, Wenck S et al (2006) The prognostic importance of sentinel lymph node biopsy in thin melanoma. Ann Surg Oncol 13:927–932
18. Wong SL, Brady MS, Busam KJ et al (2006) Results of sentinel lymph node biopsy in patients with thin melanoma. Ann Surg Oncol 13:302–309
19. Hinz T, Ahmadzadehfar H, Wierzbicki A et al (2012) Prognostic value of sentinel lymph node biopsy in 121 low-risk melanomas (tumour thickness <1.00 mm) on the basis of a long-term follow-up. Eur J Nucl Med Mol Imaging 39:581–588
20. Cecchi R, Buralli L, Innocenti S et al (2007) Sentinel lymph node biopsy in patients with thin melanomas. J Dermatol 34:512–515
21. Karakousis GC, Gimotty PA, Botbyl JD et al (2006) Predictors of regional nodal disease in patients with thin melanomas. Ann Surg Oncol 13:533–541
22. Azzola MF, Shaw HM, Thompson JF et al (2003) Tumor mitotic rate is a more powerful prognostic indicator than ulceration in patients with primary cutaneous melanoma: an analysis of 3,661 patients from a single center. Cancer 97:1488–1498

23. Francken AB, Shaw HM, Thompson JF et al (2004) The prognostic importance of tumor mitotic rate confirmed in 1317 patients with primary cutaneous melanoma and long follow-up. Ann Surg Oncol 11:426–433
24. Brogelli L, Reali UM, Moretti S et al (1992) The prognostic significance of histologic regression in cutaneous melanoma. Melanoma Res 2:87–91
25. Olah J, Gyulai R, Korom I et al (2003) Tumour regression predicts higher risk of sentinel node involvement in thin cutaneous melanomas. Br J Dermatol 149:662–663
26. Kelly JW, Sagebiel RW, Blois MS (1985) Regression in malignant melanoma. A histologic feature without independent prognostic significance. Cancer 56:2287–2291
27. Wong SL, Balch CM, Hurley P et al (2012) Sentinel lymph node biopsy for melanoma: American society of clinical oncology and society of surgical oncology joint clinical practice guideline. Ann Surg Oncol 19:3313–3324
28. Wong SL, Balch CM, Hurley P et al (2012) Sentinel lymph node biopsy for melanoma: American society of clinical oncology and society of surgical oncology joint clinical practice guideline. J Clin Oncol 30:2912–2918
29. Morton DL, Thompson JF, Cochran AJ et al (2014) Final trial report of sentinel-node biopsy versus nodal observation in melanoma. N Engl J Med 370:599–609
30. Kim SH, Garcia C, Rodriguez J et al (1999) Prognosis of thick cutaneous melanoma. J Am Coll Surg 188:241–247
31. Gershenwald JE, Mansfield PF, Lee JE et al (2000) Role for lymphatic mapping and sentinel lymph node biopsy in patients with thick (> or = 4 mm) primary melanoma. Ann Surg Oncol 7:160–165
32. Balch CM (1980) Surgical management of regional lymph nodes in cutaneous melanoma. J Am Acad Dermatol 3:511–524
33. Balch CM, Soong SJ, Milton GW et al (1982) A comparison of prognostic factors and surgical results in 1,786 patients with localized (stage I) melanoma treated in Alabama, USA, and New South Wales. Australia. Ann Surg 196:677–684
34. Ferrone CR, Panageas KS, Busam K et al (2002) Multivariate prognostic model for patients with thick cutaneous melanoma: importance of sentinel lymph node status. Ann Surg Oncol 9:637–645
35. van Akkooi AC, Nowecki ZI, Voit C et al (2008) Sentinel node tumor burden according to the Rotterdam criteria is the most important prognostic factor for survival in melanoma patients: a multicenter study in 388 patients with positive sentinel nodes. Ann Surg 248:949–955
36. van der Ploeg AP, van Akkooi AC, Rutkowski P et al (2012) Prognosis in patients with sentinel node-positive melanoma without immediate completion lymph node dissection. Br J Surg 99:1396–1405
37. Wong SL, Morton DL, Thompson JF et al (2006) Melanoma patients with positive sentinel nodes who did not undergo completion lymphadenectomy: a multi-institutional study. Ann Surg Oncol 13:809–816
38. Kingham TP, Panageas KS, Ariyan CE et al (2010) Outcome of patients with a positive sentinel lymph node who do not undergo completion lymphadenectomy. Ann Surg Oncol 17:514–520
39. van Akkooi AC, de Wilt JH, Verhoef C et al (2006) Clinical relevance of melanoma micrometastases (<0.1 mm) in sentinel nodes: are these nodes to be considered negative? Ann Oncol 17:1578–1585
40. Starz H, Siedlecki K, Balda BR (2004) Sentinel lymphonodectomy and s-classification: a successful strategy for better prediction and improvement of outcome of melanoma. Ann Surg Oncol 11:162S–168S
41. Dewar DJ, Newell B, Green MA et al (2004) The microanatomic location of metastatic melanoma in sentinel lymph nodes predicts nonsentinel lymph node involvement. J Clin Oncol 22:3345–3349

42. Nagaraja V, Eslick GD (2013) Is complete lymph node dissection after a positive sentinel lymph node biopsy for cutaneous melanoma always necessary? A Meta-Anal Eur J Surg Oncol 39:669–680
43. van der Ploeg AP, van Akkooi AC, Rutkowski P et al (2011) Prognosis in patients with sentinel node-positive melanoma is accurately defined by the combined Rotterdam tumor load and Dewar topography criteria. J Clin Oncol 29:2206–2214
44. Bilimoria KY, Balch CM, Bentrem DJ et al (2008) Complete lymph node dissection for sentinel node-positive melanoma: assessment of practice patterns in the United States. Ann Surg Oncol 15:1566–1576
45. Cormier JN, Xing Y, Ding M et al (2005) Population-based assessment of surgical treatment trends for patients with melanoma in the era of sentinel lymph node biopsy. J Clin Oncol 23:6054–6062
46. Cascinelli N (1998) Margin of resection in the management of primary melanoma. Semin Surg Oncol 14:272–275
47. Veronesi U, Cascinelli N, Adamus J et al (1988) Thin stage I primary cutaneous malignant melanoma. Comparison of excision with margins of 1 or 3 cm. N Engl J Med 318:1159–1162
48. Veronesi U, Cascinelli N (1991) Narrow excision (1-cm margin). A safe procedure for thin cutaneous melanoma. Arch Surg 126:438–441
49. Balch CM, Urist MM, Karakousis CP et al (1993) Efficacy of 2-cm surgical margins for intermediate-thickness melanomas (1–4 mm). Results of a multi-institutional randomized surgical trial. Ann Surg 218:262–267 (discussion 267–269)
50. Balch CM, Soong SJ, Smith T et al (2001) Long-term results of a prospective surgical trial comparing 2 cm vs. 4 cm excision margins for 740 patients with 1–4 mm melanomas. Ann Surg Oncol 8:101–108
51. Thomas JM, Newton-Bishop J, A'Hern R et al (2004) Excision margins in high-risk malignant melanoma. N Engl J Med 350:757–766
52. Khayat D, Rixe O, Martin G et al (2003) Surgical margins in cutaneous melanoma (2 cm versus 5 cm for lesions measuring less than 2.1-mm thick). Cancer 97:1941–1946
53. Cohn-Cedermark G, Rutqvist LE, Andersson R et al (2000) Long term results of a randomized study by the Swedish melanoma study group on 2-cm versus 5-cm resection margins for patients with cutaneous melanoma with a tumor thickness of 0.8–2.0 mm. Cancer 89:1495–1501
54. Hudson LE, Maithel SK, Carlson GW et al (2013) 1 or 2 cm margins of excision for T2 melanomas: do they impact recurrence or survival? Ann Surg Oncol 20:346–351
55. Gillgren P, Drzewiecki KT, Niin M et al (2011) 2-cm versus 4-cm surgical excision margins for primary cutaneous melanoma thicker than 2 mm: a randomised, multicentre trial. Lancet 378:1635–1642
56. Zalaudek I, Horn M, Richtig E et al (2003) Local recurrence in melanoma in situ: influence of sex, age, site of involvement and therapeutic modalities. Br J Dermatol 148:703–708
57. Harwood AR (1982) Conventional radiotherapy in the treatment of lentigo maligna and lentigo maligna melanoma. J Am Acad Dermatol 6:310–316
58. Rao NG, Yu HH, Trotti A 3rd et al (2011) The role of radiation therapy in the management of cutaneous melanoma. Surg Oncol Clin N Am 20:115–131
59. Lee RJ, Gibbs JF, Proulx GM et al (2000) Nodal basin recurrence following lymph node dissection for melanoma: implications for adjuvant radiotherapy. Int J Radiat Oncol Biol Phys 46:467–474
60. Shen P, Guenther JM, Wanek LA et al (2000) Can elective lymph node dissection decrease the frequency and mortality rate of late melanoma recurrences? Ann Surg Oncol 7:114–119
61. Burmeister BH, Smithers BM, Davis S et al (2002) Radiation therapy following nodal surgery for melanoma: an analysis of late toxicity. Anz J Surg 72:344–348
62. Burmeister BH, Henderson MA, Ainslie J et al (2012) Adjuvant radiotherapy versus observation alone for patients at risk of lymph-node field relapse after therapeutic lymphadenectomy for melanoma: a randomised trial. Lancet Oncol 13:589–597

63. Guadagnolo BA, Zagars GK (2009) Adjuvant radiation therapy for high-risk nodal metastases from cutaneous melanoma. Lancet Oncol 10:409–416
64. Starritt EC, Joseph D, McKinnon JG et al (2004) Lymphedema after complete axillary node dissection for melanoma: assessment using a new, objective definition. Ann Surg 240:866–874
65. Beadle BM, Guadagnolo BA, Ballo MT et al (2009) Radiation therapy field extent for adjuvant treatment of axillary metastases from malignant melanoma. Int J Radiat Oncol Biol Phys 73:1376–1382
66. Ballo MT, Zagars GK, Gershenwald JE et al (2004) A critical assessment of adjuvant radiotherapy for inguinal lymph node metastases from melanoma. Ann Surg Oncol 11:1079–1084
67. Burmeister BH, Mark Smithers B, Burmeister Burmeister E et al (2006) A prospective phase II study of adjuvant postoperative radiation therapy following nodal surgery in malignant melanoma-trans tasman radiation oncology group (TROG) study 96.06. Radiother Oncol 81:136–142
68. Douglas JG, Margolin K (2002) The treatment of brain metastases from malignant melanoma. Semin Oncol 29:518–524
69. Sperduto PW, Chao ST, Sneed PK et al (2010) Diagnosis-specific prognostic factors, indexes, and treatment outcomes for patients with newly diagnosed brain metastases: a multi-institutional analysis of 4,259 patients. Int J Radiat Oncol Biol Phys 77:655–661
70. Sampson JH, Carter JH Jr, Friedman AH et al (1998) Demographics, prognosis, and therapy in 702 patients with brain metastases from malignant melanoma. J Neurosurg 88:11–20
71. Broadbent AM, Hruby G, Tin MM et al (2004) Survival following whole brain radiation treatment for cerebral metastases: an audit of 474 patients. Radiother Oncol 71:259–265
72. Meier S, Baumert BG, Maier T et al (2004) Survival and prognostic factors in patients with brain metastases from malignant melanoma. Onkologie 27:145–149
73. Margolin K, Atkins B, Thompson A et al (2002) Temozolomide and whole brain irradiation in melanoma metastatic to the brain: a phase II trial of the cytokine working group. J Cancer Res Clin Oncol 128:214–218
74. Atkins MB, Sosman JA, Agarwala S et al (2008) Temozolomide, thalidomide, and whole brain radiation therapy for patients with brain metastasis from metastatic melanoma: a phase II cytokine working group study. Cancer 113:2139–2145
75. Asai A, Matsutani M, Kohno T et al (1989) Subacute brain atrophy after radiation therapy for malignant brain tumor. Cancer 63:1962–1974
76. Andrews DW, Scott CB, Sperduto PW et al (2004) Whole brain radiation therapy with or without stereotactic radiosurgery boost for patients with one to three brain metastases: phase III results of the RTOG 9508 randomised trial. Lancet 363:1665–1672
77. Aoyama H, Shirato H, Tago M et al (2006) Stereotactic radiosurgery plus whole-brain radiation therapy vs stereotactic radiosurgery alone for treatment of brain metastases: a randomized controlled trial. JAMA 295:2483–2491
78. Aoyama H, Westerly DC, Mackie TR et al (2006) Integral radiation dose to normal structures with conformal external beam radiation. Int J Radiat Oncol Biol Phys 64:962–967
79. Liew DN, Kano H, Kondziolka D et al (2011) Outcome predictors of gamma knife surgery for melanoma brain metastases. Clinical Article J Neurosurg 114:769–779
80. Gold JS, Jaques DP, Busam KJ et al (2007) Yield and predictors of radiologic studies for identifying distant metastases in melanoma patients with a positive sentinel lymph node biopsy. Ann Surg Oncol 14:2133–2140
81. Aloia TA, Gershenwald JE, Andtbacka RH et al (2006) Utility of computed tomography and magnetic resonance imaging staging before completion lymphadenectomy in patients with sentinel lymph node-positive melanoma. J Clin Oncol 24:2858–2865
82. Miranda EP, Gertner M, Wall J et al (2004) Routine imaging of asymptomatic melanoma patients with metastasis to sentinel lymph nodes rarely identifies systemic disease. Arch Surg 139:831–836 (discussion 836–837)
83. National Comprehensive Cancer Center Network. Melanoma (version 4.2014). http://www.nccn.org/professional/physician_gls/pdf/melanoma.pdf

63. Guadagnolo BA, Zagars GK (2009) Adjuvant radiation therapy for high-risk nodal metastases from cutaneous melanoma. Lancet Oncol 10:409–416
64. Spratt BC, Joseph D, McKinnon JG et al (2004) Lymphedema after complete axillary node dissection for melanoma: assessment using a new, objective definition. Ann Surg 240:564–571
65. Beadle BM, Guadagnolo BA, Ballo MT et al (2009) Radiation therapy field extent for adjuvant treatment of axillary metastases from malignant melanoma. Int J Radiat Oncol Biol Phys 73:1376–1382
66. Ballo MT, Zagars GK, Gershenwald JE et al (2004) A critical assessment of adjuvant radiotherapy for inguinal lymph node metastases from melanoma. Ann Surg Oncol 11:1079–1084
[illegible]

Comparative Effectiveness Research for Sarcoma

Nabil Wasif

Abstract

Modern multidisciplinary management of sarcoma represents several opportunities for comparative effectiveness research. Focusing on the outcomes of survival, quality of life and cost-effectiveness of care, the current state of the art is summarized. Specialized/regional care for sarcoma and the utility of tumor boards or multispecialty discussion is discussed. Issues related to treatment efficacy and sequencing in relation to chemotherapy, radiation, and surgery as well as margin reporting and surveillance are also discussed. Finally, future avenues of comparative effectiveness research for sarcoma are highlighted throughout the chapter.

Keywords

Extremity sarcoma · Retroperitoneal sarcoma · Comparative effectiveness research

Contents

N. Wasif (✉)
Department of Surgery, Mayo Clinic Arizona, Phoenix, AZ, USA
e-mail: wasif.nabil@mayo.edu

K.Y. Bilimoria et al. (eds.), *Comparative Effectiveness in Surgical Oncology*,
Cancer Treatment and Research 164, DOI 10.1007/978-3-319-12553-4_4

1 Introduction

Sarcoma represents the quintessential malignancy for a surgical oncologist. Whilst other cancers such as colon and breast may fall under the purview of the general surgeon, the rare incidence, heterogeneity in histology, and surgical challenges involved with sarcoma care call for specialized training. The multidisciplinary aspect of modern sarcoma care often requires consultation with other specialists prior to initiation of therapy, which may not be possible in practice settings not conducive to such co-ordination. The clinical challenges of sarcoma care make a ready recipe for the introduction of variation in delivery of care. Although some of this variation may be attributed to the co-ordination of complex care, lack of quality data to guide clinical management is also to blame. The focus of this chapter is to explore how this variation influences outcomes for patient with sarcoma, and to suggest future avenues for study to smooth out fluctuations in care by using the methodology of comparative effectiveness research.

Meaningful comparative effectiveness research should be linked to outcomes that are biologically relevant, measurable in an objective manner and comparable between studies. For oncologists of all stripes a scorched earth policy to maximize long-term outcomes is often justified by the primacy of long-term survival, or surrogates such as recurrence-free survival, as the arbiter of treatment efficacy. An increasing focus on patient-centered outcomes means that quality of life (QOL) among survivors is considered more often before embarking on potentially toxic therapy. In the context of the overall health care system cost can be regarded as a valid outcome measure for two treatments of equal efficacy, or one of marginal efficacy. The ideal therapy is one that combines maximal efficacy with minimal morbidity and is the most economical; this 'goldilocks' mix is seldom the case in the clinical world. In the ensuing discussion, the issues of multidisciplinary consultation and guideline-oriented care, regionalization, and treatment of soft tissue extremity and retroperitoneal sarcoma will be discussed while focusing on the three outcomes of survival, QOL, and cost.

2 Multidisciplinary Consultation and Guideline-Oriented Care

Current national comprehensive cancer network (NCCN) guidelines suggest that 'all patients be evaluated by a MD team with expertise and experience in sarcoma prior to initiation of therapy' [1]. The implication is that discussion in a multidisciplinary setting has the potential to improve patient outcomes for sarcoma. However, there is little data to support an improvement in survival, QOL, or cost of therapy with multidisciplinary consultation prior to initiation of therapy. Given the complexity of the disease and numerous patient and practice patterns involved in treatment, such a change may be hard to show in a direct comparison. Nevertheless, it does not invalidate the utility of such an approach. In a survey study of physicians involved in sarcoma care, 83 % had access to a multidisciplinary sarcoma tumor board and the usefulness in clinical decision-making was rated at a mean of 4.08 ± 0.05 on a Likert scale (where 1 = not helpful and 5 = always helpful) by the respondents [2].

Care outside of a multidisciplinary setting certainly has the potential to be fragmented and of potential detriment to the patient. Does this translate into worst outcomes? Although there is no direct confirmation, circumstantial evidence can be obtained from the same survey study of sarcoma specialists. When presented with an identical clinical scenario, each specialist was inclined to favor their respective treatment modality at the expense of others, suggesting a 'specialty bias' exists in treatment recommendations for soft tissue extremity sarcoma [3]. One would hope that in a multidisciplinary setting, consensus opinion would counteract the influence of individual bias on clinical decision-making. The role of multidisciplinary consultation on sarcoma survival, QOL, and cost outcomes remains an area ripe for comparative effectiveness research. Performing an observational cohort study of patients treated in a multidisciplinary setting versus those who are not, perhaps using the National Cancer Database (NCDB) to obtain the necessary information, could help demonstrate the effect of having a multidisciplinary team. Qualitative studies evaluating physicians' changes in plans before and after tumor board meetings may also help to illustrate the role of multidisciplinary care. This could both be done in an academic center as well as in community centers without multidisciplinary meetings, who would then begin to take part in academic tumor boards.

A central tenant of the NCCN guidelines is to provide providers with a set of recommendations as a reference point for the management of complex cancer patients. These guidelines are based on best available evidence with the tacit understanding that compliance with guideline-oriented care should improve outcomes. This approach is predicated on the quality of the evidence available to formulate the guidelines themselves, as well as access. The latter is usually not an issue as the guidelines are freely available on the web [1]. For sarcoma, many of the guidelines are derived not from randomized trials but Category 2 or below level evidence, leading to intentionally vague recommendations. Nevertheless, until better data becomes available, one can assume that adherence to current recommendations is not worse, and potentially better, than unstandardized care. Participation in multidisciplinary care has been shown to improve compliance with guidelines, suggesting that discussion in a group setting improves conformity to best available evidence [4].

The discussion above begs the question—does care that is compliant with current sarcoma guidelines improve the quality of clinical care compared to care that is not? There is precious little data to inform this debate. Establishment of national guidelines for soft tissue sarcoma in the Netherlands led to improvements in preoperative diagnoses and pathology reporting for patients [5]. An analysis of the SEER database looking at the stage specific use of radiation therapy for soft tissue extremity sarcoma showed that omission of radiation therapy for Stage III patients led to worse survival outcomes, although selection bias could also explain these results. [6]. A cost-effectiveness analysis from two European regions showed that noncompliance to sarcoma guidelines resulted in a cost increase of 16 % compared to patients in whom guideline-oriented care was delivered [7]. These studies notwithstanding, an unambiguous association between multidisciplinary, guideline-oriented care, and an improvement in survival outcomes, QOL, or costs has yet to be demonstrated in the United States. Use of large databases to determine the outcomes of guideline-adherent practices should be undertaken.

3 Regionalization of Sarcoma Care

The majority of sarcoma care in the United States is performed by nonspecialists or 'part-time' sarcoma physicians. As with other complex cancers, there has been a call to regionalize care of sarcoma patients to high volume or specialized centers so that outcomes can be improved. Are there any grounds to justify these claims? Guiterrez et al. [8] looked at data from the Florida Cancer Data System (FCDS) to show that both survival and functional outcomes were indeed better at high volume centers. Although the majority of patients (68 %) received care at low-volume centers, 30-day mortality at high volume centers was lower (0.7 % vs. 1.5 %, $p = 0.028$). Long-term survival was also improved at high-volume centers, with a median survival of 40 months compared to 37 months at low-volume centers ($p = 0.002$). QOL may also be impacted by treatment at a low-volume center; the amputation rate was 13.8 % compared to 9.4 % for high volume centers ($p = 0.048$). Another study from the United Kingdom showed that only 21 % of patients were adequately worked up, and only 60 % received adequate treatment after an audit of sarcoma care [9]. The majority of these patients were treated by general surgeons and the authors called for treatment to be shunted toward specialists to improve care metrics. Several studies from Europe suggest that specialized care for sarcoma results in better compliance with guidelines and less variation in care [4, 9, 10]. The weight of the evidence currently available suggests that regionalization of sarcoma care results in improved survival outcomes and QOL. How this impacts cost and timeliness of care has yet to be determined, leaving the door open for well-designed cost-effectiveness analyses. Use of databases such as the NCDB or the Surveillance,

Epidemiology, and End Results (SEER)-Medicare datasets, which have been used by other regionalization studies, could also help to evaluate oncologic outcomes as a result of regionalization.

4 Soft Tissue Extremity Sarcoma

4.1 Neoadjuvant Chemotherapy

The use of neoadjuvant chemotherapy has several theoretical advantages, especially in high-risk extremity sarcoma. With visible disease an in vivo tumor response model is available. Shrinkage of a large tumor can potentially enhance limb salvage and decrease the morbidity associated with eventual surgery. Finally, early treatment of micrometastatic disease has the potential to improve long-term survival outcomes. Although an increase in perioperative morbidity due to myelosuppression and interference with optimal wound healing is a concern, this is not borne out by the data [11]. However, the evidence supporting the efficacy of chemotherapy alone in the neoadjuvant setting is underwhelming. Although an extensive review on the subject is beyond the purview of this chapter, some of the more pertinent studies are mentioned.

An EORTC randomized phase II trial compared neoadjuvant doxorubicin plus ifosfamide versus surgery alone in a high-risk population and failed to show better survival in the chemotherapy arm (5 years DFS 56 % vs. 52 %), and expansion into phase III study was abandoned [12]. Although a phase III study utilizing hyperthermia in combination with etoposide, ifosfamide, and doxorubicin (EIA) versus chemotherapy alone showed a relative hazard of 0.7 for the combination therapy, this approach is not currently used in the United States [13]. Besides the additional resources needed to establish hyperthermia, a major limitation of the study was that a comparison with surgery alone was not performed. The evidence to date suggests that there is no benefit to neoadjuvant chemotherapy plus surgery versus surgery alone for soft tissue sarcoma.

4.2 Neoadjuvant Chemoradiation

Although there are no randomized phase III studies on the topic of combination chemoradiation given in the neoadjuvant setting, some data suggest this may be an acceptable clinical choice. A RTOG phase II trial of the MAID regimen and interdigitated radiation therapy showed acceptable efficacy and toxicity [14]. Although no clear evidence of an improvement in cancer related survival was seen, preservation of QOL by acceptable morbidity with this approach was also confirmed in another study [11]. More data is needed with head-to-head comparisons between neoadjuvant chemoradiation versus surgery alone and neoadjuvant chemoradiation versus radiation alone.

4.3 Adjuvant Chemotherapy

There is a large body of literature on the use of adjuvant chemotherapy in soft tissue sarcoma which will not be reviewed in detail. Several meta-analyses of the published trials have been performed which are briefly discussed. In the initial study by the Sarcoma Meta-Analysis Collaboration (SMAC) group the addition of a doxorubicin-containing chemotherapeutic regimen following surgery compared to surgery alone showed a significantly longer local and distant recurrence-free survival, but not a statistically significant better overall survival (HR for death 0.89, 95 % CI 0.76–1.03). In the subset of patients with extremity and truncal sarcomas, a modest but significant benefit was seen for adjuvant chemotherapy, (HR 0.80, $p = 0.029$), which translates into a 7 % absolute benefit in overall survival at 10 years [15]. An updated meta-analysis conducted in 2008 showed an OR for local recurrence of 0.73 (95 % CI 0.56–0.94) and for distant recurrence of 0.67 (95 % CI 0.56–0.82) both in favor of chemotherapy. In contrast to the prior meta-analysis, the use of doxorubicin with ifosfamide was associated with a statistically significant overall survival benefit (HR 0.56, 95 % CI 0.36–0.85) [16]. Current consensus opinion is that adjuvant chemotherapy is not routinely recommended for patients with soft tissue sarcoma, but may be used in select cases for modest benefit [1].

4.4 Neoadjuvant Radiation

The advantages of using radiation in the neoadjuvant setting include downstaging of the tumor to increase chances of a margin negative resection, limitation of radiation dose to a smaller volume and minimizing long-term radiation-related morbidity. This has to be balanced against the risk of an increase in wound complications following surgery. What is the quality of the data to guide treatment sequencing for radiation use in extremity sarcoma? O'Sullivan et al. [20] conducted a randomized trial comparing preoperative with postoperative radiation in patients with extremity sarcoma with the primary endpoint being the rate of wound complications within 120 days of surgery. Wound complications occurred in 35 % of the preoperative group compared to 17 % in the postoperative group ($p = 0.01$). On follow up at 2 years after treatment, patients in the postoperative arm had greater rates of fibrosis, joint stiffness, and wound edema [21]. Generally, early complications were reversible with minimal impact on QOL while late radiation associated complications were not. Perhaps due to these findings an increase in the use of neoadjuvant radiation from 6.4 to 11.6 % from 2000 to 2009 was seen in a study of the National Cancer Database, with a corresponding decrease in postoperative radiation (34.3–29.2 %) during the same time period [22]. In a survey study of sarcoma specialists, we showed that radiation oncologists, physicians with >75 % of their practice devoted to sarcoma care, and those in practice <5 years had a preference for neoadjuvant radiation therapy [2]. Taken together, these data suggest that there is a trend toward an increasing use of neoadjuvant radiation for extremity sarcoma due to equivalent local control and a decrease in irreversible late radiation associated morbidity. To date, no study on the cost-effectiveness of this approach has been conducted.

4.5 Adjuvant Radiation

The current standard of limb sparing surgery for the majority of extremity sarcomas is established based on evidence from randomized trials. The initial trials compared amputation alone versus limb sparing surgery plus adjuvant radiation therapy and showed equivalent rates of long-term survival [17]. Although there were no local recurrences in the amputation group compared to four in the limb sparing group, disease-free survival at 5 years was equivalent (71 % vs. 78 %, $p = 0.75$). This suggested that aggressive attempts at local control with amputation did not improve long-term survival and came at the expense of considerable physical limitation to the patient. Consequently, most modern series of extremity sarcoma have an amputation rate of <5 %.

Subsequent studies confirmed that limb sparing surgery alone had higher rates of local recurrence compared with limb sparing surgery plus radiation therapy. Yang et al. [18] randomized 91 patients with extremity sarcoma into two groups following surgery; external beam radiation versus no radiation. Following a median follow-up of 9.6 years, a significant decrease in the probability of a local recurrence but no difference in overall survival was seen. Although an improvement in local control was seen for both high-grade and low-grade tumors, the effect was more pronounced for high-grade tumors. A concurrent QOL study showed that patients who received radiation had significantly worse limb strength, edema, and range of motion. Although these deficits were mostly transient, further work is needed to identify a subset of patients at low risk for local recurrence who can undergo limb sparing surgery without adjuvant radiation therapy. A review of patients with T1 soft tissue sarcoma treated at the Memorial Sloan Kettering Cancer Center between 1996 and 2002 showed that in patients with a microscopically negative (R0) margin following surgery who did not receive radiation therapy, the cumulative incidence of local recurrence at 5 and 10 years was 7.9 and 10.6 % [19]. In this subset, surgery alone provided excellent local control rates without adjuvant radiation therapy, thus minimizing morbidity without compromising recurrence outcomes.

4.6 Brachytherapy

Advantages of brachytherapy over conventional external beam radiation include minimization of the radiation dose to the surrounding tissue and shorter treatment times. A phase III trial comparing the use of brachytherapy and surgery versus brachytherapy alone showed an improvement in local control with the use of brachytherapy [23]. After 76 months of median follow up, 5-year actuarial local control rates were 82 % in the brachytherapy group and 69 % in the surgery alone group ($p = 0.04$). There was no difference in disease-specific survival rates. However, this improvement in local control was seen only for high-grade tumors and not for low-grade ones, with no improvement in long-term survival even in the high-grade subset [24]. To date there has not been a head-to-head comparison for brachytherapy versus external beam radiation in terms of local control, morbidity, or cost.

4.7 Surgery for Local Recurrence

Local failure in management of soft tissue extremity sarcoma manifests clinically as a local recurrence. Local recurrence is generally a poor prognostic sign and is associated with distant metastasis in a significant proportion of patients [25]. Once confirmed by physical exam or imaging subsequent management can be challenging. If resectable, then further surgery represents an attempt to re-establish local control. However, should aggressive re-resection be pursued in patients who are at high risk of dying from distant disease, especially in the absence of options for effective systemic control? Although there is no direct comparison between patients with local recurrence undergoing re-resection compared to those treated nonsurgically, we can use some published data to inform the debate. Ramanathan et al. [26] developed a prognostic index in patients developing a local recurrence to identify initial tumor size, histologic grade, and time to recurrence as the primary determinants of distant metastases and survival. This suggests that surgical re-resection for locally recurrent disease should be limited to patients at low risk for the development of synchronous or metachronous systemic metastases.

5 Retroperitoneal Sarcoma

5.1 Biopsy Versus No Biopsy

The question of a preoperative biopsy for a suspicious retroperitoneal mass is a vexing one for the nonspecialist. Often biopsies carried out target the wrong part of the tumor, violate oncological principles, and do not provide information that would result in a change in management. Generally agreed on indications for biopsy include presentation with metastatic disease and confirmation of the diagnosis in the neoadjuvant setting prior to initiation of chemotherapy [27]. Routine biopsy for a retroperitoneal mass felt to be a sarcoma after adequate work-up is not recommended. Some advocate performance of an intraoperative biopsy at the time of definitive surgery to confirm the diagnosis prior to radical surgery [27].

Open biopsy involves general anesthesia and a second operation for definitive treatment. CT-guided core biopsy is less invasive and costly but runs the risk of seeding of the needle tract [28]. An adequately performed core biopsy has been shown to be 95 % accurate for diagnostic purposes, but less so for detailed information such as grade, and can be considered the modality of choice if a biopsy is indicated [29]. In general, if the information gained by a preoperative biopsy is not going to change management, then it is not routinely recommended.

5.2 Radical Compartment Surgery Versus Complete Resection

The basic principles of surgery for retroperitoneal sarcomas involve complete removal of the tumor with negative margins. Violation of the pseudocapsule often results in a marginal resection and is to be avoided. The best outcomes are obtained in series that have achieved an R0 or microscopically negative resection. Macroscopically incomplete resection (R2) does not result in better survival outcomes than biopsy alone [30]. These facts have led to increasingly radical surgery to improve margin negative rates and long-term survival. Multivisceral resections and vascular reconstruction are techniques used to accomplish this. Theoretically, this should also lead to increased morbidity, yet there is little data to show this, likely because of publication bias. Analysis of the American College of Surgeons National Surgical Quality Improvement Program (ACS-NSQIP) showed that multivisceral resection of contiguous organs in patients undergoing surgery for retroperitoneal sarcoma did not lead to an increase in 30-day or overall morbidity [31].

More recently radical compartment surgery has been proposed as a surgical technique to improve local control and possibly survival outcomes. This involves complete en bloc removal of organs present in the compartment of the abdomen containing the tumor, even if the organs themselves are not involved directly. Bonvalot et al. [30] reported a 93 % complete macroscopic resection rate when the median number of organs resected with the tumor was 2. At 5 years, overall survival was 65.4 % and local and distant recurrence cumulative incidences were 22.3 and 24.2 %, respectively. These results come at the expense of serious morbidity in 18 % and surgical reintervention in 12 % of patients. The same group has previously shown that compartmental resection predicted a 3.29-fold lower rate of abdominal recurrence compared with complete resection on multivariable analysis [32]. However, compartmental resection was not associated with an improvement in overall survival, which has led to criticism of this technique [33]. Until the role of selection bias can be eliminated by a head-to-head randomized comparison with complete resection, the jury is still out on whether compartment surgery can be considered as standard of care for improving local recurrence. The relative impact on QOL and cost of treatment will also need to be further studied.

5.3 Radiation Therapy

The utility of radiation to improve locoregional control as an adjunct therapy to surgery for retroperitoneal sarcoma is yet to be clearly defined, with no randomized trials to demonstrate efficacy. Nevertheless, local recurrence remains the main cause of death even in patients with radical compartmental resection, suggesting that further improvement in local control will not be achieved by surgery alone. The American College of Surgeons Oncology Group (ACOSOG) attempted a phase III randomized trial (Z9031) to address the role of radiation in retroperitoneal sarcoma. Accrual to the trial was poor, leading to early closure [34]. Leaving asides issues of efficacy, treatment sequencing and modality of radiation delivery also need to be clarified for retroperitoneal sarcoma.

Retroperitoneal sarcomas present an unique challenge for radiation therapy, in which the area of the body to be covered may be quite large and potential benefit balanced against the morbidity of scatter damage to adjacent organs. Radiation has been used in the pre-, intra- and postoperative setting for these tumors. Potential advantages for preoperative radiation include shielding of adjacent organs by the tumor mass itself, better assessment of tumor volume, and a better response to radiation due to improved oxygenation. Resection of the tumor often results in displacement of normal tissue into the tumor bed, potentially increasing the dose of radiation delivered to tissue such as bowel in the postoperative setting [35]. The ideal sequence with surgery should be determined either by an improvement in local recurrence, overall survival or improvement in QOL as manifested by a reduction in complications.

Data on treatment sequencing to date is equivocal, although comparable survival and local recurrence results have been seen for preoperative radiotherapy when compared with 'traditional' postoperative therapy. Pawlik et al. [36] reported on the results from two prospective trials that showed a 5-year disease free survival rate of 46 %. This was even higher in patients who had a macroscopically negative resection after completing radiotherapy; 5-year local recurrence free survival of 60 %. Currently, preoperative radiotherapy is considered for intermediate or high-grade retroperitoneal sarcomas likely to have close or positive margins following resection. In most cases, a preoperative biopsy is needed to verify histology prior to initiation of therapy. Toxicity and impact on quality of QOL has been variable in the reported series but, in general, appear to be less with preoperative radiation [35, 37].

Modality of radiation delivery also remains unsettled. Attempts have been made to minimize toxicity by alternative targeting methods. Intensity modulated radiation therapy (IMRT) is an approach which has shown promise in minimizing delivery of high-dose radiation to regions of the body with low radiation tolerance, such as small bowel [38]. Intraoperative radiotherapy (IORT) can be delivered alone or in combination with pre- or postoperative external beam radiotherapy. This technique is limited by the need for a specialized operating room and equipment. Nevertheless, the use of IORT does appear to augment local control, albeit at the cost of additional toxicity. In one trial looking at long-term outcome in patients with retroperitoneal sarcoma treated by preoperative radiation, surgical resection and IORT, patients who underwent resection only had worse overall survival (30 % vs. 70 %) and local control (61 % vs. 83 %) compared to patients who had both resection and IORT [39]. Additional toxicity that has been reported with IORT is likely due to the exposure of tissue to the high doses employed and includes neuropathy, ureteral fistula, and bowel obstruction [40]. Brachytherapy is an alternative technique that has been looked at for increasing the dose of radiation delivered to the tumor bed. Again, although the local control rates are promising, toxicity remains substantial, with reoperation rates of 21.5 % reported in one series in addition to long-term issues [41]. At this time, more prospective studies with long-term follow up are needed to establish the modality of choice to deliver radiotherapy for retroperitoneal sarcoma.

5.4 Margin Reporting

Current NCCN guidelines recommend that pathologists with expertise in STS should review pathological assessment of biopsies and resected specimens, especially to establish the initial diagnosis. Ancillary techniques such as cytogenetics, immunohistochemistry, electron microscopy, and molecular genetic testing should be available as needed. The report itself should include details about the primary, depth, size, histologic grade, presence or absence of necrosis, status of the excision margins, tumor, node, and metastases (TNM) stage. Additional features are mitotic rate, presence or absence of vascular invasion and the type and extent of inflammatory infiltration [1]. In particular, the margin status of the resected specimen should be clearly delineated, as this has direct bearing on the need for additional therapy and local recurrence.

No well-publicized study to date has looked at the completeness of pathology reporting for sarcoma following surgical resection. Audits of national registries in the Netherlands and in Scandinavia show considerable variability in reporting of margins following surgery for sarcoma [10, 42]. Margin status has direct bearing on decisions about adjuvant treatment and local recurrence, which in turn may influence long-term survival. How variability of margin reporting influences comparability of outcomes in the United States is essentially unknown.

5.5 Surveillance Imaging

Surveillance following multidisciplinary treatment of sarcoma is an issue with little research to guide management. A study conducted by Whooley et al. [43] of 141 patients with extremity sarcoma showed that 20 patients developed local recurrence on follow up, of which only one was detected by imaging and the rest by physical examination. Furthermore, 45 % of these recurrences were detected by the patient in between scheduled doctor visits. The conclusion was that a thorough history and physical combined with surveillance chest Xray was cost effective, whereas routine laboratory testing and imaging of the primary tumor site were not. Others have recommended a more intensive surveillance regimen for high-risk extremity sarcomas with more frequent chest imaging and abdominopelvic CT scan for retroperitoneal sarcoma [44]. Does more intense surveillance improve outcomes for patients with recurrent sarcomas? How does this influence QOL and cost of care? These questions are currently unanswered.

In sum, we have a smattering of data that makes it difficult to establish evidence-based treatment guidelines. In part, this is due to the nature of this disease; it is rare, with a considerable amount of histological variation, making timely accrual to large trial difficult. The time needed to enroll patients, test an intervention, and determine recurrence/survival would probably be largely outstripped by the evolution of medical advances. Instead, we need to mine large databases to get sufficient numbers; since trials have been so difficult to carry out in this disease, observation studies or decision analyses would be the best way to determine the best course of treatment for extremity and retroperitoneal sarcomas. Cost-effectiveness studies and meta-analyses also have a place in further developing the realm of sarcoma studies.

6 Conclusions and Future Directions

Sarcoma care involves multidisciplinary collaboration and the use of several treatment modalities. Questions about treatment efficacy and sequencing lead to varying approaches in clinical management. Further research is needed to identify ideal treatment sequencing for chemotherapy and radiation with surgery. For interventions that do not improve local recurrence or overall survival, additional outcomes such as quality of life and cost should be considered when considering clinical use. The table below summarizes the discussion in this chapter and highlights areas of further research needed on the subject.

	Outcome		
Clinical area	Local recurrence/overall survival	Quality of life	Cost
Multidisciplinary consultation	?	NA	?
Guideline oriented care	?	NA	Lower
Regionalization of sarcoma care	Improved	Improved	?
Soft tissue extremity sarcoma			
Neoadjuvant chemotherapy	Not improved	Similar	?
Neoadjuvant chemoradiation	Not improved	Similar	?
Adjuvant chemotherapy	Modest improvement in selected patients	?	?
Adjuvant radiation	Improved local control	Worse	Higher
Neoadjuvant radiation	Equivalent local control	Improved	?
Brachytherapy	Improved local control	?	?
Radiation modality	?	?	?
Surgery for local recurrence	Improved	?	?
Retroperitoneal sarcoma			
Preoperative biopsy	NA	NA	?

(continued)

(continued)

	Outcome		
Radical compartment surgery	?	?	?
Radiation	?	?	?
Surveillance	?	?	?

References

1. NCCN clinical practice guidelines in oncology (NCCN)—soft tissue sarcoma 2013. Available at www.nccn.org
2. Wasif N, Tamurian RM, Christensen S et al (2012) Influence of specialty and clinical experience on treatment sequencing in the multimodal management of soft tissue extremity sarcoma. Ann Surg Oncol 19(2):504–510
3. Wasif N, Smith CA, Tamurian RM et al (2013) Influence of physician specialty on treatment recommendations in the multidisciplinary management of soft tissue sarcoma of the extremities. JAMA Surg 148(7):632–639
4. Ray-Coquard I, Thiesse P, Ranchere-Vince D et al (2004) Conformity to clinical practice guidelines, multidisciplinary management and outcome of treatment for soft tissue sarcomas. Ann Oncol Official J Eur Soc Med Oncol/ESMO 15(2):307–315
5. Jansen-Landheer ML, Krijnen P, Oostindier MJ et al (2009) Improved diagnosis and treatment of soft tissue sarcoma patients after implementation of national guidelines: a population-based study. Eur J Surg Oncol J Eur Soc Surg Oncol Brit Assoc Surg Oncol 35(12):1326–1332
6. Bagaria SP, Ashman JB, Daugherty LC et al (2014) Compliance with national comprehensive cancer network guidelines in the use of radiation therapy for extremity and superficial trunk soft tissue sarcoma in the United States. J Surg Oncol 109(7):633–638
7. Perrier L, Buja A, Mastrangelo G et al (2012) Clinicians' adherence versus non adherence to practice guidelines in the management of patients with sarcoma: a cost-effectiveness assessment in two European regions. BMC Health Serv Res 12:82
8. Gutierrez JC, Perez EA, Moffat FL et al (2007) Should soft tissue sarcomas be treated at high-volume centers? An analysis of 4205 patients. Ann Surg 245(6):952–958
9. Clasby R, Tilling K, Smith MA et al (1997) Variable management of soft tissue sarcoma: regional audit with implications for specialist care. Br J Surg 84(12):1692–1696
10. Nijhuis PH, Schaapveld M, Otter R et al (2001) Soft tissue sarcoma–compliance with guidelines. Cancer 91(11):2186–2195
11. Meric F, Milas M, Hunt KK et al (2000) Impact of neoadjuvant chemotherapy on postoperative morbidity in soft tissue sarcomas. J Clin Oncol Official J Am Soc Clin Oncol 18 (19):3378–3383
12. Gortzak E, Azzarelli A, Buesa J et al (2001) A randomised phase II study on neo-adjuvant chemotherapy for 'high-risk' adult soft-tissue sarcoma. Eur J Cancer 37(9):1096–1103
13. Issels RD, Lindner LH, Verweij J et al (2010) Neo-adjuvant chemotherapy alone or with regional hyperthermia for localised high-risk soft-tissue sarcoma: a randomised phase 3 multicentre study. Lancet Oncol 11(6):561–570
14. Kraybill WG, Harris J, Spiro IJ et al (2006) Phase II study of neoadjuvant chemotherapy and radiation therapy in the management of high-risk, high-grade, soft tissue sarcomas of the extremities and body wall: radiation therapy oncology group trial 9514. J Clin Oncol Official J Am Soc Clin Oncol 24(4):619–625
15. Adjuvant chemotherapy for localised resectable soft-tissue sarcoma of adults: meta-analysis of individual data. Sarcoma Meta-analysis Collaboration. Lancet 1997 350(9092):1647–1654

16. Pervaiz N, Colterjohn N, Farrokhyar F et al (2008) A systematic meta-analysis of randomized controlled trials of adjuvant chemotherapy for localized resectable soft-tissue sarcoma. Cancer 113(3):573–581
17. Rosenberg SA, Tepper J, Glatstein E et al (1982) The treatment of soft-tissue sarcomas of the extremities: prospective randomized evaluations of (1) limb-sparing surgery plus radiation therapy compared with amputation and (2) the role of adjuvant chemotherapy. Ann Surg 196 (3):305–315
18. Yang JC, Chang AE, Baker AR et al (1998) Randomized prospective study of the benefit of adjuvant radiation therapy in the treatment of soft tissue sarcomas of the extremity. J Clin Oncol Official J Am Soc Clin Oncol 16(1):197–203
19. Pisters PW, Pollock RE, Lewis VO et al (2007) Long-term results of prospective trial of surgery alone with selective use of radiation for patients with T1 extremity and trunk soft tissue sarcomas. Ann Surg 246(4):675–681 discussion 681–682
20. O'Sullivan B, Davis AM, Turcotte R et al (2002) Preoperative versus postoperative radiotherapy in soft-tissue sarcoma of the limbs: a randomised trial. Lancet 359(9325):2235–2241
21. Davis AM, O'Sullivan B, Turcotte R et al (2005) Late radiation morbidity following randomization to preoperative versus postoperative radiotherapy in extremity soft tissue sarcoma. Radiother Oncol J Eur Soc Ther Radiol Oncol 75(1):48–53
22. Sherman KL, Wayne JD, Chung J et al (2013) Assessment of multimodality therapy use for extremity sarcoma in the United States. J Surg Oncol 109(5):395–404
23. Pisters PW, Harrison LB, Woodruff JM et al (1994) A prospective randomized trial of adjuvant brachytherapy in the management of low-grade soft tissue sarcomas of the extremity and superficial trunk. J Clin Oncol Official J Am Soc Clin Oncol 12(6):1150–1155
24. Pisters PW, Harrison LB, Leung DH et al (1996) Long-term results of a prospective randomized trial of adjuvant brachytherapy in soft tissue sarcoma. J Clin Oncol Official J Am Soc Clin Oncol 14(3):859–868
25. Lewis JJ, Leung D, Heslin M et al (1997) Association of local recurrence with subsequent survival in extremity soft tissue sarcoma. J Clin Oncol Official J Am Soc Clin Oncol 15 (2):646–652
26. Ramanathan RC, A'Hern R, Fisher C et al (2001) Prognostic index for extremity soft tissue sarcomas with isolated local recurrence. Ann Surg Oncol 8(4):278–289
27. Hueman MT, Herman JM, Ahuja N (2008) Management of retroperitoneal sarcomas. Surg Clin N Am 88(3):583–597 vii
28. Schwartz HS, Spengler DM (1997) Needle tract recurrences after closed biopsy for sarcoma: three cases and review of the literature. Ann Surg Oncol 4(3):228–236
29. Hoeber I, Spillane AJ, Fisher C et al (2001) Accuracy of biopsy techniques for limb and limb girdle soft tissue tumors. Ann Surg Oncol 8(1):80–87
30. Bonvalot S, Miceli R, Berselli M et al (2010) Aggressive surgery in retroperitoneal soft tissue sarcoma carried out at high-volume centers is safe and is associated with improved local control. Ann Surg Oncol 17(6):1507–1514
31. Tseng WH, Martinez SR, Tamurian RM et al (2011) Contiguous organ resection is safe in patients with retroperitoneal sarcoma: an ACS-NSQIP analysis. J Surg Oncol 103(5):390–394
32. Bonvalot S, Rivoire M, Castaing M et al (2009) Primary retroperitoneal sarcomas: a multivariate analysis of surgical factors associated with local control. J Clin Oncol Official J Am Soc Clin Oncol 27(1):31–37
33. Mullinax JE, Zager JS, Gonzalez RJ (2011) Current diagnosis and management of retroperitoneal sarcoma. Cancer Control J Moffitt Cancer Cent 18(3):177–187
34. Kane JM 3rd (2006) At the crossroads for retroperitoneal sarcomas: the future of clinical trials for this "orphan disease". Ann Surg Oncol 13(4):442–443
35. Kaushal A, Citrin D (2008) The role of radiation therapy in the management of sarcomas. Surg Clin N Am 88(3):629–646 viii

36. Pawlik TM, Pisters PW, Mikula L et al (2006) Long-term results of two prospective trials of preoperative external beam radiotherapy for localized intermediate- or high-grade retroperitoneal soft tissue sarcoma. Ann Surg Oncol 13(4):508–517
37. Ballo MT, Zagars GK, Pollock RE et al (2007) Retroperitoneal soft tissue sarcoma: an analysis of radiation and surgical treatment. Int J Radiat Oncol Biol Phys 67(1):158–163
38. Bossi A, De Wever I, Van Limbergen E et al (2007) Intensity modulated radiation-therapy for preoperative posterior abdominal wall irradiation of retroperitoneal liposarcomas. Int J Radiat Oncol Biol Phys 67(1):164–170
39. Gieschen HL, Spiro IJ, Suit HD et al (2001) Long-term results of intraoperative electron beam radiotherapy for primary and recurrent retroperitoneal soft tissue sarcoma. Int J Radiat Oncol Biol Phys 50(1):127–131
40. Bobin JY, Al-Lawati T, Granero LE et al (2003) Surgical management of retroperitoneal sarcomas associated with external and intraoperative electron beam radiotherapy. Eur J Surg Oncol J Eur Soc Surg Oncol Br Assoc Surg Oncol 29(8):676–681
41. Dziewirski W, Rutkowski P, Nowecki ZI et al (2006) Surgery combined with intraoperative brachytherapy in the treatment of retroperitoneal sarcomas. Ann Surg Oncol 13(2):245–252
42. Trovik CS, Skjeldal S, Bauer H et al (2012) Reliability of margin assessment after surgery for extremity soft tissue sarcoma: the SSG experience. Sarcoma 2012:290698
43. Whooley BP, Gibbs JF, Mooney MM et al (2000) Primary extremity sarcoma: what is the appropriate follow-up? Ann Surg Oncol 7(1):9–14
44. Kane JM 3rd (2004) Surveillance strategies for patients following surgical resection of soft tissue sarcomas. Curr Opin Oncol 16(4):328–332

Comparative Effectiveness in Thyroid Cancer: Key Questions and How to Answer Them

Elliot A. Asare and Tracy S. Wang

Abstract

Controversies in treatment of thyroid cancer remain despite numerous published studies. Robust comparative effectiveness studies examining: (1) the role of prophylactic central compartment neck dissection (pCCND) in patients with papillary thyroid cancer (PTC); (2) the use of post-operative radioactive iodine (RAI) ablation therapy following total thyroidectomy; (3) use of low versus high doses of I-131 in RAI therapy; (4) thyroid hormone withdrawal (THW) versus recombinant thyroid stimulating hormone (rhTSH) prior to RAI; and (5) the role of routine measurement of serum calcitonin levels are needed to help strengthen existing treatment recommendations. Reasons for the controversies and suggestions for quality comparative effectiveness studies are discussed.

Keywords

Thyroid cancer · Prophylactic central compartment neck dissection · Recombinant thyroid stimulating hormone · Radioactive iodine ablation · Thyroid hormone withdrawal · Calcitonin · Thyroid nodules

Contents

E.A. Asare · T.S. Wang (✉)
Department of Surgery, Medical College of Wisconsin, Milwaukee, WI, USA
e-mail: tswang@mcw.edu

E.A. Asare
e-mail: easare@mcw.edu

K.Y. Bilimoria et al. (eds.), *Comparative Effectiveness in Surgical Oncology*,
Cancer Treatment and Research 164, DOI 10.1007/978-3-319-12553-4_5

1 Comparative Effectiveness in Thyroid Cancer: Key Questions and How to Answer Them

In the United States (U.S.), the prevalence of clinically palpable thyroid nodules in adults over age 50 is approximately 5 % [1]. Autopsy, intraoperative and ultrasound findings estimate the prevalence of thyroid nodules in adults in the U.S. at near 50 % [2–4]. The female to male prevalence ratio of thyroid nodules is 4:1, with most nodules being benign [1].

Thyroid cancer is the 9th most common cancer in the United States, with an incidence of 12.2 per 100,000 per year and a mortality rate of 0.5 per 100,000 [5]. The estimated lifetime risk of being diagnosed with thyroid cancer is 1.1 % and the relative 5-year survival is 97.7 % [5]. The three primary histologic types are differentiated (papillary, follicular, Hurthle cell), medullary, and anaplastic thyroid cancer. Papillary thyroid cancer (PTC) accounts for over 80 % of all cases of thyroid cancer [1, 6].

The absolute increase in the incidence of thyroid cancer is estimated to be 9.4 per 100,000 individuals, with PTC accounting for the majority of these cases [7]. With such a significant increase in the incidence of thyroid nodules and thyroid cancer, robust evidence-based guidelines to provide all providers with a framework for the management of the patient with thyroid cancer is critical. Topics in the treatment of differentiated thyroid cancer (DTC) where comparative effectiveness studies would help strengthen the level of evidence-based recommendations include: (1) the role of prophylactic central compartment neck dissection (pCCND) in patients with PTC; (2) the use of post-operative radioactive iodine (RAI) ablation therapy following total thyroidectomy; (3) use of low versus high doses of I-131 in RAI therapy; and (4) thyroid hormone withdrawal (THW) versus recombinant thyroid stimulating hormone (rhTSH) prior to RAI. The role of routine measurement of serum calcitonin levels in patients with thyroid nodules also will be discussed.

2 Prophylactic Central Compartment Neck Dissection (pCCND) for Papillary Thyroid Cancer

The incidence of macroscopic cervical lymph node metastases, detectable by physical examination, cervical ultrasonography, or visual inspection at the time of surgery, in patients with PTC is between 20 and 50 %, while the incidence of micrometastasis approaches 90 % [2]. The central neck compartment (level VI) is the most common site of lymph node metastases in patients with PTC [8, 9]. The central compartment is bounded by the hyoid bone (superior), carotid artery (lateral), sternal notch or innominate artery (inferior), Fig. 1 [10].

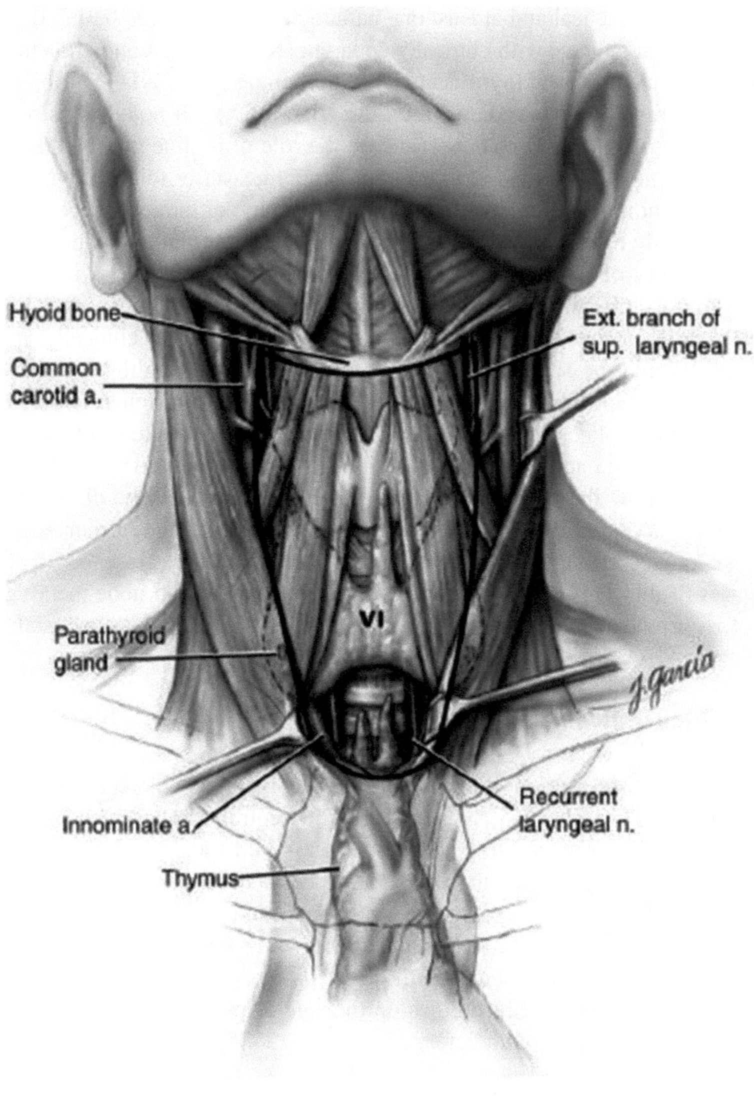

Fig. 1 The central compartment of the neck (reprinted with permission from Carty et al.) [10]

Table 1 Common prognostic factors for differentiated thyroid carcinoma [12, 37, 88]

Name of prognostic grouping	Components
AMES	**A**ge, **M**etastases, **E**xtent of disease, **S**ize of tumor
AGES	**A**ge, **G**rade, **E**xtent of disease, **S**ize of tumor
MACIS	**M**etastases, **A**ge, **C**ompleteness of resection, **I**nvasion, **S**ize of tumor
TNM	**T**umor, **N**ode, **M**etastasis, Age

The American Thyroid Association (ATA) defines central compartment neck dissection (CCND) as "the comprehensive, compartment-oriented removal of the prelaryngeal, pretracheal and at least one paratracheal lymph node basin" [2]. There is consensus that patients with clinically apparent (N1a) central compartment lymph nodes should undergo total thyroidectomy with therapeutic CCND [2]. However, in view of the prevailing contradictions on the effect of lymph node status on recurrence and survival, there is no consensus on the role of routine pCCND in patients with PTC and no clinical evidence of lymph node metastases (clinically N0), either by physical examination, preoperative ultrasonography, or intraoperative inspection at the time of thyroidectomy. As level C evidence, the current ATA guidelines on the management of patients with DTC recommends that patients with advanced primary tumors (T3 or T4) with clinically negative lymph nodes may undergo pCCND while patients with small tumors (T1 or T2) with no clinically apparent lymph nodes may be spared CCND [2]. This section will highlight some of the pros and cons of pCCND with regards to locoregional recurrence, survival, and postoperative complications based on studies from various single institution, multi-institution and large administrative databases. The reasons for the persistent controversies and how they could be effectively resolved will also be discussed.

Generally accepted prognostic factors for PTC include age, tumor size, completeness of resection, extrathyroidal extension, and the presence of distant metastases (Table 1) [11–14]. The effect of locoregional lymph node metastases on rates of recurrence and survival in patients with PTC remains controversial.

2.1 Recurrence

Single and multi-institution studies estimate the locoregional recurrence rate of patients with PTC to be 6–59 % [15–18]. The central compartment is the most common site of recurrence [16]. There is increased cost and morbidity in patients with recurrent disease, given that reoperative cervical surgery is associated with higher rates of recurrent laryngeal nerve injury and hypoparathyroidism, both transient and permanent [19–21]. The probability of recurrence is influenced by the lymph node status of the patient, with clinically node-positive patients having a higher rate of recurrence [22]. Studies on the role of pCCND in decreasing tumor recurrence have yielded contradictory results [9, 23–25].

The sensitivity of high-resolution ultrasonography in detecting cervical lymph node metastases is reported to be 52 % with a false negative rate of 58 % [26]. While ultrasonography has a higher detection rate than physical exam alone in the detection of metastatic lymphadenopathy, the overall detection rate remains low. Given the difficulty in predicting the presence of metastatic lymphadenopathy preoperatively, one would expect that reliance on only therapeutic CCND at the time of thyroidectomy would miss a significant number of patients with micrometastatic lymphadenopathy [27]. As a result, failure to remove microscopic metastases at the time of initial thyroidectomy would theoretically place patients at a higher risk for recurrent DTC and need for further treatment, including reoperative surgery [22, 28].

Early locoregional recurrence of DTC may be due to existing nodal metastases which was not recognized pre- or intraoperatively and thus not removed at the index operation, if routine pCCND was not performed [28]. In addition, routine pCCND and resection of micrometastatic nodal disease may influence the need for, and dosage of I-131 given at the time of subsequent RAI, although data are conflicting [27, 29, 30]. Some studies have found that patients in whom the true nodal status is unknown because they did not undergo pCCND may be under-treated and subsequently are more likely to have a locoregional recurrence; this is in part due to the fact that identification of micrometastasis 'upstages' PTC from Nx to N1a disease, in the American Joint Committee on Cancer (AJCC) staging system and N1a PTC is considered "Stage III" PTC in patients >45 years [27, 29, 31, 32]. Other studies, however, suggest that performance of pCCND and identification of micrometastasis may preclude the need for RAI in patients with undetectable serum thyroglobulin levels and no evidence of disease on whole body prescans performed at the time of RAI [30].

Serum thyroglobulin is a postoperative marker for recurrent PTC and higher rates of athyroglobulinemia have been reported among patients who underwent total thyroidectomy with ipsilateral pCCND [33]. A meta-analysis of 11 published studies with a total of 2,318 patients revealed a lower trend toward recurrence in patients treated with total thyroidectomy and prophylactic central neck dissection, although statistical significance was not reached, OR 0.59 (95 % CI 0.33–1.07) in favor of total thyroidectomy with pCCND [34]. The pooled recurrence rate for total thyroidectomy with pCCND was 4.7 % compared to 7.9 % in the total thyroidectomy group [34].

Contrary to the studies reporting favorably on the effect of pCCND on recurrence, some studies have not found more aggressive surgery to correlate with decreased recurrence [16, 35]. A single institution, retrospective cohort review of patients with PTC over a 60 year period found the recurrence rate among clinically node negative patients to be 0.8 % compared to a recurrence rate of 16 % in patients who had clinically positive lymph nodes at presentation [16]. There was no increased risk of mortality from thyroid cancer in the cohort that experienced tumor recurrence. Another single institution study in which all surgeries were performed by a single surgeon, did not find any central neck recurrence in patients who received total thyroidectomy with CCND, however, lateral neck recurrences were observed in 5 patients who had more than 5 metastatic central neck lymph nodes on therapeutic CCND only [36]. These findings would suggest that pCCND offers no benefit to patients with clinical N0 disease [36].

Contrary to other studies, another single institution retrospective cohort study in which both groups received post-operative 131-I therapy found similar levels of serum thyroglobulin levels at 1-year follow-up in both patients who underwent total thyroidectomy alone versus total thyroidectomy with pCCND [27].

2.2 Survival

Both single-institution, retrospective cohort studies and those using larger administrative databases, such as Surveillance, Epidemiology, and End Results (SEER) have reported no effect of metastatic cervical lymph nodes on survival [26, 37, 38]. In one study using the SEER database, multivariable analysis of the factors predictive of survival in patients with PTC did not find the effect of cervical lymph node metastasis to be statistically significant [38].

In contrast, a separate study also utilizing the SEER database reported a relative risk of 1.3 (1.20–1.5) in patients with positive cervical lymph node metastasis when multivariable analysis was performed for prognostic factors of survival [39]. The role of pCCND on survival is hard to evaluate given the relatively long-term survival in patients with PTC. A prospective cohort study of patients with PTC who received total thyroidectomy with microdissection in the city of Göteborg showed that over a median follow-up of 13 years, 1.6 % died from thyroid cancer compared to 8.4 and 11.1 % with median follow-up of 10 and 11.4 years from Bergen and Helsinki respectively where patients underwent "node picking" or no information on lymph node dissection was provided [40]. In a thorough systematic review evaluating the effect of CCND on survival [23], studies from various institutions across the world reported conflicting results. A retrospective cohort study from Hannover, Germany in which 342 patients with PTC were analyzed, found improved survival in the cohort who received systematic compartment oriented dissection compared to the cohort who received selective node removal [24]. On the contrary, another single institution retrospective cohort review of 139 patients with DTC did not find lymphadenectomy to improve survival [41]. No higher level evidence exists to conclusively settle on the effect of pCCND on survival among patients with DTC [23].

2.3 Morbidity

The potential complications of CCND include hypoparathyroidism (transient or permanent), recurrent laryngeal nerve injury (transient or permanent), esophageal injury, tracheal injury, seroma, hematoma and wound infection [42]. Transient hypoparathyroidism is the most common complication of both thyroidectomy and CCND, whether performed as a therapeutic or prophylactic procedure [9, 43].

Table 2 Complications and incidence rates for total thyroidectomy with or without central compartment neck dissection [42]

Complication	Incidence (%)
Permanent hypoparathyroidism	1.2
Transient vocal cord palsy	1.1
Permanent vocal cord paralysis	3.4
Hemorrhage	1–2

In a meta-analysis of 5 studies with a total of 1,132 patients with DTC, transient hypoparathyroidism was an increased adverse event in patients undergoing thyroidectomy and CCND compared to thyroidectomy alone [42]. The reported incidence of transient hypocalcemia for thyroidectomy with or without CCND ranges from 1.6 to 53.6 % [20]. The rates of permanent hypoparathyroidism (1.2 %), transient vocal cord palsy (3.4 %), permanent vocal cord paralysis (1.1 %) and hemorrhage (1–2 %) were similar between those who underwent total thyroidectomy alone compared to recipients of total thyroidectomy with CCND, Table 2 [42]. Furthermore, different single institution studies report increased risk of hypoparathyroidism and recurrent laryngeal nerve injury in reoperative CCNDs, suggesting that prevention of reoperative surgery, perhaps by performing prophylactic CCND at the time of initial surgery, may be appropriate [23, 28, 44].

Still other studies, both single institution retrospective and prospective cohort studies, have found the complication rates of initial pCCND to be comparable to reoperative CCND [9, 45], thus suggesting that if patients experience a recurrence, they can be operated on safely and therefore they should not undergo CCND at first operation if cervical nodes are clinically negative. A large single institution retrospective review of 295 patients at a high-volume center in which 189 patients had initial total thyroidectomy with pCCND and 106 patients underwent reoperative surgery reported the following rates of complications when comparing the two cohorts: permanent hypoparathyroidism (0.5 % vs. 0.9 %), neck hematoma (1.1 % vs. 0.9 %), permanent hoarseness (2.6 % vs. 1.9 %) [9]. Furthermore, in contrast to the previously discussed meta-analysis by Chisholm et al. [42] in which patients undergoing total thyroidectomy and pCCND had only transient hypoparathyroidism as a worse outcome compared to total thyroidectomy alone, others have reported increased rates of permanent hypoparathyroidism [23, 46]. A systematic review of multiple single institution cohort studies by White et al. concluded that the rate of permanent hypoparathyroidism may be higher in patients who undergo CCND [23]. The sub-samples analyzed in the cohort studies to derive the incidence of permanent hypoparathyroidism were small and the reported rates of permanent hypoparathyroidism ranged from 1.4 to 4 % among the cohort who underwent total thyroidectomy with CCND [23]. These data would suggest that pCCND may place patients at higher risk of postoperative morbidity.

The majority of previous studies investigating the issue of pCCND in patients with PTC have been case reports, case series, prospective, or retrospective review of single or national databases, although some meta-analyses have recently been performed. Another weakness of the single institution studies is that, they are usually done at high-volume centers where surgeries are done by very experienced surgeons; hence the findings may not be generalizable. Furthermore, much of the existing literature comparing postoperative morbidity in patients undergoing total thyroidectomy with or without CCND do not accurately distinguish between prophylactic and therapeutic CCND and the extent of lymphadenectomy performed is difficult to assess in a retrospective manner. None of the studies on this controversial issue has a level of evidence better than III, Grade C. Despite the benefit of large sample size in studies using Surveillance, Epidemiology and End Results (SEER) data, the lack of a robust randomized controlled clinical trial to effectively compare thyroidectomy alone versus thyroidectomy with pCCND has left this controversy unresolved. A randomized, controlled study examining postoperative calcium supplementation in patients following total thyroidectomy did not identify patients undergoing CCND, prophylactic or therapeutic, to be at higher risk of postoperative hypoparathyroidism, although this study was not designed to look specifically at the issue of CCND [47].

2.4 Challenges to Obtaining a Higher Level of Evidence

There are several challenges to conducting a randomized controlled trial to address the role of pCCND in patients with PTC. The low incidence of PTC, the overall low morbidity associated with pCCND and the favorably long survival necessitates a very large sample size and long follow-up time in order to detect statistically significant differences in outcome [45]. The feasibility of a multicenter randomized controlled trial is also constrained by the high budgetary estimate of $20 million [45]. Existing studies are limited by multiple factors. First, there is heterogeneity of the histology of study participants. In some studies, there are no separate subgroup analyses between PTC and follicular thyroid cancer; follicular thyroid cancer does not typically spread via the lymphatic channels and therefore, pCCND has little clinical utility in this subset of patients. Second, earlier studies may not meet the current ATA definition of a pCCND, making the extent of lymphadenectomy difficult to determine. Next, most existing studies did not have a control group of patients who did not undergo CCND and there is wide variability in inclusion/exclusion criteria and confounding factors, thus making it difficult to examine the direct effect of pCCND. Finally, temporal trends in knowledge, imaging, diagnosis, surgical technique and patient preferences call for a more robust, contemporary study.

2.5 How High Quality Evidence May Be Obtained

Large healthcare systems with integrated electronic health records such as American College of Surgeons National Surgical Quality Improvement Program (ACS NSQIP) regional collaboratives may be able to implement a prospective cohort study to compare patients with cN0 who receive total thyroidectomy with age-matched patients with cN0 who undergo total thyroidectomy with pCCND. In such a study, standardized definitions of variables would be used thus decreasing the variability that has characterized most existing studies. Given the favorable long-term survival in patients with PTC, these cohort studies would examine short to medium term outcomes such as complications and recurrence. Also, the findings are likely to be more generalizable since the spectrum of hospital volume and surgeon experience will reflect the real world as opposed to a single institution. While this type of prospective cohort study may not be as robust as RCT, it may not be hampered by the same barriers that make RCT infeasible [45].

3 Postoperative Radioactive Iodine Therapy for Papillary Thyroid Cancer

RAI using 131-I is an important adjunct in the treatment of patients with PTC. Given the high avidity of thyroid tissue for iodine, administered 131-I enters remnant thyroid tissue where it kills tissues. Controversy exists regarding: (1) whom should undergo additional postoperative treatment with RAI; (2) THW versus recombinant TSH (rhTSH) stimulation prior to remnant ablation; and (3) the optimal dose of 131-I.

3.1 Indications for Administration of RAI in Patients with PTC

RAI is used for remnant thyroid tissue ablation resulting in the [2, 48] (i) destruction of microscopic remnants of thyroid tissue with the goal to decreasing tumor recurrence (ii) facilitation of follow-up and early detection of persistent or recurrent disease based on serum thyroglobulin levels (iii) facilitation in identifying previously undiagnosed or persistent disease when the post-ablation therapy scan is performed. ^{131}I may also be used for adjuvant therapy after complete surgical resection [2].

There remains debate about the use of postoperative RAI in patients with PTC, particularly in patients at low-risk for disease recurrence. Factors predictive of low-risk versus high-risk for disease recurrence and mortality are shown in Table 3 [49].

The ATA has made recommendations for use of RAI ablation based on the AJCC TNM staging criteria for PTC, Table 4 [2]. With the exception of patients with metastatic disease, no level A evidence exists to guide the recommendations, hence the persistent variation in the use of RAI therapy, although studies have shown an increasing trend in RAI usage [50]. A recent retrospective review of the SEER database found that for every 3 years, there is an average increase in RAI use by 1.5 % [50].

Table 3 Factors predictive of high versus low risk of recurrence and mortality (adopted and modified from Mazzaferri and Kloos) [49]

High risk features	Low risk features
Age <15 years or >45 years	Age 15–45 years
Male sex	Female sex
Family history of thyroid cancer	
Size >4 cm in diameter	Size <4 cm
Bilateral disease	Unilateral disease
Vascular invasion	No vascular invasion
Extrathyroidal extension	No extrathyroidal extension
Cervical/mediastinal lymph node metastasis	No lymph node metastasis
High histologic grade	Low histologic grade
Poor concentration of radioiodine in tumors or metastasis	Tumors with high radioiodine avidity
Distant metastasis	No metastasis

Table 4 Factors, recommendations and level of evidence regarding radioiodine remnant ablation (adopted and modified from ATA guidelines) [2]

Factors	Description	Recommendation	Strength of evidence
T1	1 cm or less, intrathyroidal or microscopic multifocal	No	E
	1–2 cm, intrathyroidal	Selective use	I
T2	>2–4 cm, intrathyroidal	Selective use	C
T3	>4 cm		
	<45 years old	Yes	B
	≥45 years old	Yes	B
	Any size, any age, minimal extrathyroidal extension	Selective use	I
T4	Any size with gross extrathyroidal extension	Yes	B
Nx, N0	No metastatic nodes documented	No	I
N1	<45 years old	Selective use	C
	>45 years old	Selective use	C
M1	Distant metastatic disease	Yes	A

3.2 Does RAI Decrease Recurrence and Improve Survival?

The effect of RAI on recurrence and survival has been debated. Some cohort studies and case series have reported decreased recurrence and improved disease-specific mortality in patients treated with RAI after thyroidectomy [2, 15, 51, 52]. Decreased rates of pulmonary metastases has been reported in patients treated with surgery and 131-I compared to those treated with surgery alone [49]. Also, a single institution cohort study found decreased rates of recurrence in patients with microscopic residual disease treated with RAI [53]. A review of a single institution data by Mazzaferri and Kloos [49], in which recurrences were examined in a large cohort over a 40 year period revealed that patients who received total thyroidectomy with RAI and L-thyroxine therapy had fewer recurrences compared to those who had total thyroidectomy with L-thyroxine but without RAI. An older single institution study which reviewed a large cohort of patients with well DTC in which 736 patients received surgery and RAI therapy versus 863 who received surgery only, concluded that RAI treatment was the single most important prognostic factor for recurrence ($p < 0.0001$) [52].

However, there is no higher level evidence based on robust randomized controlled trials to support the claim of decreased disease recurrence and improved disease specific survival among patients who receive post-surgical RAI ablation [48]. A thorough systematic review and meta-analysis has not found consistent benefit of RAI therapy in decreasing disease recurrence and disease specific mortality.

Due to the inconsistent results from single institution studies on the benefits of RAI use on disease-specific survival and tumor recurrence, some have questioned if RAI therapy for some risk groups with PTC are necessary [54, 55]. Increased rate of secondary malignancies (absolute risk of 2 % for second primary malignancy, absolute risk of 0.4 % for leukemia) [56], sialoadenitis (estimated incidence of 2.8–33 %) [57, 58] and decreased quality-of-life are some of the adverse effects of RAI therapy [54, 59]. Studies reporting these negative effects of postoperative RAI therapy are single institution retrospective reviews, case reports or case series and hence lack the strength of evidence to sway proponents of RAI therapy.

3.3 Thyroid Hormone Withdrawal Versus Recombinant TSH Prior to Remnant Ablation

TSH stimulation is required before postoperative RAI ablation of the remnant thyroid tissue. TSH stimulation could be either via withholding of exogenous thyroid hormone (withdrawal) or administration of exogenous rhTSH [2]. rhTSH is a synthetic analog of endogenous TSH, which is produced by the anterior pituitary gland. Unlike endogenous TSH, which is both sialylated and sulfated, rhTSH is only sialylated [60]. rhTSH binds to the TSH receptor on normal thyroid follicular cells or well-differentiated thyroid cells where the adenylate cyclase and the phosphatidylinositol signaling pathways are activated and therefore mimics the hypothyroid state [60].

THW induces hypothyroidism in patients, which may lead to symptoms such as decreased cognitive function, altered emotional state, and physical discomfort. Randomized controlled trials and a number of prospective cohort studies have demonstrated the decreased quality-of-life in patients who undergo THW prior to postoperative RAI [61–64]. In a single institution randomized controlled trial, there was a statistically significant difference in a quality-of-life survey comparing use of rhTSH versus THW prior to RAI. Patients in the rhTSH arm demonstrated better scores on each of the following measures: symptoms and signs of hypothyroidism, duration of symptoms, impact on daily and social life, mood changes and cognitive dysfunction and genital dysfunction [61]. Furthermore, use of rhTSH avoids the need to induce hypothyroidism and is invaluable in clinical situations where THW is contraindicated prior to postoperative RAI therapy, such as congestive heart failure, hyponatremia, and adrenal insufficiency [65]. Initial doubts about the effectiveness of rhTSH on successful tumor ablation have been answered by a number of studies using randomized controlled, prospective cohort and retrospective study designs [66–68]. A retrospective review of a single institution study comparing 74 patients who underwent THW before remnant ablation versus 320 patients treated with rhTSH before remnant ablation reported similar time to recurrence in the two groups as well as similar rates of disease recurrence (4 % in rhTSH group vs. 7 % in the THW group, $p = 0.1$) [68].

Questions remain about the appropriate dose of 131-I to utilize when administering postoperative RAI with rhTSH. Some studies have reported comparable outcomes with low-dose RAI after TSH stimulation using rhTSH or THW in patients at low-risk for recurrent PTC [61, 67, 69]. A single institution prospective study of 162 patients with DTC followed for 10 years after post-surgical therapy with rhTSH or THW before remnant ablation with 1.1 GBq (30 mCi) found no statistically significant difference in disease recurrence between those who received rhTSH and the THW group [69]. This result differs from that done by a prospective cohort study with a control group in which patients treated with 30 mCi (low dose) of RAI had significantly lower ablation rates [70]. This was a prospective cohort study with controls that compared the success of remnant ablation (assessed by 131-I WBS) in a cohort treated with rhTSH before remnant ablation versus cohort who underwent THW before remnant ablation. Findings showed successful remnant ablation rate of 54 % in the group who received rhTSH compared to 84 % in the THW group [70].

Initial concerns about the cost-effectiveness of using rhTSH compared to THW have recently been addressed. Cost-effectiveness studies have concluded that despite the high cost of rhTSH, avoidance of hypothyroidism and associated decreased quality-of-life which may impair productivity and safety afforded by rhTSH make the cost equivalent to THW [62, 71]. A study in which 236 patients were surveyed (61 % response rate) examined comparative cost-effectiveness of rhTSH versus THW withdrawal using a pharmacoeconomic model on the following measures; medical cost, missed work time or decreased productivity and accident and concluded that costs to society associated with THW exceeded that of rhTSH by 25 % [62]. Another cost- effectiveness study found that differences in societal cost between rhTSH and THW were dependent on days of work lost, cost of rhTSH, duration of THW, rates of failure of remnant ablation and patient's utility in the first 12 weeks after thyroidectomy [71].

Current ATA guidelines on the management of patients with DTC state that "remnant ablation can be performed following thyroxine withdrawal or rhTSH stimulation" [2].

3.4 Low- Versus High-Doses of 131-I in Administration of RAI for Patients with DTC

The optimal dosage of 131-I to use for remnant ablation continues to be an area of controversy. Because of increased side-effects such as sialoadenitis and increased second primary tumors with "high" doses of 131-I [56, 58], as well as the long-term risk of developing pulmonary fibrosis with large cumulative doses of RAI, some have questioned the use of "high" doses of 131-I by citing studies in which "low" doses have achieved similar outcome as "high" doses [72, 73]. A meta-analysis of 9 randomized controlled trials concluded that remnant ablation with 30 mCi was as successful as 100 mCi with associated fewer adverse events [73]. However, some of the individual randomized controlled trials included in the study had different thresholds for "low-dose" versus "high-dose", as well as different criteria for evaluating success of ablation, making interpretation of the results difficult to generalize [73]. Additionally, the individual studies had relatively low sample sizes (range 40–752 patients). On the contrary, a double blind randomized controlled trial from a single institution in which 341 patients were randomized to treatment with 100 mCi ("high") versus 30 mCi ("low") showed that patients in the "low" dose group often required a second dose, leading to increased cumulative activity (median dose of 130 mCi vs. 100 mCi, $p < 0.0001$) and had longer inpatient stay (median of 4 days vs. 3 days) [74].

3.5 Challenges to Obtaining a Higher Level of Evidence

The controversy regarding post-surgical RAI use persists due to some issues that affect the quality of previously published studies. Some of the prospective cohort studies and retrospective cohort studies from single institutions did not have control arms to allow for effective comparison of treatment effect. Also, in studies comparing surgical therapy alone versus surgical therapy plus RAI, some participants in the latter group may have received additional therapy such as hormonal therapy thus making it difficult to attribute treatment effect to RAI therapy only. Further, the degree of surveillance for recurrence may vary from institution to institution and thus the reported recurrence rates may not be generalizable. Additionally, variation in RAI dosage among various institutions does not allow for accurate comparison of studies to allow for a definitive conclusion to be drawn. Finally, different methods of assessing success of remnant ablation have been used in different studies thus affecting their comparability.

3.6 How High Quality Evidence May Be Obtained

A large, multicenter randomized controlled trial comparing outcomes in patients who receive low-dose RAI with high-dose RAI may help resolve this controversy. The ideal study protocol would use generally agreed upon standard definitions and end-points in order to avoid ambiguity which would decrease the validity of the results; it would be particularly important to utilize standard definitions of disease persistence and recurrence. Participating centers would agree on a single dosage for "low" and "high" respectively and on use of rhTSH versus THW. Short- and intermediate-term outcomes such as success of remnant ablation, based on serum thyroglobulin and/or follow-up radiographic studies, salivary gland dysfunction, lacrimal gland dysfunction, and patient quality-of-life could be assessed with a multicenter RCT.

Given the favorably long-term survival among patients with PTC, a prospective cohort study of patients in an ideal geographic region with easy access to healthcare and well established follow-up system may enable an assessment of the effect of post-operative RAI therapy on recurrence and disease specific survival. The quality of such a prospective cohort study will be improved if standards for "low-dose", "high-dose", and methods of assessing response to treatment are determined before start of study.

Also, to address the controversy surrounding appropriate dosing of 131-I in patients stimulated with rhTSH, a large multicenter randomized controlled trial with well-defined inclusion and exclusion criteria, as well as standard defined "low dose" versus "high dose", and end-points that can be assessed with standard techniques or lab measurements would be ideal.

4 Routine Serum Calcitonin Screening for Thyroid Nodules

Medullary thyroid carcinoma (MTC) comprises 2–4 % of the incidence of all thyroid cancers [75, 76]. Among patients with thyroid nodules, the prevalence of medullary thyroid cancer is estimated between 0.4 and 1.4 % [77–80]. It is relatively more aggressive than PTC and has a reported overall relative survival of 75 % at 10 years [75]. MTC may be inherited as autosomal dominant in 20–25 % of cases or occur sporadically in the rest of cases [81]. Prognostic factors for medullary thyroid cancer include age at diagnosis, extent of tumor, nodal disease, extent of surgical resection and distant metastases [81, 82]. Given the poor prognosis associated with late stage MTC, efforts to aid early diagnosis are being pursued.

Routine serum calcitonin levels in all patients with thyroid nodules in order to screen for possible MTC is common practice in most European countries, [77] in large part because of the inability to appropriately interpret indeterminate values [2]. While serum calcitonin levels <10 pg/mL is considered normal and >100 pg/mL is nearly diagnostic for MTC, serum calcitonin levels can be elevated in patients with elevated serum gastrin levels, follicular neoplasms, Hashimoto's thyroiditis, renal failure, and with alcohol or tobacco use. In Europe, indeterminate serum calcitonin levels (20–100 pg/mL) can be stimulated with pentagastrin to determine the risk of MTC. However, in the United States, pentagastrin is not available and calcium stimulation is a far less reliable method. As a result, current ATA guidelines do not endorse routine screening of serum calcitonin levels in patients with thyroid nodules [2, 81].

A number of prospective, non-randomized studies have shown that serum calcitonin is the most sensitive screening test for diagnosing occult medullary thyroid cancer in thyroid nodules [83–86]. Some of the reasons for the difference in practice patterns on the use of routine serum calcitonin screening in the United States include: lack of a robust randomized controlled trial, the reliance of screening on pentagastrin to increase specificity in patients with indeterminate levels, questions about assay performance, and the cost-effectiveness of screening for a rare disease [2]. A cost-effectiveness study from North America concluded that routine serum calcitonin screening was appropriate and comparable to colonoscopy and mammography [87]. A limitation of this study was the inclusion of patients with micromedullary carcinoma and C-cell hyperplasia in the prevalence estimate [2]. Barriers to conducting a randomized controlled trial to evaluate the role of routine serum calcitonin screening on early detection of MTC include: (i) rarity of MTC, leading to difficulties with accrual and adequate power; (ii) unavailability of pentagastrin in North America; and (iii) variability in assay preparation.

A randomized controlled trial in the United States does not appear to be feasible, given the lack of an accurate way to interpret serum calcitonin levels and the relative rarity of this disease. Any attempt to evaluate the effectiveness of routine calcitonin screening in human subjects in the US is limited by the unavailability of pentagastrin. While some of the European studies evaluating the role of routine calcitonin in diagnosing MTC are of high quality, comparable studies cannot be conducted in the U.S. due to Food and Drug Administration (FDA) regulation and hence this issue will remain unresolved for a while.

References

1. Tuttle RM, Ball DW, Byrd D, Dilawari RA, Doherty GM, Duh QY et al (2010) Thyroid carcinoma. J Nat Compr Cancer Netw 8(11):1228–1274. PubMed PMID: 21081783. Epub 2010/11/18. eng
2. American Thyroid Association Guidelines Taskforce on Thyroid nodules, Differentiated Thyroid cancer, Cooper DS, Doherty GM, Haugen BR, Kloos RT et al (2009) Revised American Thyroid Association management guidelines for patients with thyroid nodules and differentiated thyroid cancer. Thyroid 19(11):1167–1214. PubMed PMID: 19860577
3. Ezzat S, Sarti DA, Cain DR, Braunstein GD (1994) Thyroid incidentalomas. Prevalence by palpation and ultrasonography. Arch Intern Med 154(16):1838–1840. PubMed PMID: 8053752. Epub 1994/08/22. eng
4. Stark DD, Clark OH, Gooding GA, Moss AA (1983) High-resolution ultrasonography and computed tomography of thyroid lesions in patients with hyperparathyroidism. Surgery 94 (6):863–868. PubMed PMID: 6648798. Epub 1983/12/01. eng

5. Kim MS, Lee SY, Cho WH, Song WS, Koh JS, Lee JA et al (2008) Tumor necrosis rate adjusted by tumor volume change is a better predictor of survival of localized osteosarcoma patients. Ann Surg Oncol 15(3):906–914
6. Sherman SI (2003) Thyroid carcinoma. Lancet 361(9356):501–511. PubMed PMID: 12583960. Epub 2003/02/14. eng
7. Davies L, Welch HG (2014) Current Thyroid cancer trends in the United States. JAMA Otolaryngol—Head Neck Surg. PubMed PMID: 24557566. Epub 2014/02/22. eng
8. Kouvaraki MA, Shapiro SE, Fornage BD, Edeiken-Monro BS, Sherman SI, Vassilopoulou-Sellin R et al (2003) Role of preoperative ultrasonography in the surgical management of patients with thyroid cancer. Surgery 134(6):946–954; discussion 54-5. PubMed PMID: 14668727
9. Shen WT, Ogawa L, Ruan D, Suh I, Kebebew E, Duh QY et al (2010) Central neck lymph node dissection for papillary thyroid cancer: comparison of complication and recurrence rates in 295 initial dissections and reoperations. Arch Surg 145(3):272–275. PubMed PMID: 20231628. Epub 2010/03/17. eng
10. American Thyroid Association Surgery Working Group, American Association of Endocrine Surgeons, American Academy of O-H, Neck S, American H, Neck S et al (2009) Consensus statement on the terminology and classification of central neck dissection for thyroid cancer. Thyroid 19(11):1153–1158. PubMed PMID: 19860578
11. Stephen B, Edge CCC, Fritz AG, Greene FL, Trotti III A, Byrd D (eds) (2011) AJCC cancer staging manual, 7th edn. Springer, New York
12. Cady B, Sedgwick CE, Meissner WA, Wool MS, Salzman FA, Werber J (1979) Risk factor analysis in differentiated thyroid cancer. Cancer 43(3):810–820. PubMed PMID: 427722. Epub 1979/03/01. eng
13. Roh JL, Kim JM, Park CI (2011) Central compartment reoperation for recurrent/persistent differentiated thyroid cancer: patterns of recurrence, morbidity, and prediction of postoperative hypocalcemia. Ann Surg Oncol 18(5):1312–1318. PubMed PMID: 21140230. Epub 2010/12/09. eng
14. Gimm O, Rath FW, Dralle H (1998) Pattern of lymph node metastases in papillary thyroid carcinoma. Br J Surg 85(2):252–254. PubMed PMID: 9501829. Epub 1998/03/21. eng
15. Mazzaferri EL, Jhiang SM (1994) Long-term impact of initial surgical and medical therapy on papillary and follicular thyroid cancer. Am J Med 97(5):418–428. PubMed PMID: 7977430. Epub 1994/11/01. eng
16. Hay ID, Hutchinson ME, Gonzalez-Losada T, McIver B, Reinalda ME, Grant CS et al (2008) Papillary thyroid microcarcinoma: a study of 900 cases observed in a 60-year period. Surgery 144(6):980–987; discussion 7-8. PubMed PMID: 19041007. Epub 2008/12/02. eng
17. McConahey WM, Hay ID, Woolner LB, van Heerden JA, Taylor WF (1986) Papillary thyroid cancer treated at the Mayo Clinic, 1946 through 1970: initial manifestations, pathologic findings, therapy, and outcome. Mayo Clinic Proceed 61(12):978-96. PubMed PMID: 3773569. Epub 1986/12/01. eng
18. Cranshaw IM, Carnaille B (2008) Micrometastasis in thyroid cancer. An important finding? Surg Oncol 17(3):253–258. PubMed PMID: 18504121. Epub 2008/05/28. eng
19. Chao TC, Jeng LB, Lin JD, Chen MF (1997) Reoperative thyroid surgery. World J Surg 21(6):644–647. PubMed PMID: 9230664. Epub 1997/07/01. eng
20. Pattou F, Combemale F, Fabre S, Carnaille B, Decoulx M, Wemeau JL et al (1998) Hypocalcemia following thyroid surgery: incidence and prediction of outcome. World J Surg 22(7):718–724. PubMed PMID: 9606288. Epub 1998/06/20. eng
21. Kim MK, Mandel SH, Baloch Z, Livolsi VA, Langer JE, Didonato L et al (2004) Morbidity following central compartment reoperation for recurrent or persistent thyroid cancer. Arch Otolaryngol–Head Neck Surg 130(10):1214–1216. PubMed PMID: 15492172. Epub 2004/10/20. eng
22. Conzo G, Docimo G, Pasquali D, Mauriello C, Gambardella C, Esposito D et al (2013) Predictive value of nodal metastases on local recurrence in the management of differentiated

thyroid cancer. Retrospective Clin Study. BMC Surg 13(2):S3. PubMed PMID: 24267409. Pubmed Central PMCID: Pmc3851192. Epub 2013/12/07. eng
23. White ML, Gauger PG, Doherty GM (2007) Central lymph node dissection in differentiated thyroid cancer. World J Surg 31(5):895–904. PubMed PMID: 17347896. Epub 2007/03/10. eng
24. Scheumann GF, Gimm O, Wegener G, Hundeshagen H, Dralle H (1994) Prognostic significance and surgical management of locoregional lymph node metastases in papillary thyroid cancer. World J Surg 18(4):559-67; discussion 67-8. PubMed PMID: 7725745. Epub 1994/07/01. eng
25. Shah MD, Hall FT, Eski SJ, Witterick IJ, Walfish PG, Freeman JL (2003) Clinical course of thyroid carcinoma after neck dissection. Laryngoscope 113(12):2102–2107. PubMed PMID: 14660910. Epub 2003/12/09. eng
26. Shaha AR, Shah JP, Loree TR (1996) Risk group stratification and prognostic factors in papillary carcinoma of thyroid. Ann Surg Oncol 3(6):534–538. PubMed PMID: 8915484. Epub 1996/11/01. eng
27. Hughes DT, White ML, Miller BS, Gauger PG, Burney RE, Doherty GM (2010) Influence of prophylactic central lymph node dissection on postoperative thyroglobulin levels and radioiodine treatment in papillary thyroid cancer. Surgery 148(6):1100-6; discussion 006-7. PubMed PMID: 21134539. Epub 2010/12/08. eng
28. Simon D, Goretzki PE, Witte J, Roher HD (1996) Incidence of regional recurrence guiding radicality in differentiated thyroid carcinoma. World J Surg 20(7):860-6; discussion 6. PubMed PMID: 8678963. Epub 1996/09/01. eng
29. Moo TA, McGill J, Allendorf J, Lee J, Fahey T, 3rd Zarnegar R (2010) Impact of prophylactic central neck lymph node dissection on early recurrence in papillary thyroid carcinoma. World J Surg 34(6):1187–1191. PubMed PMID: 20130868. Epub 2010/02/05. eng
30. Wang TS, Evans DB, Fareau GG, Carroll T, Yen TW (2012) Effect of prophylactic central compartment neck dissection on serum thyroglobulin and recommendations for adjuvant radioactive iodine in patients with differentiated thyroid cancer. Ann Surg Oncol 19(13):4217–4222. PubMed PMID: 23010732. Epub 2012/09/27. eng
31. Popadich A, Levin O, Lee JC, Smooke-Praw S, Ro K, Fazel M et al (2011) A multicenter cohort study of total thyroidectomy and routine central lymph node dissection for cNo papillary thyroid cancer. Surgery 150(6):1048–1057. PubMed PMID: 22136820. Epub 2011/12/06. eng
32. Laird AM, Gauger PG, Miller BS, Doherty GM (2012) Evaluation of postoperative radioactive iodine scans in patients who underwent prophylactic central lymph node dissection. World J Surg 36(6):1268–1273. PubMed PMID: 22270997. Epub 2012/01/25. eng
33. Sywak M, Cornford L, Roach P, Stalberg P, Sidhu S, Delbridge L (2006) Routine ipsilateral level VI lymphadenectomy reduces postoperative thyroglobulin levels in papillary thyroid cancer. Surgery 140(6):1000–1005; discussion 5-7. PubMed PMID: 17188149. Epub 2006/12/26. eng
34. Wang TS, Cheung K, Farrokhyar F, Roman SA, Sosa JA (2013) A meta-analysis of the effect of prophylactic central compartment neck dissection on locoregional recurrence rates in patients with papillary thyroid cancer. Ann Surg Oncol 20(11):3477–3483. PubMed PMID: 23846784. Epub 2013/07/13. eng
35. Gyorki DE, Untch B, Tuttle RM, Shaha AR (2013) Prophylactic central neck dissection in differentiated thyroid cancer: an assessment of the evidence. Ann Surg Oncol 20(7):2285–2289. PubMed PMID: 23417435. Epub 2013/02/19. eng
36. Pereira JA, Jimeno J, Miquel J, Iglesias M, Munne A, Sancho JJ et al (2005) Nodal yield, morbidity, and recurrence after central neck dissection for papillary thyroid carcinoma. Surgery 138(6):1095–1100, discussion 100-1. PubMed PMID: 16360396. Epub 2005/12/20. eng
37. Hay ID, Bergstralh EJ, Goellner JR, Ebersold JR, Grant CS (1993) Predicting outcome in papillary thyroid carcinoma: development of a reliable prognostic scoring system in a cohort of 1779 patients surgically treated at one institution during 1940 through 1989. Surgery 114 (6):1050–1057; discussion 7-8. PubMed PMID: 8256208. Epub 1993/12/01. eng

38. Bhattacharyya N (2003) A population-based analysis of survival factors in differentiated and medullary thyroid carcinoma. Otolaryngol–Head Neck Surg (official journal of American Academy of Otolaryngology-Head and Neck Surgery) 128(1):115–123. PubMed PMID: 12574769. Epub 2003/02/08. eng
39. Podnos YD, Smith D, Wagman LD, Ellenhorn JD (2005) The implication of lymph node metastasis on survival in patients with well-differentiated thyroid cancer. Am Surg. 71(9):731–734. PubMed PMID: 16468507. Epub 2006/02/14. eng
40. Tisell LE, Nilsson B, Molne J, Hansson G, Fjalling M, Jansson S et al (1996) Improved survival of patients with papillary thyroid cancer after surgical microdissection. World J Surg 20(7):854–859. PubMed PMID: 8678962. Epub 1996/09/01. eng
41. Steinmuller T, Klupp J, Rayes N, Ulrich F, Jonas S, Graf KJ et al (2000) Prognostic factors in patients with differentiated thyroid carcinoma. Euro J Surg = Acta Chir 166(1):29–33. PubMed PMID: 10688213. Epub 2000/02/25. eng
42. Chisholm EJ, Kulinskaya E, Tolley NS (2009) Systematic review and meta-analysis of the adverse effects of thyroidectomy combined with central neck dissection as compared with thyroidectomy alone. Laryngoscope 119(6):1135–1139. PubMed PMID: 19358241. Epub 2009/04/10. eng
43. Cheah WK, Arici C, Ituarte PH, Siperstein AE, Duh QY, Clark OH (2002) Complications of neck dissection for thyroid cancer. World J Surg 26(8):1013–1016. PubMed PMID: 12045861. Epub 2002/06/05. eng
44. Segal K, Friedental R, Lubin E, Shvero J, Sulkes J, Feinmesser R (1995) Papillary carcinoma of the thyroid. Otolaryngol–Head Neck Surg (official journal of American Academy of Otolaryngology-Head and Neck Surgery) 113(4):356–363. PubMed PMID: 7567004. Epub 1995/10/01. eng
45. Carling T, Carty SE, Ciarleglio MM, Cooper DS, Doherty GM, Kim LT et al (2012) American Thyroid Association design and feasibility of a prospective randomized controlled trial of prophylactic central lymph node dissection for papillary thyroid carcinoma. Thyroid (official journal of the American Thyroid Association) 22(3):237–244. PubMed PMID: 22313454. Epub 2012/02/09. eng
46. Conzo G, Pasquali D, Bellastella G, Esposito K, Carella C, De Bellis A et al (2013) Total thyroidectomy, without prophylactic central lymph node dissection, in the treatment of differentiated thyroid cancer. Clinical retrospective study on 221 cases. Endocrine 44(2):419–425. PubMed PMID: 23334946. Epub 2013/01/22. eng
47. Cayo AK, Yen TW, Misustin SM, Wall K, Wilson SD, Evans DB et al (2012) Predicting the need for calcium and calcitriol supplementation after total thyroidectomy: results of a prospective, randomized study. Surgery 152(6):1059–1067. PubMed PMID: 23068088. Epub 2012/10/17. eng
48. Sawka AM, Brierley JD, Tsang RW, Thabane L, Rotstein L, Gafni A et al (2008) An updated systematic review and commentary examining the effectiveness of radioactive iodine remnant ablation in well-differentiated thyroid cancer. Endocrinol Metab Clin North Am 37(2):457–480, x. PubMed PMID: 18502337. Epub 2008/05/27. eng
49. Mazzaferri EL, Kloos RT (2001) Clinical review 128: Current approaches to primary therapy for papillary and follicular thyroid cancer. J Clin Endocrinol Metab 86(4):1447–1463. PubMed PMID: 11297567. Epub 2001/04/12. eng
50. Goffredo P, Roman SA, Sosa JA. Have 2006 ATA practice guidelines affected the treatment of differentiated Thyroid cancer in the United States? Thyroid 24(3):463–471. PubMed PMID: 23978295. Epub 2013/08/28. eng
51. DeGroot LJ, Kaplan EL, McCormick M, Straus FH. Natural history, treatment, and course of papillary thyroid carcinoma. J Clin Endocrinol Metab 71(2):414–424. PubMed PMID: 2380337. Epub 1990/08/01. eng
52. Samaan NA, Schultz PN, Hickey RC, Goepfert H, Haynie TP, Johnston DA et al (1992) The results of various modalities of treatment of well differentiated thyroid carcinomas: a

retrospective review of 1599 patients. J Clin Endocrinol Metab 75(3):714–720. PubMed PMID: 1517360. Epub 1992/09/01. eng

53. Tsang RW, Brierley JD, Simpson WJ, Panzarella T, Gospodarowicz MK, Sutcliffe SB (1998) The effects of surgery, radioiodine, and external radiation therapy on the clinical outcome of patients with differentiated thyroid carcinoma. Cancer 82(2):375–388. PubMed PMID: 9445196. Epub 1998/01/28. eng
54. Nixon IJ, Shah JP (2014) Well differentiated thyroid cancer: are we over treating our patients? Euro J Surg Oncol (the journal of the European Society of Surgical Oncology and the British Association of Surgical Oncology) 40(2):129–132. PubMed PMID: 24373300. Epub 2014/01/01. eng
55. Hay ID, Thompson GB, Grant CS, Bergstralh EJ, Dvorak CE, Gorman CA et al (2002) Papillary thyroid carcinoma managed at the Mayo clinic during six decades (1940–1999): temporal trends in initial therapy and long-term outcome in 2444 consecutively treated patients. World J Surg 26(8):879–885. PubMed PMID: 12016468. Epub 2002/05/23. eng
56. Sawka AM, Thabane L, Parlea L, Ibrahim-Zada I, Tsang RW, Brierley JD et al (2009) Second primary malignancy risk after radioactive iodine treatment for thyroid cancer: a systematic review and meta-analysis. Thyroid (official journal of the American Thyroid Association) 19 (5):451–457. PubMed PMID: 19281429. Epub 2009/03/14. eng
57. Almeida JP, Sanabria AE, Lima EN, Kowalski LP (2011) Late side effects of radioactive iodine on salivary gland function in patients with thyroid cancer. Head Neck 33(5):686–690. PubMed PMID: 21484917. Epub 2011/04/13. eng
58. Alexander C, Bader JB, Schaefer A, Finke C, Kirsch CM (1998) Intermediate and long-term side effects of high-dose radioiodine therapy for thyroid carcinoma. J Nucl Med: (official publication, Society of Nuclear Medicine) 39(9):1551–1554. PubMed PMID: 9744341. Epub 1998/09/23. eng
59. Lang BH, Wong IO, Wong KP, Cowling BJ, Wan KY (2012) Risk of second primary malignancy in differentiated thyroid carcinoma treated with radioactive iodine therapy. Surgery 151(6):844–850. PubMed PMID: 22341041. Epub 2012/02/22. eng
60. Gramza A, Schuff KG (2009) Recombinant human thyroid stimulating hormone in 2008: focus on thyroid cancer management. Onco Targets Ther 1:87–101. PubMed PMID: 21127756. Pubmed Central PMCID: Pmc2994210. Epub 2009/01/01. eng
61. Lee J, Yun MJ, Nam KH, Chung WY, Soh EY, Park CS (2010) Quality of life and effectiveness comparisons of thyroxine withdrawal, triiodothyronine withdrawal, and recombinant thyroid-stimulating hormone administration for low-dose radioiodine remnant ablation of differentiated thyroid carcinoma. Thyroid (official journal of the American Thyroid Association) 20(2):173–179. PubMed PMID: 20151824. Epub 2010/02/16. eng
62. Luster M, Felbinger R, Dietlein M, Reiners C (2005) Thyroid hormone withdrawal in patients with differentiated thyroid carcinoma: a one hundred thirty-patient pilot survey on consequences of hypothyroidism and a pharmacoeconomic comparison to recombinant thyrotropin administration. Thyroid (official journal of the American Thyroid Association) 15 (10):1147–1155. PubMed PMID: 16279848. Epub 2005/11/11. eng
63. Dow KH, Ferrell BR, Anello C (1997) Quality-of-life changes in patients with thyroid cancer after withdrawal of thyroid hormone therapy. Thyroid (official journal of the American Thyroid Association) 7(4):613–619. PubMed PMID: 9292951. Epub 1997/08/01. eng
64. Taieb D, Sebag F, Cherenko M, Baumstarck-Barrau K, Fortanier C, Farman-Ara B et al (2009) Quality of life changes and clinical outcomes in thyroid cancer patients undergoing radioiodine remnant ablation (RRA) with recombinant human TSH (rhTSH): a randomized controlled study. Clin Endocrinol 71(1):115–23. PubMed PMID: 18803678. Epub 2008/09/23. eng
65. Roberts CG, Ladenson PW (2004) Hypothyroidism. Lancet 363(9411):793–803. PubMed PMID: 15016491. Epub 2004/03/16. eng
66. Robbins RJ, Driedger A, Magner J (2006) Recombinant human thyrotropin-assisted radioiodine therapy for patients with metastatic thyroid cancer who could not elevate endogenous thyrotropin or be withdrawn from thyroxine. Thyroid (official journal of the

American Thyroid Association) 16(11):1121–1130. PubMed PMID: 17123339. Epub 2006/11/25. eng
67. Barbaro D, Boni G, Meucci G, Simi U, Lapi P, Orsini P et al (2006) Recombinant human thyroid-stimulating hormone is effective for radioiodine ablation of post-surgical thyroid remnants. Nucl Med Comm 27(8):627–632. PubMed PMID: 16829763. Epub 2006/07/11. eng
68. Tuttle RM, Brokhin M, Omry G, Martorella AJ, Larson SM, Grewal RK et al (2008) Recombinant human TSH-assisted radioactive iodine remnant ablation achieves short-term clinical recurrence rates similar to those of traditional thyroid hormone withdrawal. J Nucl Med (official publication, Society of Nuclear Medicine) 49(5):764–770. PubMed PMID: 18413378. Epub 2008/04/17. eng
69. Molinaro E, Giani C, Agate L, Biagini A, Pieruzzi L, Bianchi F et al (2013) Patients with differentiated thyroid cancer who underwent radioiodine thyroid remnant ablation with low-activity (1)(3)(1)I after either recombinant human TSH or thyroid hormone therapy withdrawal showed the same outcome after a 10-year follow-up. J Clin Endocrinol Metab 98(7):2693–2700. PubMed PMID: 23626005. Epub 2013/04/30. eng
70. Pacini F, Molinaro E, Castagna MG, Lippi F, Ceccarelli C, Agate L et al (2002) Ablation of thyroid residues with 30 mCi (131)I: a comparison in thyroid cancer patients prepared with recombinant human TSH or thyroid hormone withdrawal. J Clin Endocrinol Metab 87 (9):4063–4068. PubMed PMID: 12213846. Epub 2002/09/06. eng
71. Wang TS, Cheung K, Mehta P, Roman SA, Walker HD, Sosa JA. To stimulate or withdraw? A cost-utility analysis of recombinant human thyrotropin versus thyroxine withdrawal for radioiodine ablation in patients with low-risk differentiated thyroid cancer in the United States. J Clin Endocrinol Metab 95(4):1672–1680. PubMed PMID: 20139234. Epub 2010/02/09. eng
72. Caglar M, Bozkurt FM, Akca CK, Vargol SE, Bayraktar M, Ugur O et al (2012) Comparison of 800 and 3700 MBq iodine-131 for the postoperative ablation of thyroid remnant in patients with low-risk differentiated thyroid cancer. Nucl Med Commun 33(3):268–274. PubMed PMID: 22205241. Epub 2011/12/30. eng
73. Cheng W, Ma C, Fu H, Li J, Chen S, Wu S et al (2013) Low- or high-dose radioiodine remnant ablation for differentiated thyroid carcinoma: a meta-analysis. J Clin Endocrinol Metab 98(4):1353–1360. PubMed PMID: 23436920. Epub 2013/02/26. eng
74. Fallahi B, Beiki D, Takavar A, Fard-Esfahani A, Gilani KA, Saghari M et al (2012) Low versus high radioiodine dose in postoperative ablation of residual thyroid tissue in patients with differentiated thyroid carcinoma: a large randomized clinical trial. Nucl Med Commun 33 (3):275–282. PubMed PMID: 22124360. Epub 2011/11/30. eng
75. Hundahl SA, Fleming ID, Fremgen AM, Menck HR (1998) A National Cancer data base report on 53,856 cases of thyroid carcinoma treated in the U.S. 1985–1995 (see commetns). Cancer 83(12):2638–2648. PubMed PMID: 9874472. Epub 1999/01/05 21:59. eng
76. Enewold L, Zhu K, Ron E, Marrogi AJ, Stojadinovic A, Peoples GE et al (2009) Rising thyroid cancer incidence in the United States by demographic and tumor characteristics, 1980–2005. Cancer Epidemiol, Biomark Prev (a publication of the American Association for Cancer Research, cosponsored by the American Society of Preventive Oncology) 18(3):784–791. PubMed PMID: 19240234. Pubmed Central PMCID: Pmc2676561. Epub 2009/02/26. eng
77. Elisei R (2008) Routine serum calcitonin measurement in the evaluation of thyroid nodules. Best Pract Res Clin Endocrinol Metab 22(6):941–953. PubMed PMID: 19041824. Epub 2008/12/02. eng
78. Bondeson L, Ljungberg O (1981) Occult thyroid carcinoma at autopsy in Malmo, Sweden. Cancer 47(2):319–323. PubMed PMID: 7459819. Epub 1981/01/15. eng
79. Bondeson L, Ljungberg O (1984) Occult papillary thyroid carcinoma in the young and the aged. Cancer 53(8):1790–1792. PubMed PMID: 6697317. Epub 1984/04/15. eng
80. Bergholm U, Adami HO, Telenius-Berg M, Johansson H, Wilander E (1990) Incidence of sporadic and familial medullary thyroid carcinoma in Sweden 1959 through 1981. A nationwide study in 126 patients. Swedish MCT study group. Acta Oncol (Stockholm, Sweden) 29(1):9–15. PubMed PMID: 2310607. Epub 1990/01/01. eng

81. Kloos RT, Eng C, Evans DB, Francis GL, Gagel RF, Gharib H et al (2009) Medullary thyroid cancer: management guidelines of the American Thyroid Association. Thyroid (official journal of the American Thyroid Association) 19(6):565–612. PubMed PMID: 19469690. Epub 2009/05/28. eng
82. Baloch ZW, LiVolsi VA (2001) Prognostic factors in well-differentiated follicular-derived carcinoma and medullary thyroid carcinoma. Thyroid (official journal of the American Thyroid Association) 11(7):637–645. PubMed PMID: 11484892. Epub 2001/08/04. eng
83. Daniels GH (2011) Screening for medullary thyroid carcinoma with serum calcitonin measurements in patients with thyroid nodules in the United States and Canada. Thyroid (official journal of the American Thyroid Association) 21(11):1199–1207. PubMed PMID: 21936671. Epub 2011/09/23. eng
84. Vierhapper H, Niederle B, Bieglmayer C, Kaserer K, Baumgartner-Parzer S (2005) Early diagnosis and curative therapy of medullary thyroid carcinoma by routine measurement of serum calcitonin in patients with thyroid disorders. Thyroid (official journal of the American Thyroid Association) 15(11):1267–1272. PubMed PMID: 16356091. Epub 2005/12/17. eng
85. Costante G, Meringolo D, Durante C, Bianchi D, Nocera M, Tumino S et al (2007) Predictive value of serum calcitonin levels for preoperative diagnosis of medullary thyroid carcinoma in a cohort of 5817 consecutive patients with thyroid nodules. J Clin Endocrinol Metab 92(2):450–455. PubMed PMID: 17119000. Epub 2006/11/23. eng
86. Pacini F, Fontanelli M, Fugazzola L, Elisei R, Romei C, Di Coscio G et al (1994) Routine measurement of serum calcitonin in nodular thyroid diseases allows the preoperative diagnosis of unsuspected sporadic medullary thyroid carcinoma. J Clin Endocrinol Metab 78(4):826–829. PubMed PMID: 8157706. Epub 1994/04/01. eng
87. Cheung K, Roman SA, Wang TS, Walker HD, Sosa JA (2008) Calcitonin measurement in the evaluation of thyroid nodules in the United States: a cost-effectiveness and decision analysis. J Clin Endocrinol Metab 93(6):2173–2180. PubMed PMID: 18364376. Epub 2008/03/28. eng
88. Hay ID, Grant CS, Taylor WF, McConahey WM (1987) Ipsilateral lobectomy versus bilateral lobar resection in papillary thyroid carcinoma: a retrospective analysis of surgical outcome using a novel prognostic scoring system. Surgery 102(6):1088–1095. PubMed PMID: 3686348. Epub 1987/12/01. eng

Comparative Effectiveness in Head and Neck Malignancies

Carol M. Lewis, Katherine A. Hutcheson and Michael E. Kupferman

Abstract

To date, there is limited comparative effectiveness research (CER) in head and neck surgical oncology. Several barriers exist, the most common of which include low patient accrual, selection bias inherent to observational studies, and the difficulty of integrating both clinical and functional outcomes. Areas in need of meaningful CER range from initial evaluation to post-treatment surveillance, as well as the identification and evaluation of significant quality metrics and patient-reported outcomes. Despite existing hurdles, careful study design and statistical analyses can address current gaps in head and neck cancer care.

Keywords

Head and neck cancer · Head and neck surgery · Otolaryngology · Functional outcomes · HPV

Contents

C.M. Lewis (✉) · K.A. Hutcheson · M.E. Kupferman
Department of Head and Neck Surgery, University of Texas MD Anderson Cancer Center, Houston, TX, US
e-mail: CMLewis@mdanderson.org

K.Y. Bilimoria et al. (eds.), *Comparative Effectiveness in Surgical Oncology*,
Cancer Treatment and Research 164, DOI 10.1007/978-3-319-12553-4_6

1 Introduction

Medical literature is classified based on the strength of study design to assist in evaluating the impact of a particular study; in each of these, randomized controlled trials (RCTs) or systematic reviews of RCTs provide the highest level of evidence, with observational studies considered less cogent [1]. Recently, there has been increasing emphasis on comparative effectiveness research (CER), the role of which is to identify and validate diagnostic and treatment options for physicians, patients, payers, and policymakers in an attempt to provide the best medical care for patients while containing costs [2, 3]. The Institute of Medicine defines CER as "the generation and synthesis of evidence that compares the benefits and harms of alternative methods to prevent, diagnose, treat, and monitor a clinical condition, or to improve the delivery of care" [4]. CER aims to achieve this in a way that applies to the general population; fundamental to this is that the study population is diverse and assembled from a primary care practice setting with outcomes that include decisions based on patients' values [5]. With these goals in mind, RCTs do not necessarily represent the best study design; some authors argue that RCTs determine efficacy, not effectiveness [5].

In head and neck oncology, RCTs do not generally compare different treatment modalities. However, one pivotal RCT changed the approach to advanced laryngeal cancer by comparing surgery and postoperative radiation to induction chemotherapy followed by radiation for advanced laryngeal cancer. Finding no difference in overall survival, this study promoted organ preservation approaches to head and neck cancer [6]. Subsequently, the organ preservation approach to hypopharyngeal cancers was evaluated in a RCT comparing surgery with postoperative radiation to induction chemotherapy followed by radiation; both groups were found to have similar median survivals [7]. These studies lead to widespread acceptance of organ preservation management of advanced laryngeal and hypopharyngeal cancers, as reflected by longitudinal clinical registry data [8, 9]. Surprisingly, this change in treatment paradigm has been accompanied by a decrease in survival, especially at low-volume community medical centers [8, 9]. This potentially reflects the danger of generalizing the findings of RCTs, which have clearly outlined patient eligibility. For example, a RCT comparing induction chemotherapy to concurrent chemotherapy for advanced laryngeal cancers exclude those patients who present with cartilage destruction; [10] this criterion may not be appropriately recognized when recommending organ-preserving treatments. Additionally, patients included in most head and neck oncology RCTs are younger and healthier than this general patient population [2]. The majority of the otolaryngology literature consists of a low level of evidence, with the majority of studies containing level 4 evidence, but this landscape is changing [11]. Carefully-designed observational studies, which represent lower echelons of evidence strength, may complement RCTs and provide meaningful CER in head and neck oncology [2].

2 Major Barriers to Comparative Effectiveness Research

2.1 Powering Meaningful Studies

In 2014, the projected incidence of head and neck cancer is 55,070 people or 3.3 % of all cancers, and the projected mortality is 12,000 deaths or 2.0 % of all cancer deaths [12]. With such a small portion of the general population affected, it is difficult to accrue enough patients to studies to have meaningful results, especially as compared to a more prevalent medical condition, such as otitis media [13]. Without enough patients for appropriate power, negative results do not necessarily mean that a significant difference does not exist.

A meta-analysis of prophylactic antibiotic use in head and neck surgery patients identified 7 RCTs between 1981 and 2003 that compared 24 h of peri-operative antibiotics to a longer course (3–4 days in some trials, 5 days in others). Each of these studies were underpowered, so the result of no difference between the treatment groups was not particularly reliable; by pooling these results in a meta-analysis, the authors were able to achieve adequate power to conclude that no difference exists [14]. Even within this group of studies, the surgical procedure ranged from upper aerodigestive tract surgery to pedicled myocutaneous flaps to combined composite resections with free flap reconstructions. In addition, little information was provided about patient characteristics that might affect outcomes, such as smoking history, comorbidities, or previous radiation therapy, for a subset analysis [14]. This meta-analysis evaluated perioperative antibiotic use without addressing specific subsites of disease; considering that the treatment for head and neck cancer varies by each subsite (e.g., paranasal sinuses, nasopharynx, oropharynx, oral cavity, hypopharynx, larynx, skin, and thyroid), assessing head and neck cancer patients by subsite of disease even further reduces the ability to achieve adequate power.

Multicenter clinical trials may accrue enough patients to answer CER questions prospectively, whereas clinical registry data may be appropriate to evaluate existing gaps. A common limitation to tumor registries is the lack of detailed information, such as clinical indications, tobacco history, TNM staging, test results, and treatment-related complications, to name a few [2]. Despite these limitations, there are certain questions within head and neck oncology that could be appropriately addressed. The Longitudinal Outcomes Registry of Head and Neck Carcinoma was built to address these shortcomings [15], but has since closed due to insufficient funding; developing similarly motivated registries would be worthwhile. As more sophisticated electronic health records bridge medical centers and health systems, such detailed data may be accessible on adequate numbers of patients.

2.2 Selection Bias

Selection bias occurs when patients are assigned to one intervention or another in a way that confounds the study outcomes. In retrospective cohort studies, for example, patients were likely chosen to receive one treatment or another based upon patient or tumor characteristics. Majoufre et al. [16] evaluated a historical cohort of patients who presented with clinically N0 oral cavity cancer and underwent either a type 3 modified radical neck dissection or a supraomohyoid neck dissection, finding no significant difference in recurrence or survival. Interestingly, however, the group that underwent supraomohyoid neck dissections had a better 2-year and 5-year survival when compared to the modified radical neck dissection group (85.8 % vs. 73.6 %, and 70.2 % vs. 57.2 %, respectively); [16] although these differences did not reach statistical significance, they suggest that there was a selection bias involved in surgical planning such that the patients who underwent the less extensive neck dissection had a favorable 5-year survival. This same question of whether a modified radical neck dissection or supraomohyoid neck dissection is more appropriate for N0 oral cavity cancer patients was addressed by the Brazilian Head and Neck Cancer Study Group in a RCT [17]. Randomizing patients to one type of neck dissection or another removes selection bias; accordingly, the 5-year survival for the modified radical neck dissection group was 63 and 67 % for the supraomohyoid neck dissection group ($p = 0.72$) [17]. Although the majority of the otolaryngology literature has a low level of evidence, [11] careful study design, and data analyses can adjust for biases inherent in observational studies to generate meaningful CER.

2.3 Evaluating Clinical and Functional Outcomes

Head and neck cancer and its treatment can be functionally debilitating. However, most studies focus either on clinical outcomes, such as survival and recurrence, or on functional outcomes and quality of life; rarely do studies prioritize both outcomes. To further complicate this issue, few studies use accepted, validated instruments to evaluate patients' function.

When comparing endoscopic resection versus radiation therapy for early (T1) glottic cancer, a recent systematic review identified 1,045 studies, 888 of which were dismissed after a review of their abstracts [18]. After reviewing, the complete manuscripts for the remaining 146 studies, 127 were subsequently excluded. The review then focused on 2 systematic reviews and 17 articles, the majority of which were retrospective comparative and cross-sectional studies. After reviewing this literature, the authors were unable to pool the data because of poor study designs, heterogeneity among study populations, and inherent period bias from the years covered (e.g., changes in radiation technique and dosing). Of the 17 primary studies, 3 did not report length of follow-up. Only 11 of the 17 studies reported survival outcomes; of these, 2 did not report overall survival, 9 did not report disease-free survival, and 6 did not report disease-specific survival. Only 7 studies reported a functional evaluation, which ranged from clinician-ratings to patient perception ratings to acoustic and aerodynamic analysis. Of the validated patient perception instruments used, 2 studies used the Voice Handicap Index, 1 used head and neck quality of life questionnaires, and 2 used the voice-related quality of life scale [18]. In an attempt to organize these best available data for clinical practice guideline recommendations, the authors conclude that there is not enough evidence to demonstrate a difference between these treatment modalities [19]. The issues faced by these authors are fairly representative of the quality of head and neck surgical oncology literature.

Standards surrounding clinical and functional outcomes need to be established for successful and meaningful CER; these might be best determined by specialty society efforts. Ideally, both types of outcomes would be evaluated and reported in the same study, with the use of validated instruments to assess patient function at baseline and in short- and long-term post-treatment intervals. One such example is in the realm of laryngeal preservation. The premise of laryngeal preservation is to achieve locoregional control but maintain a functioning larynx for natural breathing, speaking, and swallowing. Landmark RCTs (as previously discussed in this chapter) established equivalent survival after frontline chemoradiation in lieu of complete surgical removal of the larynx (i.e., total laryngectomy) for locally advanced stage laryngeal cancer. With broad application of nonsurgical laryngeal preservation, it became clear that structural preservation of the larynx does not equate to functional laryngeal preservation. A pooled analysis of three RTOG chemoradiation trials reported an alarming crude rate of 43 % of patients with adequate baseline functioning developing late grade 3–4 laryngopharyngeal dysfunction after aggressive nonsurgical therapy [20]. This largely constituted chronic gastrostomy dependence related to dysphagia (difficulty swallow). Bearing in mind these outcomes, an international consensus panel developed a combined endpoint to account for both survival and functioning in phase III clinical trials of laryngeal preservation strategies—"laryngoesophageal dysfunction (LED)-free survival, which includes the events of death, local relapse, total or partial laryngectomy, tracheotomy at ≥2 years, or feeding tube at ≥2 years". Secondary endpoints were also defined including patient-centered outcomes contributing to QOL in survivorship [21].

Functional outcomes are considered a key measure of success in contemporary management of head and neck malignancies. Among these outcomes, swallowing emerges as a top functional priority of patients and a driver of post-treatment quality of life [22, 23]. When rated subjectively in the clinical setting (e.g., per CTCAE), grade 3 dysphagia is essentially a marker of feeding tube dependence. The clinical literature has a preponderance of studies using grade 3 dysphagia (i.e., feeding tube-dependent dysphagia) as the sole functional outcome. It is clear, however, that alone feeding tube dependence is not a sensitive marker of swallowing impairment. Many survivors with substantial and clinically meaningful levels of swallowing impairment (such as tracheal aspiration) continue to eat without a feeding tube, albeit with great effort and risk of secondary complications (i.e., aspiration pneumonia).

For instance, we have previously demonstrated in observational studies that only 33–45 % of chronic aspirators are feeding tube dependent [24]. Looking beyond gastrostomy-dependent dysphagia, swallowing abilities can be quantified from the patient's perspective using a validated patient-reported outcome inventory developed specifically for the head and neck population—the MD Anderson Dysphagia Inventory (MDADI) [25]. Opportunities for CER using meta-analysis or pooled datasets are ripe with now widespread adoption of the MDADI in published single institutional series using various treatment modalities (e.g., MDADI after robotic surgery for TORS in oropharyngeal cancer, [26–30] and MDADI scores after nonsurgical therapy for oropharyngeal cancer [31–34]). Consistent reporting of confounding factors like precise tumor subsite, TNM, and therapeutic details will be required to pool data for comparative purposes.

3 Important Target Areas for Comparative Effectiveness Research

3.1 Pre-treatment Evaluation

Human papillomavirus (HPV)-associated head and neck cancers have been found to confer favorable survival [35] and are presenting with increasing incidence [36]. Given the higher treatment response rate, lower risk oropharyngeal squamous cell carcinomas may respond just as well to deescalated therapy, which may limit treatment-associated morbidity while providing similar clinical outcomes. The Radiation Therapy Oncology Group has an on-going RCT (1016) that is evaluating how concurrent cetuximab and radiation compare to the traditional regimen of cisplatin and radiation in patients with HPV-positive tumors [37]. The European Cooperative Oncology Group has also conducted a RCT offering induction chemotherapy followed by concurrent cetuximab and radiation, with patients randomized to receive either high or low doses of radiotherapy [38]. Prospective studies and RCTs address these questions well, but long-term survival and functional outcomes take longer to obtain. These studies may be complemented by carefully designed observational studies.

Just as HPV-positivity is associated with a favorable prognosis and response to treatment, other biomarkers reflecting etiology or molecular expression hold promise as important predictive markers, including the epidermal growth factor receptor, p53, B cell lymphoma-2 (Bcl-2), cyclin D1, and vascular endothelial growth factor, to name a few [39]. None of these have yet been established in routine clinical management because of problems with consistency and study design [40]. CER has great potential in evaluating the clinical utility of these markers for personalized treatment approaches [41]. Identifying the predictive capabilities of biomarkers may lead to more targeted treatment choices with possible reduction in treatment-related toxicity.

3.2 Treatment

Subsites of head and neck cancer in which radiation and surgery are both considered valid approaches are in need of meaningful CER to compare treatment modalities. As illustrated by the earlier discussion of endoscopic surgery versus radiotherapy for T1 glottic cancers [18, 19], the literature that exists on this subject is of questionable quality. Although most data indicate that radiation and minimally invasive surgery have similar effectiveness for early glottic cancers, there has not been an adequate prospective trial allowing for direct comparison of clinical and functional outcomes.

There has been renewed interest in surgery for oropharyngeal cancers with the advent of robotic surgery; transoral robotic surgery (TORS) is becoming more commonly accepted for early stage oropharyngeal cancers. CER comparing TORS to traditional open surgical approaches and to radiation-based therapy is needed. Currently, there are five independent TORS trials on-going, each with a single arm of TORS at a single institution [42]. The feasibility of TORS at multiple institutions was previously reported by Weinstein et al. [43] Given the low incidence of TORS-appropriate cases, a multicenter trial with standardized functional assessments and multiple study arms has been opened, although the primary study group are intermediate-risk, who are randomized to either standard (60 Gy) versus low-dose (50 Gy) adjuvant radiotherapy. A more robust RCT is necessary that would directly compare TORS to radiotherapy.

CER would also be helpful in overcoming the barriers to fully evaluating the clinical benefit of neoadjuvant therapy in head and neck cancers. Induction chemotherapy is used in the management of many solid tumors, but its role in head and neck cancer is less clear. In 2000, the Meta-Analysis of Chemotherapy on Head and Neck Cancer (MACH-NC) collaborative group evaluated 31 clinical trials, finding no improvement in survival. However, this group also reported that there was a small but significant benefit when analysis was limited to trials using cisplatin and fluorouracil (FU) [44]. Subsequent clinical trials have been hampered largely by low accrual, which translates into an underpowered study; unfortunately, this makes it difficult to determine whether there is an actual clinical benefit from the addition of neoadjuvant chemotherapy despite negative results [45, 46]. Larger multicenter trials may address this issue, although the use of clinical registries may need to be developed in order to achieve adequate power for conclusive findings.

3.3 Post-treatment Surveillance

Clinical practice guidelines for post-treatment surveillance of head and neck cancer patients lack strong evidence in the medical literature [47]. The clinical effectiveness of imaging strategies (e.g., one post-treatment imaging and then as-needed for symptoms vs. only as-needed for symptoms vs. routine imaging) with regard to identifying asymptomatic recurrences and second primary tumors is an area that warrants CER. Broad variability exists in the oncology community vis-à-vis the interval and type of surveillance imaging (PET-CT, CT, MRI, chest X-ray) necessary in the post-treatment setting. Most challenging is that these strategies and imaging choices may differ by disease subsite and treatment modality utilized.

Additionally, although the National Comprehensive Cancer Network (NCCN) formally prescribes a post-treatment surveillance schedule of office visits, [48] this is not evidence-based. In fact, the United Kingdom's National Institute of Health and Care Excellence (NICE), which also creates evidence-based guidelines, simply emphasizes that follow-up is important in the first two post-treatment year, since the risk of recurrence is higher during that time, with increasing intervals between visits as time goes on [49]. As with post-treatment imaging, these follow-up strategies may be impacted by disease subsite and treatment modality.

3.4 Quality of Care Metrics

There has been a great deal of interest in identifying quality metrics for head and neck cancer care; [50–52] in most cases, these metrics are identified from the best available evidence [53] but their impact on clinical and functional outcomes is largely unknown. With appropriate statistical modeling, CER could identify which process metrics impact patient outcomes. These standards would include technical aspects of radiation therapy, treatment breaks, and peri-operative complications. Endpoints would include patient-reported outcomes, functional outcomes, and clinical outcomes, such as survival and recurrence, both in short- and long-term follow-up.

4 Conclusion

CER has the potential to reform the care head and neck cancer patients. Current barriers include low-powered studies limited by the low incidence of this disease, selection bias in clinical trials, and few established standards for reporting clinical and functional outcomes in comparative studies. All of these have workable solutions that will improve the quality of head and neck cancer studies in the areas of pretreatment evaluation, treatment, posttreatment surveillance, and the identification and validation of quality metrics.

References

1. Shin JJ, Randolph GW, Rauch SD (2010) Evidence-based medicine in otolaryngology, part 1: the multiple faces of evidence-based medicine. Otolaryngol Head Neck Surg 142:637–646
2. Goulart BH, Ramsey SD, Parvathaneni U (2014) Observational study designs for comparative effectiveness research: an alternative approach to close evidence gaps in head-and-neck cancer. Int J Radiat Oncol Biol Phys 88:106–114

3. Mushlin AI, Ghomrawi H (2010) Health care reform and the need for comparative-effectiveness research. N Engl J Med 362:e6
4. Haut ER, Pronovost PJ (2011) Surveillance bias in outcomes reporting. JAMA 305:2462–2463
5. Neely JG, Paniello RC, Graboyes EM et al (2014) Practical guide to understanding clinical research compliance. Otolaryngol Head Neck Surg 150:716–721
6. Induction chemotherapy plus radiation compared with surgery plus radiation in patients with advanced laryngeal cancer. The Department of Veterans Affairs Laryngeal Cancer Study Group. N Engl J Med 324:1685–1690 (1991)
7. Lefebvre JL, Chevalier D, Luboinski B et al (1996) Larynx preservation in pyriform sinus cancer: preliminary results of a European organization for research and treatment of cancer phase III trial. EORTC head and neck cancer cooperative group. J Natl Cancer Inst 88:890–899
8. Chen AY, Fedewa S, Pavluck A, Ward EM (2010) Improved survival is associated with treatment at high-volume teaching facilities for patients with advanced stage laryngeal cancer. Cancer 116:4744–4752
9. Hoffman HT, Porter K, Karnell LH et al (2006) Laryngeal cancer in the United States: changes in demographics, patterns of care, and survival. Laryngoscope 116:1–13
10. Forastiere AA, Goepfert H, Maor M et al (2003) Concurrent chemotherapy and radiotherapy for organ preservation in advanced laryngeal cancer. N Engl J Med 349:2091–2098
11. Wasserman JM, Wynn R, Bash TS, Rosenfeld RM (2006) Levels of evidence in otolaryngology journals. Otolaryngol Head Neck Surg 134:717–723
12. American Cancer Society (2014) Cancer Facts and Figures 2014. American Cancer Society
13. Marchisio P, Chonmaitree T, Leibovitz E et al (2013) Panel 7: treatment and comparative effectiveness research. Otolaryngol Head Neck Surg 148:E102–E121
14. Shin JJ, Johnson JT (2008) Prophylaxis in head and neck surgery: one-day versus longer-course perioperative antibiotics: impact on postoperative surgical-site infections. In: Shin JJ, Hartnick CJ, Randolph GW (eds) Evidence-Based Otolaryngology. Springer, Berlin, pp 587–598
15. Wong SJ, Harari PM, Garden AS et al (2011) Longitudinal oncology registry of head and neck carcinoma (LORHAN): analysis of chemoradiation treatment approaches in the United States. Cancer 117:1679–1686
16. Majoufre C, Faucher A, Laroche C et al (1999) Supraomohyoid neck dissection in cancer of the oral cavity. Am J Surg 178:73–77
17. Results of a prospective trial on elective modified radical classical versus supraomohyoid neck dissection in the management of oral squamous carcinoma. Brazilian Head and Neck Cancer Study Group. Am J Surg 176:422–427 (1998)
18. Yoo J, Lacchetti C, Hammond JA et al (2013) Role of endolaryngeal surgery (with or without laser) versus radiotherapy in the management of early (T1) glottic cancer: a systematic review. Head Neck 12:1807–1819
19. Yoo J, Lacchetti C, Hammond JA et al (2013) Role of endolaryngeal surgery (with or without laser) compared with radiotherapy in the management of early (T1) glottic cancer: a clinical practice guideline. Curr Oncol 20:e132–e135
20. Machtay M, Moughan J, Trotti A et al (2008) Factors associated with severe late toxicity after concurrent chemoradiation for locally advanced head and neck cancer: an RTOG analysis. J Clin Oncol 26:3582–3589
21. Ang KK (2010) Larynx preservation clinical trial design: summary of key recommendations of a consensus panel. Oncologist 15(Suppl 3):25–29
22. Wilson JA, Carding PN, Patterson JM (2011) Dysphagia after nonsurgical head and neck cancer treatment: patients' perspectives. Otolaryngol Head Neck Surg 145:767–771
23. Hunter KU, Schipper M, Feng FY et al (2013) Toxicities affecting quality of life after chemo-IMRT of oropharyngeal cancer: prospective study of patient-reported, observer-rated, and objective outcomes. Int J Radiat Oncol Biol Phys 85:935–940

24. Hutcheson KA, Barringer DA, Rosenthal DI et al (2008) Swallowing outcomes after radiotherapy for laryngeal carcinoma. Arch Otolaryngol Head Neck Surg 134:178–183
25. Chen AY, Frankowski R, Bishop-Leone J et al (2001) The development and validation of a dysphagia-specific quality-of-life questionnaire for patients with head and neck cancer: the M. D. Anderson dysphagia inventory. Arch Otolaryngol Head Neck Surg 127:870–876
26. More YI, Tsue TT, Girod DA et al (2013) Functional swallowing outcomes following transoral robotic surgery vs primary chemoradiotherapy in patients with advanced-stage oropharynx and supraglottis cancers. JAMA Otolaryngol Head Neck Surg 139:43–48
27. de Almeida JR, Park RC, Villanueva NL et al (2014) Reconstructive algorithm and classification system for transoral oropharyngeal defects. Head Neck 36:934–941
28. Hans S, Hoffman C, Croidieu R et al (2013) Evaluation of quality of life and swallowing in patients with cancer of the oropharynx treated with assisted transoral robotic surgery. Rev Laryngol Otol Rhinol (Bord) 134:49–56
29. Sinclair CF, McColloch NL, Carroll WR et al (2011) Patient-perceived and objective functional outcomes following transoral robotic surgery for early oropharyngeal carcinoma. Arch Otolaryngol Head Neck Surg 137:1112–1116
30. Iseli TA, Kulbersh BD, Iseli CE et al (2009) Functional outcomes after transoral robotic surgery for head and neck cancer. Otolaryngol Head Neck Surg 141:166–171
31. Schwartz DL, Garden AS, Shah SJ et al (2013) Adaptive radiotherapy for head and neck cancer–dosimetric results from a prospective clinical trial. Radiother Oncol 106:80–84
32. Prestwich RJ, Teo MT, Gilbert A et al (2014) Long-term swallow function after chemoradiotherapy for oropharyngeal cancer: the influence of a prophylactic gastrostomy or reactive nasogastric tube. Clin Oncol (R Coll Radiol) 26:103–109
33. Gillespie MB, Brodsky MB, Day TA et al (2004) Swallowing-related quality of life after head and neck cancer treatment. Laryngoscope 114:1362–1367
34. Cartmill B, Cornwell P, Ward E et al (2012) Long-term functional outcomes and patient perspective following altered fractionation radiotherapy with concomitant boost for oropharyngeal cancer. Dysphagia 27:481–490
35. Ang KK, Harris J, Wheeler R et al (2010) Human papillomavirus and survival of patients with oropharyngeal cancer. N Engl J Med 363:24–35
36. Chaturvedi AK, Engels EA, Pfeiffer RM et al (2011) Human papillomavirus and rising oropharyngeal cancer incidence in the United States. J Clin Oncol 29:4294–4301
37. (ICSI) IfCSI. Health Care Guideline: Venous Thromboembolism. Institute for Clinical Systems Improvement
38. Thromboembolism NCSftPaCoV. National Quality Forum Project
39. Lothaire P, de Azambuja E, Dequanter D et al (2006) Molecular markers of head and neck squamous cell carcinoma: promising signs in need of prospective evaluation. Head Neck 28:256–269
40. Kim KY, McShane LM, Conley BA (2014) Designing biomarker studies for head and neck cancer. Head Neck 36:1069–1075
41. Lyman GH, Levine M (2012) Comparative effectiveness research in oncology: an overview. J Clin Oncol 30:4181–4184
42. Collins R, Scrimgeour A, Yusuf S, Peto R (1988) Reduction in fatal pulmonary embolism and venous thrombosis by perioperative administration of subcutaneous heparin. Overview of results of randomized trials in general, orthopedic, and urologic surgery. N Engl J Med 318:1162–1173
43. Weinstein GS, O'Malley BW Jr, Magnuson JS et al (2012) Transoral robotic surgery: a multicenter study to assess feasibility, safety, and surgical margins. Laryngoscope 122:1701–1707
44. Pignon JP, Bourhis J, Domenge C, Designe L (2000) Chemotherapy added to locoregional treatment for head and neck squamous-cell carcinoma: three meta-analyses of updated individual data. MACH-NC collaborative group. meta-analysis of chemotherapy on head and neck cancer. Lancet 355:949–955

45. Cohen EE, Karrison TG, Kocherginsky M et al (2014) Phase III randomized trial of induction chemotherapy in patients with N2 or N3 locally advanced head and neck cancer. J Clin Oncol 32:2735–2743
46. Haddad R, O'Neill A, Rabinowits G et al (2013) Induction chemotherapy followed by concurrent chemoradiotherapy (sequential chemoradiotherapy) versus concurrent chemoradiotherapy alone in locally advanced head and neck cancer (PARADIGM): a randomised phase 3 trial. Lancet Oncol 14:257–264
47. Manikantan K, Khode S, Dwivedi RC et al (2009) Making sense of post-treatment surveillance in head and neck cancer: when and what of follow-up. Cancer Treat Rev 35:744–753
48. Shortell SM, Rundall TG, Hsu J (2007) Improving patient care by linking evidence-based medicine and evidence-based management. JAMA 298:673–676
49. Campbell SM, Braspenning J, Hutchinson A, Marshall M (2002) Research methods used in developing and applying quality indicators in primary care. Qual Saf Health Care 11:358–364
50. Hessel AC, Moreno MA, Hanna EY et al (2010) Compliance with quality assurance measures in patients treated for early oral tongue cancer. Cancer 116:3408–3416
51. Weber RS, Lewis CM, Eastman SD et al (2010) Quality and performance indicators in an academic department of head and neck surgery. Arch Otolaryngol Head Neck Surg 136:1212–1218
52. Lewis CM, Weber RS, Hanna EY (2011) Quality of care in head and neck cancer. Curr Oncol Rep 13:120–125
53. Chen AY (2010) Quality initiatives in head and neck cancer. Curr Oncol Rep 12:109–114

Comparative Effectiveness Issues in Lung Cancer

Thomas K. Varghese

Abstract

Lung cancer accounts for more cancer deaths than breast, prostate, colorectal and pancreatic cancer combined. With an aging population, greater intensity of cancer care, and the need for care of the growing number of cancer survivors, comparative effectiveness research opportunities will continue to emerge for this disease. In this chapter, we focus on CER opportunities in lung cancer surgery from the vantage point of those factors directly influenced by the surgeon, patient and the healthcare system.

Keywords

Lung neoplasms · Comparative effectiveness research · Thoracic surgery

Contents

T.K. Varghese (✉)
Division of Thoracic Surgery, Department of Surgery,
Harborview Medical Center, University of Washington, Seattle, WA, USA
e-mail: tkv@uw.edu

K.Y. Bilimoria et al. (eds.), *Comparative Effectiveness in Surgical Oncology*,
Cancer Treatment and Research 164, DOI 10.1007/978-3-319-12553-4_7

1 Introduction

Comparative effectiveness research (CER) aims to generate evidence on effectiveness of strategies for diagnosis, treating or preventing disease in the "real-world" compared to the existing "standard of care" so that informed decisions can be made to improve health care [1, 2]. CER studies thus often need to account for physician (surgeon), patient and system factors that affect outcomes observed when interventions are made in the real world, away from the controlled settings of a randomized clinical trial. As CER is by definition comparative, it can address questions on both clinical utility and added clinical value compared with standard of care. With an aging population, increasing cancer incidence, greater intensity of cancer care, and the need for continuing care of the growing number of cancer survivors, there is no doubt a growing economic burden associated with cancer and cancer treatment [3]. In this chapter, we will discuss CER issues for the surgeon with respect to the most common lethal malignancy—lung cancer. There are very few randomized clinical trials with respect to surgical interventions for lung cancer. Several factors have led to this situation including difficulties with accrual (including both provider and patient bias), and expense. With increasing need to answer questions on clinical care with respect to quality, outcomes and cost-effectiveness, opportunities for CER studies will emerge for this disease now and into the future. We will address 3 types of surgeon factors, patient factors and system factors that influence outcomes and can be the genesis of CER studies in the future.

In 1953, lung cancer became the most common cause of cancer death in men, while the same occurred for women in 1985. In 2012, there were 1.8 million patients with lung cancer globally, causing an estimated 1.6 million deaths [4]. In 2014, there will be an estimated 224,000 new cases of lung cancer and 159,000 deaths [5]. Lung cancer causes more deaths than the next three most lethal common cancers combined (colon, breast and pancreatic) [6].

There are several factors that can influence whether patients receive any type of treatment for lung cancer (Fig. 1). Evidence-based treatment options for lung cancer depend on histology, stage and patient specific factors (such as age, pulmonary function and comorbidities). Approximately 95 % of all lung cancers are classified as either small cell lung cancer (SCLC) or non-small cell lung cancer (NSCLC). SCLC is distinguished from NSCLC by its rapid doubling time, and early development of widespread metastases. In light of these factors, surgical intervention is not the standard of care for SCLC. Sadly, though SCLC is initially responsive to chemotherapy and radiation therapy, it typically relapses, with subsequent resistance to treatment modalities within a few months to a year. A two-stage classification is used for SCLC derived from the Veterans' Affairs Lung Study Group (VALG) in the late 1950s [7]:

- Limited disease (Tumor confined to ipsilateral hemithorax and regional nodes)
- Extensive disease (Tumor beyond the borders of limited disease, including malignant pleural and pericardial effusions)

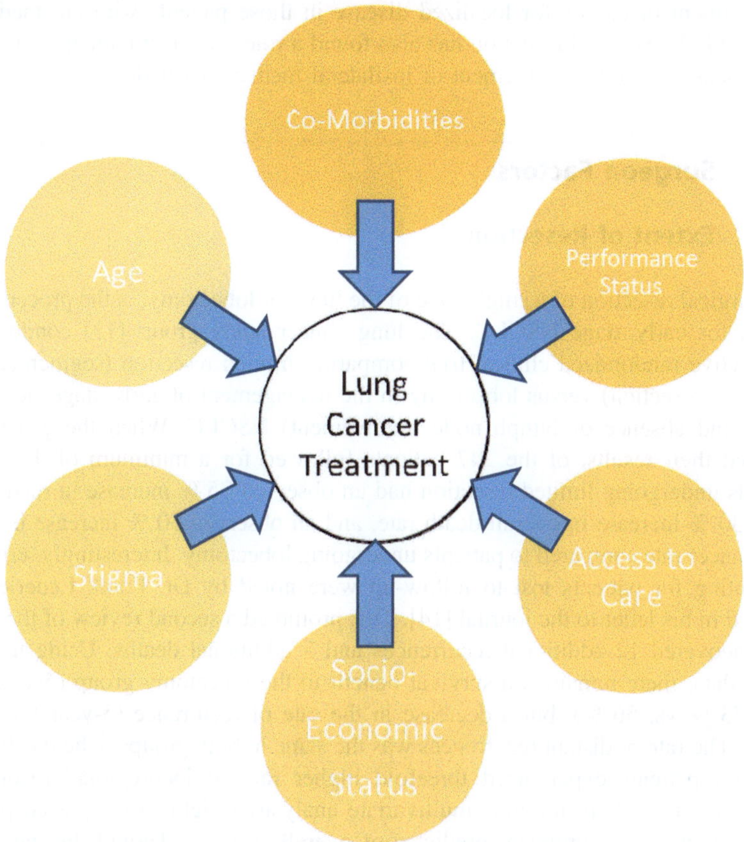

Fig. 1 Non-disease factors that influence receipt of lung cancer treatment

Limited disease is treated with chemotherapy and radiation therapy, while extensive disease is often treated with chemotherapy. Five-year survival rates for limited and extensive disease are poor (10–13 % vs. 1–2 %) with the median time of survival 15–20 months and 8–13 months respectively [8–10].

The remainder of this chapter will be focused on CER for NSCLC, where surgical intervention plays a role in early stage disease.

NSCLC accounts for the majority (approximately 85 %) of lung cancers. Localized disease is where the cancer is limited to one lobe of the lung, and does not involve the mediastinum. Stage I disease (small lesion, without involvement of any lymph nodes) and Stage II disease (larger lesion without lymph node involvement, involvement of structures that can be resected such as the chest wall or diaphragm, or involvement of hilar lymph nodes) makes up about a third of patients with NSCLC [11]. Although validation hasn't occurred with randomized clinical trials, good results and long-term survival data have established surgery as the treatment of choice for localized disease in those patients who are medically operable [12]. Surgical resection has also found a role for select patients with stage IIIA disease as well (involvement of ipsilateral mediastinal nodes).

2 Surgeon Factors

2.1 Extent of Resection

The surgical resection of a single lobe of the lung, or lobectomy, is the procedure of choice for early stage NSCLC. The lung cancer study group [13] conducted a prospective randomized clinical trial comparing limited resection (segmentectomy or wedge resection) versus lobectomy in the management of early stage (less than 3 cm, and absence of lymph node involvement) NSCLC. When the group first reported their results, of the 247 patients followed for a minimum of 4.5 years, patients undergoing limited resection had an observed 75 % increase in recurrence rates, 30 % increase in overall death rate, and an observed 50 % increase in death with cancer rate compared to patients undergoing lobectomy. Interestingly, errors in accounting for patients lost to follow-up were noted by Dr. Frank Lederle, and detailed in his letter to the journal [14]. This prompted a second review of the study that uncovered 12 additional recurrences and 3 additional deaths. Using the corrected data, there remained a survival benefit to the lobectomy group (5-year survival 73 % vs. 56 %), but a decrease in the rate of recurrence (5-year 63 % vs. 78 %). The rate of distant recurrences was the same in both groups, whereas limited resection patients experienced threefold higher rate of locoregional recurrence (5.4 % vs. 1.9 %). In the new multivariate analysis, weight loss replaced performance status as a significant predictor of overall survival. Though the numbers, graphs and multivariate findings changed slightly, the overall conclusions of the lung cancer study group study were not altered by the corrected data [15].

Lobectomy became the norm for those patients with adequate pulmonary reserve. Additional observational studies demonstrated improved survival in individuals with earlier stage disease who undergo resection (lobectomy) [16–18]. Most surgical series demonstrated five-year survival for stage I NSCLC in the range from 55 to 72 % [19, 20], with even more favorable results reported for those with small (less than 3 cm) peripheral lesions [21, 22]. In contrast, the 5-year survival of patients with Stage I lung cancer not treated surgically is reported to be from 4 to 14 % [23–25]. The role of surgery for Stage IIIA disease is limited. If previously unsuspected microscopic disease is found in the mediastinal nodes at the time of resection, then proceeding with lobectomy followed by adjuvant therapy is recommended [26]. In those patients where the mediastinal nodes are prospectively identified with sampling and imaging, then multimodality treatment is recommended, with concurrent chemotherapy and radiation therapy. Surgical resection can subsequently be an option in a subset of these patients after chemoradiation with low volume or microscopic mediastinal nodal disease involvement, where resection is technically feasible [26].

Proximal tumors with endobronchial involvement traditionally were treated with pneumonectomies. In the modern era, sleeve resection of the involved airway with lobectomy is preferred over pneumonectomy as a result of similar oncologic results, better preservation of pulmonary function, and avoidance of the complications associated with pneumonectomy [27].

There has been a renewed interest in the role of sublobar (limited) resection. Sublobar resection may be performed either as the removal of one or more anatomical segments (segmentectomy) or as a non-anatomical wedge resection. Sublobar resections can be an option for those patients with early stage disease who cannot tolerate a lobectomy due to decreased pulmonary reserve, or medical comorbidities. Several prospective studies have reported favorable outcomes in those patients undergoing segmentectomies or wedge resections for peripheral <2 cm in size, N0 lung cancers [28–30]. There are two ongoing clinical trials focusing on this issue. The Cancer and Leukemia Group B (CALGB) trial 140503 [31] has had a difficult time accruing patients since its launch in 2007, and aims to directly compare lobectomy versus limited resection among patients with peripheral tumors measuring <2 cm in size. In Japan, the nearly accrued JCOG 0802/WJOG 4607 L 1,100 trial is comparing the outcomes of peripheral invasive adenocarcinomas of less than or equal to 2 cm in size treated by lobectomy or segmentectomy. Another Japanese study (JCOG 0804/WJOG 4507L) has completed accrual evaluating the role of limited resections in the management of non-invasive adenocarcinomas. Results from these Japanese studies are awaited [32, 33]. Even after findings from these studies are released, CER opportunities will be present (Table 1).

Table 1 Surgeon factors—extent of resection

Dimension of care	Opportunities for CER study
Extent of lung resection for early stage lung cancer	• Can the findings from recent randomized clinical trials on lobectomy versus sublobar resection be replicated in real-world settings?
	• What is the cost-effectiveness of performing segmentectomies (which is not a direct focus of training in today's environment and thus require a learning curve) if indeed it is proven to be equivalent in outcomes to lobectomy?
	• What are the quality-of-life implications for patients with respect to lobectomy, segmentectomy, and wedge resections? Should quality of life be the driving factor in decisions in how much lung to resect in contrast to cancer survival times, and for which patient populations is this relevant?

2.2 Video-Assisted Thoracoscopic Surgery (VATS) Versus Open Lobectomy

VATS is a minimally invasive thoracic surgical procedure that can be utilized for the diagnosis and treatment of intra-thoracic diseases. Many procedures that historically were performed with an open thoracotomy are now performed as VATS. Absolute contraindications for VATS are the same as for a thoracotomy including the inability to perform a complete (R0) resection with suitable residual cardiopulmonary reserve, lymph node metastasis beyond regional lymph nodes, and widely metastatic disease [34, 35].

VATS procedures use ports that for the most part are <2 cm in length, except for one access or utility incision that ranges from 4 to 8 cm in length through which instruments can be inserted and allow for removal of the resected lung at the completion of the case. The important principle that is maintained during a VATS resection procedure is that a rib-spreader is not used. By avoiding muscle splitting, and rib-spreading with a retractor, VATS is believed to result in less pain, earlier ambulation, and fewer postoperative complications [36]. VATS lobectomy was first performed in 1992, and has been rapidly adopted in the surgical management of lung cancer. Several studies have shown lower rates of postoperative complications associated with VATS when compared with open lobectomy for early stage lung cancer [37–41]. Further studies have shown improved functional outcomes and equivalent oncologic efficacy as well [42–45].

Interestingly, cost effectiveness analyses have shown variable results. A study using the Surveillance, Epidemiology, and End-Results Medicare database found that VATS lobectomy was associated with a shorter length of stay (LOS) but not with differences in costs [36]. One explanation offered in the study was that payer reimbursement was linked to episodes of care rather than LOS. Other studies using the all-payer Nationwide Inpatient Sample [44, 45] described lower complication rates and LOS for VATS lobectomy, but no differences in costs. In contrast, an all-payer Premier Perspective database study [41] found that adjusted inpatients costs were $700 lower for VATS. A study from our group using the MarketScan database examined whether VATS lobectomy was associated with lower 90-day costs—thus assessing for costs and complications beyond the index hospitalization [46]. We found that the biggest driver of cost was prolonged LOS (PLOS) at the index hospitalization, VATS lobectomy was associated with lower rates of PLOS, and that the cost difference of the VATS approach extends only minimally into the period after discharge (i.e., health care use after discharge was only minimally different between the VATS and open thoracotomy groups). Outpatient use and readmissions accounted for approximately 16 % of the total 90-day costs of care after lobectomy. Emerging evidence suggests that the pressure to discharge patients earlier after lung resection may be driving readmission rates, independent of the surgical approach [47, 48].

Although use of VATS has increased over time, open thoracotomy is still the most widely used procedure for lobectomy with less than 50 % of lobectomies in the US performed using VATS [49]. Factors that have been proposed to explain this finding include insufficient training or experience, difficulty to achieve competency with minimally invasive approaches in low volume centers, and a belief that there remains an insufficient level of evidence for safety and efficacy. However, there are now two large institutional prospective cohort studies involving 1,100 and 500 patients respectively [50, 51], a randomized clinical trial [52] and two meta-analyses [53, 54] that have demonstrated safety and efficacy of the approach. The Cancer and Leukemia Group B (CALGB) 39802 trial [55] was a novel multi-institutional safety and feasibility study that not only standardized the definition of VATS lobectomy, but also standardized surgeon credentialing. The rigorous credentialing process had participating surgeons attend a course to review technique; submission of an unedited video tape, operative and pathology reports from a VATS lobectomy for central review; and participation in an animal laboratory. Surgeons were required to perform at least five VATS lobectomies before being credentialed. Eleven surgeons at six centers underwent credentialing, and the subsequent success rate, morbidity and mortality observed in the study achieved or surpassed prior levels cited in the literature. The study demonstrated a method for surgeons who had no prior experience with the technique to attain sufficient training and expertise in a supervised real-world environment.

Robotic-assisted thoracoscopic surgery (RATS) approaches for lobectomy have recently emerged as an alternative to traditional VATS. Initial results of robotic lobectomy have shown the same benefits achieved with VATS approaches as compared to open thoracotomy can be maintained [56–58]. Additionally, advocates for RATS cite benefits of improved ergonomics, three-dimensional optics, and wristed instrument motions. On the other hand, opponents of robotic surgery have cited increased costs and longer procedure times [59]. It is still to early to tell whether RATS is truly an advance in surgical technique, or as nay-sayers are fond of stating—a marketing gimmick. Cost analyses can be challenging for robotic programs as the cost of the robotic platform varies between institutions (purchase of a new robot versus incorporation of RATS into a facility with an existing platform), and that theoretic costs include the price of the robotic system divided by the total number of robotic cases (all specialties) performed. However, this shouldn't deter us from assessing the impact of RATS into practice, as similar issues are raised when assessing the introduction of any new surgical technology. Even if one is not convinced that RATS is a significant advance as compared to VATS lobectomy, there may be other reasons for surgeons to transition to robotic surgery, including the performance of other thoracic surgical procedures such as a thymectomy, robotic technology will continue to evolve, and more clearly delineated benefits of robotic surgery may become the reality in the future. What is missing till date is a standardized detailed credentialing process for RATS similar to that which was outlined in CALGB 39802. CER opportunities with respect to minimally invasive approaches are outlined in Table 2.

Table 2 Surgeon factors—type of surgical approach

Dimension of care	Opportunities for CER study
Minimally invasive lung surgery	• If PLOS at index hospitalization is the main driver of cost difference, are there evidence-based strategies to mitigate the frequency of PLOS that can be incorporated into systematic practice? Can these strategies be found from programs that incorporate VATS approaches as part of their practice?
	• VATS lobectomies are more commonly performed by high-volume surgeons working at high-volume or teaching hospitals. Are the lower 90-day costs only associated with VATS (i.e. more attributable to environment of practice) or directly attributable to VATS?
	• Can a standardized credentialing process be implemented for Robotic VATS lobectomy, accounting for feasibility, safety, efficacy and cost-effectiveness?
	• Can a prospective, pragmatic multi-institutional study be performed comparing robotic VATS, traditional VATS and open thoracotomy approaches for lobectomy for short-term outcomes, oncologic efficacy, and cost-effectiveness?

2.3 Specialty Training

The issue of who should provide care has led to considerable debate about access, and healthcare disparities. Surgeon specialty has been shown to be associated with better post-operative outcomes among high-risk operations [60–62]. In the United States, the majority of lung resections are performed by general surgeons [63]. However, there have been several studies demonstrating that board-certified thoracic surgeons have lower rates of operative mortality with lung resections compared to general surgeons [64–66]. In a study conducted by our group in the SEER-Medicare population [67], we extended the analysis to compare the results of board-certified general thoracic surgeons (GTS), board-certified cardiothoracic surgeons (CTS) (those who performed both cardiac and thoracic procedures as part of their practice), and those treated by general surgeons (GS). After adjustment for several well-known prognostic factors for survival, patients under the care of GTS had an 11 % lower risk of death compared with those treated by GS. General thoracic surgeons used preoperative and intraoperative staging procedures more often than GS or CTS, more often applied video-assisted thoracoscopic techniques, and less often performed bi-lobectomy (precision of resection).

Common themes in these studies were influence of provider volume on the overall effect, as well as more consistent process-of-care measures by specialty surgeons. As there is a trend towards increasing specialization amongst surgeons, other factors that may have influenced decision-making include training in the modern era, with inclusion of evidence-based protocols, and multi-disciplinary participation in tumor boards amongst specialists. The results however of all these studies are relevant to the overriding issue of how best to improve the quality of

Table 3 Surgeon factors—specialist care

Dimension of care	Opportunities for CER study
Surgeon specialty (general thoracic surgery [GTS] vs. cardiothoracic surgery [CTS] vs. general surgery [GS])	• What are the workforce implications if a policy was created to selectively refer patients with early-stage lung cancer to only board-certified GTS? For both GTS and CTS?
	• If the workforce implications were not practical, how can CTS or GS predominantly serving an underserved population gain additional expertise to mitigate against some of the factors leading to disparity in outcomes?
	• Should there be a central credentialing process for those surgeons who wish to perform surgical resections for lung cancer?

thoracic surgical care. One option might be to encourage referral of potentially resectable lung cancer patients to GTS. This of course would need to be accompanied by the addressing of issues such as barriers to access, especially amongst low-income patients and those that live in rural areas, as well as workforce issues. Attempting to improve outcomes by selective referral without addressing infrastructure and workforce issues could lead to vast segments of the population without access to surgical resection for an otherwise uniformly fatal disease. Opportunities for CER are detailed in Table 3.

3 Patient Factors

As overall outcomes for lung cancer treatment are poor, opportunities exist to explore the impact of treatment choices on the patient. When one traditionally thinks of patient factors, the focus has been on co-morbidities. In surgery, the decision-making process is often situational. Patient autonomy and participation can be influenced by medical condition, surgeon factors, patient educational level, and availability of evidence-based information on the particular condition. The degree of decisional authority assumed by patients can lead to three types of surgeon-patient relationships—the surgeon as agent, shared decision-making, and informed decision-making. Large-scale studies on decision-making have not been performed till date for lung cancer, but are anticipated to increase in the years ahead alongside the patient-centered movement.

The surgeon as agent occurs when the surgeon acts as an expert adviser who incorporates the values of the patient when making a treatment recommendation. In this model, the patient role is passive, as the surgeon assumes the values of the patient, and has total command over the decision-making process. Patients may be subjected to biased treatment if the surgeon only gives or delivers limited treatment options. In contrast, the informed decision-making model is one where the surgeon is recognized as the one who has technical expertise, but the patient plays an active role eliciting and understanding information about their treatment choices. The surgeon in this model doesn't volunteer their opinions, but rather presents the patient with various treatment options, allowing the patients to arrive at their own conclusions. In between these two extremes is shared decision-making. Here the surgeon and patient are equal partners, where each freely exchanges information and preferences about treatment options to arrive at a mutually acceptable decision. This works especially in those situations where there is ambiguity in treatment of choice, and helps to align the decision-making with patient's preferences and values.

Though surgeons may profess to always include patient-centered values in their discussions, there are plenty of opportunities for improvement. Some of these issues and opportunities for CER are detailed in Table 4.

4 Healthcare System Factors Related to Clinical Decision Making

4.1 Impact of Practice Environment

In principle, the Patient Protection and Affordable Care Act (ACA) signed into law in March 2010 seeks to improve health care delivery. The goal of ACA is to create a movement of payment reforms, in which private insurance companies would follow the lead of successful government payment reforms, such as bundled payments, and ultimately create system-wide changes for reimbursement [68]. Changing the reimbursement structure for providers will inevitably create new issues for surgeons who are making decisions for their patients. Payment reforms began in 2011 and 2012, and will continue through 2016. Two programs designed to restructure the way health care is delivered have been proposed under ACA, namely Patient-Centered Medical Homes (PCMHs) and Accountable Care Organizations (ACOs). These programs are designed to improve care coordination by encouraging use of electronic medical records, changing providers' financial incentives by including quality measures in reimbursement, and ultimately moving away from a fee-for-service to one where quality of care is valued [69].

The ACO movement has led to increased consolidation and integration in the medical marketplace. Hospitals are buying practices to keep their market share intact and to have access to electronic record systems and other infrastructure that are expensive to capitalize. Awareness emerges for surgeons that their medical decisions can potentially negatively influence their income. This is not necessarily unethical, as cost containment has been recognized as an important circumstance in

Table 4 Patient factors

Dimension of care	Patient perspective	Opportunities for study
Determination of patient's values, preferences and expressed needs	• Short-term and long-term goals of care	Can identification of health beliefs, practices and specific ethnic and cultural groups lead to better decision-making for the lung cancer patient population?
	• Level of involvement in decision making (surgeon as agent, shared decision-making, informed decision-making)	
	• Expectations of clinic visit and healthcare team	Can clinical interview protocols elicit patients' perceptions about their illness and their expectations of treatment?
Coordination of care and integration of services within a clinical setting	Coordination of delivery of care by a multidisciplinary team	Does the patient get consistent information from different clinicians?
		Do dedicated patient navigators have an impact on the delivery of care for lung cancer?
		How can one improve efficiencies in the diagnostic and staging work-up of a potentially resectable lung cancer patient?
		Are there evidence-based interventions that can be performed to optimize patients' health prior to elective surgical intervention?
		Can a set of processes of care be delivered as a guaranteed value bundle for each and every patient, all the time?
Communication between patient and providers	Dissemination of accurate, timely and appropriate information	Are treatment decisions aligned with patient-preferences and values at each point of contact with the health system?
	Education about the long-term implications of disease and illness	Will electronic medical records, and open access to records for patients lead to better communication for members of the healthcare team, referring providers and patients?
Cancer survivorship plans	Transition and continuity from one locus of care to another	What is the best method for delivery of a cancer survivorship plan for patients, family members and primary care providers that outline treatment summary, surveillance plans, any ongoing treatments, and health risks that are now in play as a result of past treatment?

good decision-making [70]. There will be the introduction penalties for lack of delivery of quality care, which could affect physician reimbursement. Adoption of rigid guidelines for the treatment of patients is anticipated in years to come, as well as expansion of care plans. All of these are attempts at decreasing variation in care, decreasing length of stay, and reducing use of resources.

A method of performance with a powerful impact on outcomes is participation in large national or regional databases with inclusion of all patients and frequent provider feedback with comparisons to peer norms. Surgeons in the Veterans Administration hospital system have participated for more than a decade in a systematic data-gathering and feedback system of outcomes for major surgery [71]. The National Surgical Quality Improvement Project (NSQIP) works to decrease variation in clinical outcomes by demonstrating to surgeons when their center is an "outlier" in performance. This system allows hospitals to target QI activities that may influence components of care, and subsequently decision-making. The Society of Thoracic Surgeons (STS) in 1989 created a national voluntary cardiac surgery database as a means of supporting national quality improvement efforts. In 2003, a separate database was launched by the STS encompassing procedures specific to general thoracic surgery—the General Thoracic Surgery Database (GTSD) [72]. GTSD provides participants risk-adjusted benchmarks as well as data for research that can be used to improve patient care processes and clinical outcomes. On 30 July 2008, the National Quality Forum endorsed participation in a systematic national database for general thoracic surgery [73]. Unfortunately in 2012, only 8 % of all lung cancer resection cases in the US were accounted for in GTSD, with most of the participants high-volume centers with dedicated general thoracic surgeons [74].

4.2 Impact of Political Environment

The reporting of surgeon-specific outcome data is another example of the influence of the political environment. Outcome data were rarely reported prior to the mid-1980s [75]. The first release of hospital open heart surgery risk-adjusted mortality rates in December 1990 [76] and the first formal public report in December 1992 [77], marked the start of a new era. These performance reports, or physician report cards, have increased in recent years [78], and many believe will increase in frequency and across specialties in the years to come. Advocates believe that increased transparency of information on the quality of care help consumers, employers, and health plans to improve their decision-making and to stimulate quality improvement among providers. However, physicians are concerned that risk adjustment strategies in these reports are not adequate. Without this confidence, publication of procedural mortality rates may result in physicians withholding procedures in high-risk patients. Unintended consequence of scorecards might be to adversely affect healthcare decisions for especially high-risk patients. Scorecards may also impair the development of new treatments because of the more restrictive clinical practice environment.

In light of these drawbacks, many have proposed revamping the current system to facilitate rapid and accurate access to outcome data in the local practice environment. Adoption of these efforts is often embraced as this occurs on a voluntary basis rather than in response to punitive restrictions. Examples of such grass-roots initiatives on a state level that are surgeon-led include those in the states of Michigan [79] and Washington [80, 81]. On a national level, data from the STS database has been used for public reporting, and thus have an impact on risk-stratification and outcomes in cardiothoracic surgery [82, 83].

Regional quality improvement (QI) efforts have succeeded in cardiac surgery, and a regional QI initiative in thoracic surgery has been proposed in Washington State [84]. Fifteen thoracic surgeons from five institutions examined the landscape of care in the state, as well as to discuss standards for a regional QI effort in lung cancer surgery. Consensus standards endorsed in this initiative include:

- GTSD participation across all hospitals performing lung resection in the state
- Limited enhancements to data collection efforts to address local concerns and survey ongoing interventions
- Quarterly performance reports
- Surgeon-led QI interventions for addressing performance gaps, quality improvement and value optimization
- and leveraging existing QI infrastructure and relationships within Washington state to rapidly and successfully implement a regional QI effort for lung cancer surgery.

Success of the regional QI initiative will likely lead to performance of several CER studies, and can ultimately serve as a model for other regional and national efforts.

An example of a national effort to reduce unnecessary tests across specialties is the Choosing Wisely® campaign. The Choosing Wisely® initiative helps physicians and patients have important conversations necessary to ensure that timely and optimal care is delivered. Launched by the American Board of Internal Medicine (ABIM) Foundation, Choosing Wisely® enables physicians and patients to engage in conversation about the overuse of tests and procedures, and helps patients make smart and effective care choices [85]. The original campaign has evolved into a multi-year initiative where the ABIM Foundation has reached out to specialty societies to identify a list of five tests or procedures that may be overused or misused. Criteria for developing these lists include limiting to items that fall within the specialty; supported by evidence; documented and publicly available upon request; frequently ordered/costly; easy for a lay person to understand; and measurable/accountable. The STS participated in the February 2013 phase II release (Table 5) [86]. Two of the five proposed measures are directly applicable to lung cancer surgery. These specialty generated lists help to empower physician-patient

Table 5 Society of thoracic surgeons choosing Wisely® list

1. Patients who have no cardiac history and good functional status do not require preoperative stress testing before noncardiac thoracic surgery
2. Do not initiate routing evaluation of carotid artery disease before cardiac surgery in the absence of symptoms or other high-risk criteria
3. Do not perform routine predischarge echocardiogram after cardiac valve replacement surgery
4. Patients with suspected or biopsy proven Stage I non-small cell lung cancer do not require brain imaging before definitive care in the absence of neurologic symptoms
5. Before cardiac surgery there is no need for pulmonary function testing in the absence of respiratory symptoms

conversations and to avoid unnecessary procedures that may harm patients while driving up health care costs. 63 specialty societies have joined the campaign since its inception in 2012.

4.3 Lung-Cancer Screening

An example of how politics can influence standards of care recently arose with respect to lung cancer screening. A large prospective randomized clinical trial, the National Lung Screening Trial (NLST), demonstrated the potential of low-dose computed tomography (LDCT) to detect lung cancer at earlier stages, thereby decreasing mortality [87]. NLST demonstrated that annual lung cancer screening in a high-risk patient population for three years with LDCT resulted in 20 % fewer lung cancer deaths as a result of early detection and treatment. Using the strict NLST criteria, this translates to 8.6 million people eligible for screening in the US, and 12,000 averted lung cancer deaths if all those individuals are screened [88]. In light of these studies, a number of non-profit, professional and federal organizations have recommended evidence-based annual LDCT screening for lung cancer in high-risk patients, including the National Comprehensive Cancer Network (NCCN), the US Preventive Services Task Force (USPSTF), the STS, American Society of Clinical Oncology, and the American Cancer Society [89]. The USPSTF decision in the setting of the Affordable Care act resulted in a mandate for coverage by private insurers for lung cancer screening. However, controversy has arisen as despite the evidence, Medicare till date has not endorsed coverage for lung cancer screening [90]. The implications are especially pertinent as nearly 70 % of lung cancers occur in the Medicare population. Time will tell if the evidence and advocacy of several specialty societies and patient advocates will correct this, but the politics surrounding the issue are puzzling to say the least. CER opportunities will arise in the coming years assessing screening practices, access to LDCT, and impact of early referral for surgical interventions for cancers detected by LDCT.

5 Summary

Although the ideal is to practice evidence-based medicine at all times, there are many factors that influence the care that we provide. There is growing interest in assessing and improving the value of health care delivery, defined as health benefits per dollar spent. Value can be increased by improving clinical outcomes, decreasing costs, or ideally doing both. CER for surgical interventions in lung cancer should be viewed through this lens, and opportunities for health services researchers and surgeons in practice will continue to emerge in the years ahead.

References

1. Institute of Medicine (2009) Initial national priorities for comparative effectiveness research. National Academies Press, Washington
2. Rich EC (2009) The policy debate over public investment in comparative effectiveness research. J Gen Intern Med 24(6):752–757
3. Yabroff KR, Lund J, Kepka D et al (2011) Economic burden of cancer in the United States: estimates, projections, and future research. Cancer Epidemiol Biomarkers Prev 20:2006–2014
4. Brambilla E, Travis WD (2014) Lung cancer. In: Stewart BW, Wild CP (eds) World cancer report. World Health Organization, Lyon
5. Siegel R, Ma J, Jemal A (2014) Cancer statistics 2014. Cancer J Clin 64(1):9
6. American Cancer Society. Cancer facts and figures 2014. Accessed http://www.cancer.org/research/cancerfactsstatistics/cancerfactsfigures2014/index
7. Murray N (1997) Treatment of small cell lung cancer: the state of the art. Lung Cancer S1: S75–S89
8. Albain KS, Crowley JJ, Livingston RB (1991) Long-term survival and toxicity in small cell lung cancer. Expanded Southwest oncology group experience. Chest 99(6):1425
9. Lassen U, Osterling K, Hansen M, Domberneowsky P, Bergman B, Hansen HH (1995) Long-term survival in small-cell lung cancer: posttreatment characteristics in patients surviving 5 to 18+ years—an analysis of 1,714 consecutive patients. J Clin Oncol 13(5):1215
10. Tai P, Tonita J, Yu E, Skarsgard D (2003) Twenty-year follow-up study of long-term survival of limited-stage small-cell lung cancer and overview of prognostic and treatment factors. Int J Radiat Oncol Biol Phys 56(3):626
11. Dettterbeck FC, Boffa DJ, Tanoue LT (2009) The new lung cancer staging system. Chest 136 (1):260–271
12. National comprehensive cancer network guidelines—non-small cell lung cancer http://www.nccn.org/professionals/physician_gls/f_guidelines.asp Accessed on 19 March 2014
13. Ginsberg RJ, Rubinstein LV (1995) Randomized trial of lobectomy versus limited resection for T1N0 non-small cell lung cancer. Lung cancer study group. Ann Thorac Surg 60(3):615
14. Lederle F (1996) Lobectomy versus limited resection in T1 N0 lung cancer. Ann Thorac Surg 62(4):1249–1250
15. Detterbeck FC (2013) Lobectomy versus limited resection in T1N0 lung Cancer. Ann Thorac Surg 96(2):742–744
16. Jones DR, Detterbeck FC (2001) Surgery for stage I non-small cell lung cancer. In: Detterbeck FC, Rivera MP, Socinski MA, Rosenman JG (eds) Diagnosis and treatment of lung cancer: an evidence based guide. WB Saunders Company, Philadelphia, pp 177–190
17. Detterbeck FC, Egan TM (2001) Surgery for stage II non-small cell lung cancer. In: Detterbeck FC, Rivera MP, Socinski MA, Rosenman JG (eds) Diagnosis and treatment of lung cancer: an evidence based guide. WB Saunders Company, Philadelphia, pp 191–197

18. Scott WJ, Howington J, Feigenberg S, Movsas B, Pisters K (2007) Treatment of non-small cell lung cancer stage I and stage II: ACCP evidence based clinical practice guidelines (2nd Edition). Chest 132:234S–242S
19. Nesbitt JC, Putman JB, Walsh GL, Roth JA, Mountain CF (1995) Survival in early stage non-small cell lung cancer. Ann Thorac Surg 60:466–472
20. Thomas P, Doddoli C, Thirion X et al (2002) Stage I non-small cell lung cancer: a pragmatic approach to prognosis after complete resection. Ann Thorac Surg 73:1065–1070
21. Reif MS, Socinski MA, Rivera MP (2000) Evidence-based medicine in the treatment of non-small cell lung cancer. Clin Chest Med 21(1):107–120
22. Ost D, Goldberg J, Ronitzky L, Rom WN (2008) Survival after surgery in stage IA and IB non-small cell lung cancer. Am J Resp Crit Care Med 177:516–523
23. Flehinger BJ, Kimmel M, Melamed MR (1992) The effect of surgical treatment on survival from early lung cancer: implications for screening. Chest 101:1013–1018
24. Sobue T, Suzuki T, Matsuda M et al (1992) Survival for clinical stage I lung cancer not surgically treated: comparison between screen-detected and symptom-detected cases. Cancer 69:685–692
25. Rowell NP, Williams C (2001) Radical radiotherapy for stage I/II non-small cell lung cancer in patients not sufficiently fit for or declining surgery (medically inoperable). Cochrane Database Syst Rev 56(1):628–638
26. Robinson LA, Ruckdeschel JC, Wanger H Jr, Stevens W (2007) Treatment of non-small cell lung cancer stage IIIA: ACCP evidence-based clinical practice guidelines (2nd edition). Chest 123(3 Suppl):243S–265S
27. Ferguson MK, Lehman AG (2003) Sleeve lobectomy or pneumonectomy: optimal strategy using decision analytic techniques. Ann Thorac Surg 76(6):1782
28. El-Sherif A, Gooding WE, Santos R et al (2006) Outcomes of sublobar resection versus lobectomy for stage I non-small cell lung cancer: a 13-year analysis. Ann Thorac Surg 82 (2):408
29. Kodama K, Doi O, Higashiyama M, Yokouchi H (1997) Intentional limited resection for selected patients with T1N0M0 non-small cell lung cancer: a single-institution study. J Thorac Cardiovasc Surg 114(3):347
30. Lee W, Daly BD, DiPetrillo TA et al (2003) Limited resection for non-small cell lung cancer: observed local control with implantation of I-125 brachytherapy seeds. Ann Thorac Surg 75 (1):237
31. CALGB NCT00499330—comparison of different types of surgery in treating patients with stage IA non-small cell lung cancer. Clinicaltrials.gov http://www.clinicaltrials.gov.offcampus.lib.washington.edu/ct2/show/NCT00499330?term=nct00499330&rank=1 Accessed 15 May 2014
32. Asamura H. Role of limited sublobar resection for early-stage lung cancer: steady progress. J Clin Oncol 2014 Jun 30 (Epub ahead of print)
33. De Ruysscher D, Nakagawa K, Asamura H (2014) Surgical and nonsurgical approaches to small-size nonsmall cell lung cancer. Eur Respir J 44(2):483–494
34. Demmy TL, James TA, Swanson SJ et al (2005) Trouble-shooting video-assisted thoracic surgery lobectomy. Ann Thorac Surg 79(5):1744–1752 discussion 1753
35. Berry MF, D'Amico TA (2007) Complications of thoracoscopic pulmonary resection. Semin Thorac Cardiovasc Surg 19(4):350–354
36. Farjah F, Wood DE, Mulligan MS et al (2009) Safety and efficacy of video-assisted versus conventional lung resection for lung cancer. J Thorac Cardiovasc Surg 137(6):1415–1421
37. Cattaneo SM, Park BJ, Wilton AS et al (2008) Use of video-assisted thoracic surgery for lobectomy in the elderly results in fewer complications. Ann Thorac Surg 85:231–236
38. Kirby TJ, Rice TW (1993) Thoracoscopic lobectomy. Ann Thorac Surg 56:784–786
39. Whitson BA, Andrade RS, Boettcher A et al (2007) Video-assisted thoracoscopic surgery is more favorable than thoracotomy that resection of clinical stage I non-small cell lung cancer. Ann Thorac Surg 83:1965–1970

40. Paul S, Altorki NK, Sheng S et al (2010) Thoracoscopic lobectomy is associated with lower morbidity than open lobectomy: a propensity-matched analysis from the STS database. J Thorac Cardiovasc Surg 139:366–378
41. Swanson SJ, Meyers BF, Gunnarsson CL et al (2012) Video-assisted thoracoscopic lobectomy is less costly and morbid than open lobectomy: a retrospective multiinstitutional database analysis. Ann Thorac Surg 93:372–379
42. Handy JR Jr, Asaph JW, Douville EC et al (2010) Does video-assisted thoracoscopic lobectomy for lung cancer provide improved functional outcomes compared with open lobectomy? Eur J Cardiothorac Surg 37:451–455
43. Scott WJ, Allen MS, Darling G et al (2010) Video-assisted thoracic surgery versus open lobectomy for lung cancer: a secondary analysis of data from the American College of Surgeons Oncology Group Z0030 randomized clinical trial. J Thorac Cardiovasc Surg 139:976–981
44. Park HS, Deterbeck FC, Boffa DJ, Kim AW (2012) Impact of hospital volume of thoracoscopic lobectomy on primary lung cancer outcomes. Ann Thorac Surg 93:372–379
45. Gopaldas RR, Bakeen FG, Dao TK et al (2010) Video-assisted thoracoscopic versus open thoracotomy lobectomy in a cohort of 13,619 patients. Ann Thorac Surg 89:1563–1570
46. Farjah F, Backhus LM, Varghese TK et al (2014) Ninety-day costs of video-assisted thoracic surgery versus open lobectomy for lung cancer. Ann Thorac Surg 98:191–196
47. Farjah F, Wood DE, Varghese TK et al (2009) Health care use among surgically treated medicare beneficiaries with lung cancer. Ann Thorac Surg 88:1749–1756
48. Freeman RK, Dilts JR, Ascioti AJ et al (2013) A comparison of length of stay, readmission rate and facility reimbursement after lobectomy of the lung. Ann Thorac Surg 96:1740–1745
49. Boffa DJ, Asslen MS, Grab JD et al (2008) Data from the society of thoracic surgeons general thoracic surgery database: the surgical management of primary lung tumors. J Thorac Cardiovasc Surg 135:247–254
50. McKenna RJ Jr, Houck W, Fuller CB (2006) Video-assisted thoracic surgery lobectomy: experience with 1,100 cases. Ann Thorac Surg 9:421–425
51. Onaitis MW, Petersen RP, Balderson SS et al (2006) Thoracoscopic lobectomy is a safe and versatile procedure: experience with 500 consecutive patients. Ann Surg 9:420–425
52. Shigemura N, Akashi A, Nakagiri T et al (2004) Complete versus assisted thoracosocpic approach: a prospective randomized trial comparing. Surg Endosc Other Intervent Tech 18:1492–1497
53. Whilston BA, Groth SS, Dival SJ et al (2008) Surgery for early-stage non-small cell lung cancer: a systematic review of the video-assisted thoracoscopic surgery versus thoracotomy approaches to lobectomy. Ann Thorac Surg 9:2008–2018
54. Yan TD, Black D, Bannon PG, McCaughan BC (2009) Systematic review and meta-analysis of randomized and nonrandomized trials on safety and efficacy of video-assisted thoracic surgery lobectomy for early-stage non-small cell lung cancer. J Clin Oncol 9:2553–2562
55. Swanson SJ, Herndon JE 2nd, D'Amico TA et al (2007) Video-assisted thoracic surgery lobectomy: report of CALGB 39802- a prospective, multi-institution feasibility study. J Clin Oncol 9:4993–4997
56. Park BJ, Melfi F, Mussi A et al (2012) Robotic lobectomy for non-small cell lung cancer (NSCLC): long-term oncologic results. J Thoracic Cardiovasc Surg 143:383–389
57. Louie BE, Farivar AS, Aye RW, Vallieres E (2012) Early experience with robotic lung resection results in similar operative outcomes and morbidity when compared with matched video-assisted thoracoscopic surgery cases. Ann Thorac Surg 93:1598–1604
58. Cerfolio RJ, Bryant AS, Skylizard L, Minnich DJ (2011) Initial consecutive experience of completely portal robotic pulmonary resection with 4 arms. J Thorac Cardiovasc Surg 142:740–746
59. Flored RM, Alam N (2008) Video-assisted thoracic surgery lobectomy (VATS), open thoracotomy, and the robot for lung cancer. Ann Thoracic Surg 85:S710–S715

60. Halm EA, Lee C, Chassin MR (2002) Is volume related to outcome in health care? A systematic review and methodologic critique of the literature. Ann Intern Med 137:511–520
61. Dudley RA, Johansen KL, Brand R et al (2000) Selective referral to high-volume hospitals: estimating potentially avoidable deaths. JAMA 283:1159–1166
62. Birkmeyer JD, Siewers AE, Finlayson EV et al (2002) Hospital volume and surgical mortality in the United States. N Engl J Med 346:1128–1137
63. Schipper PH, Diggs BS, Ungerleifer RM, Welke KF (2009) The influence of surgeon specialty on outcomes in general thoracic surgery: a national sample 1996 to 2005. Ann Thorac Surg 88:1566–1573
64. Goodney PP, Lucas FL, Stukel TA et al (2005) Surgeon specialty and operative mortality with lung resection. Ann Surg 241:179–184
65. Luchtenborg M, Riaz SP, Coupland VH, Lim E, Jakobsen E, Kransik M, Page R, Lind MJ, Peake MD, Moller H (2013) High procedure volume is strongly associated with improved survival after lung cancer surgery. J Clin Oncol 31(25):3141–3146
66. Freeman RK, Dilts JR, Ascioti AJ et al (2013) A comparision of quality and cost indicators by surgical specialty for lobectomy of the lung. J Thorac Cardiovasc Surg 145(1):68–73 discussion 73–74
67. Farjah F, Flum DR, Varghese TK Jr et al (2009) Surgeon specialty and long-term survival after pulmonary resection for lung cancer. Ann Thorac Surg 87:995–1006
68. Lee PV, Berenson RA, Tooker J (2010) Payment reform—the need to harmonize approaches in Medicare and the private sector. N Engl J Med 362:3–5
69. Ein D, Jefferson A (2014) The patient protection and affordable care act: causes and effects. Ann Allergy Asthma Immunol 112:6–8
70. Devettere RJ (2000) Making health care decisions. In: Devettere RJ (ed) Practical decision making in health care ethics. Georgetown University Press, Washington DC, p 94
71. Itani KM (2009) Fifteen years of the national surgical quality improvement program in review. Am J Surg 198(5 Suppl):S9–S18
72. Magee MJ, Wright CD, McDonald D et al (2013) External validation of the society of thoracic surgeons general thoracic surgery database. Ann Thorac Surg 96(5):1734–1739
73. National Quality Forum endorses national consensus standards promoting accountability and public reporting—National Quality Forum Endorsed Measure #0456 http://www.qualityforum.org Accessed 15 May, 2014
74. LaPar DJ, Bhamidipati CM, Lau CL et al (2012) The society of thoracic surgeons general thoracic surgery database: establishing generalizability to national lung cancer resection outcomes. Ann Thorac Surg 94:216–221
75. Topol EJ, Califf RM (1994) Scorecard cardiovascular medicine. its impact and future directions. Ann Intern Med 120:65–70
76. Hannan EL, Kilburn H Jr, O'Donnell JF et al (1990) Adult open heart surgery in New York state. An analysis of risk factors and hospital mortality rate. JAMA 264:2768–2774
77. Epstein A (1995) Performance reports on quality—prototypes, problems and prospects. N Engl J Med 333:57–61
78. Schneider EC, Epstein AM (1998) Use of public performance reports: a survey of patients undergoing cardiac surgery. JAMA 279:1638–1642
79. Prager RL, Armenti FR, Bassett JS et al (2009) Cardiac surgeons and the quality movement: the Michigan experience. Semin Thorac Cardiovasc Surg 21:20–27
80. Flum DR, Fisher N, Thompson J et al (2005) Washington state's approach to variability in surgical processes/outcomes: surgical clinical outcomes assessment program (SCOAP). Surgery 138:821–828
81. Aldea GS, Mokadam NA, Melford R et al (2009) Changing volumes, risk profiles, and outcomes of coronary artery bypass grafting and percutaneous coronary interventions. Ann Thorac Surg 87:1828–1838
82. Clark RE, The STS (1995) Cardiac surgery national database: an update. Ann Thorac Surg 59:1376–1381

83. Wright CD, Gaissert HA, Grab JD et al (2008) Predictors of prolonged length of stay after lobectomy for lung cancer: a society of thoracic surgeons general thoracic database risk-adjustment model. Ann Thorac Surg 85:1857–1865
84. Farjah F, Varghese TK, Costas K et al (2014) Lung resection outcomes and costs in Washington state: a case for regional quality improvement. Ann Thorac Surg 98(1):175–182
85. Cassel CK, Guest JA (2012) Choosing wisely: helping physicians and patients make smart decisions about their care. JAMA 307:1801–1802
86. Wood DE, Mitchell JD, Schmitz DS et al (2013) Choosing wisely: cardiothoracic surgeons partnering with patients to make good health care decisions. Ann Thorac Surg 95(3):1130–1135
87. The national lung screening trial research team (2011) Reduced lung-cancer mortality with low-dose computed tomographic screening. N Engl J Med 365:395–409
88. Qiu R, Eberth JM, Porter N et al (2013) Annual number of lung cancer deaths potentially avertable by screening in the United States. Cancer 119(7):1381–1385
89. Eberth JM, Qiu R, Adams SA et al. Lung cancer screening using low-dose CT: the current national landscape. Lung Cancer 2014 Jul 21 (Epub ahead of print)
90. Wood DE, Kazerooni EA Medicare's puzzling refusal to cover lung-cancer screening. Wall Street J 2014 June 17. http://online.wsj.com/articles/douglas-wood-andella-kazerooni-medicares-puzzling-refusal-to-cover-lung-cancer-screening-1403046693. Accessed 20 June 2014

83. Wright CD, Gaissert HA, Grab JD et al (2008) Predictors of prolonged length of stay after lobectomy for lung cancer: a Society of Thoracic Surgeons General Thoracic Database risk-adjustment model. Ann Thorac Surg 85:1857–1865
84. Farjah F, Varghese TK, Costas K et al (2014) Lung resection outcomes and costs in Washington state: a case for regional quality improvement. Ann Thorac Surg 98(1):175–181

Comparative Effectiveness in Esophagogastric Cancer

Lawrence M. Knab, Jim Belotte, Hidayatullah G. Munshi and David J. Bentrem

Abstract

Cancer of the esophagus and the gastroesophageal junction (GEJ) continues to have a dismal prognosis, with the incidence of esophageal cancer increasing in the United States. Although radical resection was initially the primary treatment for this disease process, systemic chemotherapy and radiation have been shown to play a role in prolonging survival in most patient populations. This chapter explores the evidence that guides treatment for esophageal and GEJ cancer today. Chemotherapy and radiation therapy were introduced as treatment modalities for esophageal and GEJ cancers when it became evident that surgical therapy alone provided poor long-term survival rates. A variety of treatment

L.M. Knab · J. Belotte · D.J. Bentrem (✉)
Division of Surgical Oncology, Department of Surgery, Northwestern University, Chicago, USA
e-mail: dbentrem@nmff.org

L.M. Knab
e-mail: l-knab@md.northwestern.edu

J. Belotte
e-mail: jimbelotte@gmail.com

H.G. Munshi
Division of Hematology/Oncology, Department of Medicine, Feinberg School of Medicine, Northwestern University, Chicago, IL, USA
e-mail: h-munshi@northwestern.edu

H.G. Munshi · D.J. Bentrem
Robert H. Lurie Comprehensive Cancer Center of Northwestern University, Chicago, IL, USA

H.G. Munshi · D.J. Bentrem
Jesse Brown VA Medical Center, Chicago, IL, USA

K.Y. Bilimoria et al. (eds.), *Comparative Effectiveness in Surgical Oncology*,
Cancer Treatment and Research 164, DOI 10.1007/978-3-319-12553-4_8

strategies have been explored including preoperative (neoadjuvant) and postoperative (adjuvant) chemotherapy, with and without radiation. The evidence suggests that neoadjuvant chemotherapy or chemoradiotherapy provides better outcomes compared to surgery alone for esophageal, GEJ, and gastric cancers. Studies indicate a trend towards improved survival when neoadjuvant chemoradiotherapy is compared to chemotherapy alone. When patients have undergone resection with node-positive disease without receiving neoadjuvant therapy, some form of adjuvant treatment is recommended. This chapter also explores the surgical management of esophageal, GEJ, and gastric cancers including the extent of the gastric lymph node dissection. It also includes a discussion about adherence to national guidelines in terms of gastric cancer treatment and esophageal and gastric lymph node examinations.

Contents

1 Introduction

Esophageal cancer is the eighth most common cancer worldwide with an estimated 482,000 cases diagnosed in 2008. In the United States, it was estimated that in 2013 there would be 17,990 new cases (14,440 for men and 3,550 for women) and 15,210 deaths due to esophageal cancer [1]. The incidence of esophageal adenocarcinoma (EAC) continues to increase drastically in the United States and its incidence surpassed that of squamous cell carcinoma (SqCC) in 1990 [2]. This trend has been attributed to the fact that smoking rates and alcohol consumption are decreasing leading to a decrease in SqCC while obesity is increasing leading to an increase in gastroesophageal reflux disease and therefore increased incidence of EAC. The overall survival of patients with esophageal cancer remains poor with minimal improvement in the last 30 years [3]. The 5-year survival rate for all patients with esophageal cancer during the period of 2001–2007 was 19 % [3].

Radical resection has been the mainstay of treatment for esophageal cancer although frequent local failure and distant metastases have prompted the addition of radiation and systemic chemotherapy. As is evident by the poor survival of patients with esophageal cancer who undergo radical resection and subsequently have disease recurrence, tumor dissemination occurs early in the disease process and because of this systemic chemotherapeutic agents have been the focus of many studies. Despite multiple trials investigating the efficacy of chemotherapy with or without radiation, administered preoperatively, postoperatively, or both, much controversy remains regarding the ideal treatment course. As the cost of target chemotherapeutic agents and radiation modalities rises with only marginal gains in efficacy, the cost effectiveness of treatment is under intense investigation.

Comparative effectiveness research (CER) reached a milestone in 2009 when the American Recovery and Reinvestment Act was signed into law and allotted 1.1 billion dollars to support CER [4]. Two key elements of CER include the direct comparison of effective interventions and the study of these interventions in the typical patient population encountered in typical daily clinical care [4]. CER relies not only upon randomized clinical trials which often include patients in "ideal" circumstances to control for variables, but also upon utilizing large patient databases to draw conclusions from "everyday" patients. This section will focus on the randomized control trials comparing surgery alone to either neoadjuvant or adjuvant therapy in patients with esophageal, gastroesophageal (GEJ), and gastric cancers, as well as how we have used this information in our clinical practice in the United States with our "everyday" patient population. The extent of lymph node dissection will also be addressed in patients with gastric cancer.

2 Role of Radiation Alone

There have been several studies evaluating the role of radiation in the treatment of esophageal cancer. The use of radiation alone has resulted in poor local control and survival with local recurrence rates as high as 77 % [5] and 5-year overall survival rates between 0 and 21 % [6–11]. Clinical trials have also investigated the use of neoadjuvant radiation and surgery compared to surgery alone but there has been a lack of conclusive evidence indicating superiority. A meta-analysis including 1,147 patients from 5 randomized trials evaluated patients with resectable esophageal tumors, the majority with SqCC. These trials compared neoadjuvant radiation and surgery with surgery alone. The overall hazard ratio was 0.89 which suggests a benefit for preoperative radiation although this was not a significant difference [12]. One shortcoming in extrapolating these results to the general population is that most of these trials included patients with SqCC while the incidence of EAC is rapidly increasing in the United States. Further studies would be needed with modern radiotherapy techniques used in both histologies of esophageal cancer.

Postoperative radiation has also been studied and several randomized trials have compared patients with adjuvant radiation to no adjuvant therapy [13, 14]. While these have been small studies, the patients who received radiation did not have increased survival and suffered increased radiation-related complications. In conclusion, radiation has not been shown to be beneficial when used alone pre- or post-operatively in esophageal cancer.

3 Role of Definitive Chemoradiotherapy

Due to the poor outcomes when radiation is used alone to treat esophageal cancer, chemoradiation has been extensively used as a treatment modality. The chemotherapy is thought to sensitize the tumor cells to the radiation as well as control micrometastatic disease. Most of the studies evaluating the role of chemoradiation in non-surgical patients have been on those with SqCC. Wong evaluated 19 randomized trials comparing chemoradiation to radiation alone in nonoperative esophageal cancer patients. The study demonstrated significantly improved overall survival when chemotherapy was added to the radiotherapy compared to radiotherapy alone [15]. The Eastern Cooperative Oncology Group (ECOG) used mitomycin C and 5-FU with radiation compared to radiation alone in patients with SqCC esophageal cancer, and found a statistically significant increase in survival in the chemoradiation group. The median survival for the chemoradiation group was 14.5 months compared to 9.2 months for the radiation alone group [16]. These results were replicated when the Radiation Therapy Oncology Group (RTOG 85-01) used cisplatin and 5-FU with radiation (50 Gy) and demonstrated a survival benefit compared radiation alone (60 Gy) [7]. Despite the survival benefit of the chemotherapy with the radiation, there was a 47 % incidence of local failure. Because of this, the INT 0123 trial evaluated increased radiation doses (50.4 vs. 64.8 Gy) combined with chemotherapy. The increased radiation dose did not increase survival or local control and resulted in increased treatment-related mortality, suggesting the ideal radiation dose is 50.4 Gy. The current standard of care for nonoperative patients is 50.4 Gy combined with cisplatin and 5FU [17].

4 Role of Neoadjuvant Chemoradiotherapy

For those patients in which surgical resection is an option, the role of neoadjuvant chemoradiation has been studied. There have been at least eight randomized trials evaluating concurrent use of chemotherapy and radiation (Table 1) [18–25]. Three of those trials enrolled mostly patients with SqCC while the others included a mixture of EAC and SqCC. Out of the eight trials, four demonstrated statistically significant improvement in survival [18, 22, 23, 25]. In the CROSS trial, Dutch investigators

Table 1 Neoadjuvant chemoradiation versus surgery alone

Trial	N	Histology (%)	CRT regimen (Gy)	Median survival	3 year OS (%)	*p* value
Lee et al. [20]	50 S	SqCC 100	Cisplatin, 5FU, 45.6	27.3 m	–	NS
	51 CRT			28.2 m		
Lv et al. [23]	80 S	SqCC 100	Paclitaxel, cisplastin, 40	36 m	51.3, 33.8 (5 year)	0.04 (CRT groups compared to S group at 5 years)
	80 CRT (pre-op)			53 m	63.5, 43.5 (5 year)	
	78 CRT (post-op)			48 m	62.8, 42.3 (5 year)	
Mariette et al. [89][a]	98 S	SqCC 71	Cisplatin, 5FU, 45	43.8 m	48.6	NS
	97 CRT			31.8 m	55.2	
Walsh et al. [18]	55 S	AC 100	Cisplatin, 5FU, 40	11 m	6	0.01
	58 CRT			16 m	32	
Urba et al. [19]	50 S	AC 75	Cisplatin, 5FU, vinblastine, 45	17.6 m	16	NS
	50 CRT			16.9 m	30	
Burmeister et al. [21]	128 S	AC 62	Cisplatin, 5FU, 35	19 m	–	NS
	128 CRT			22 m	–	
Tepper et al. [22]	26 S	AC 75	Cisplatin, 5FU, 50.4	1.8 year	16 (5 year)	0.002
	30 CRT			4.5 year	39 (5 year)	
van Hagen et al. [25]	188 S	AC 75	Carboplatin, paclitaxel, 41.4	24 m	44	0.003
	178 CRT			49.4 m	58	

N number, *CRT* chemoradiation, *S* surgery, *m* months, *OS* overall survival, *NS* not significant, *SqCC* squamous cell carcinoma, *AC* adenocarcinoma, *Gy* gray, *FU* fluorouracil, [a]indicates an abstract

randomly assigned patients with resectable esophageal or gastroesophageal junction (GEJ) tumors (75 % with adenocarcinoma) to surgery alone versus carboplatin, paclitaxel, and concurrent radiotherapy followed by surgery [25]. This study demonstrated similar post-operative complications and in-hospital mortality between the two groups as well as a 29 % pathological complete response in the chemoradiation group. Significantly, there was an overall survival increase in the chemoradiation group with a median survival of 49 months compared to 24 months in the surgery alone group [25]. Walsh et al. [18] also demonstrated a significant survival benefit in the chemoradiation group with a 3-year survival of 32 % compared to 6 % in the surgery alone group. While the two trials mentioned above were mostly EAC, Lv et al. [23] conducted a study in China with only SqCC patients. In this study patients were randomized to one of three arms: preoperative chemoradiation, postoperative chemoradiation, or surgery alone. There was a statistically significant improvement in survival in both the pre- and post-operative chemoradiation groups compared to the surgery alone group [23]. The largest meta-analysis conducted evaluating neoadjuvant chemoradiation included 1,854 patients and found the all-cause mortality HR to be 0.78 ($p < 0.0001$). The study included 12 randomized trials evaluating sequential and concurrent treatment, as well as SqCC and EAC [26]. When the patients were divided into histologic subtypes, the HR for SqCC was 0.80 ($p = 0.004$) and the HR for AC was 0.75 ($p = 0.02$).

In summary, for patients with potentially resectable localized esophageal and GEJ cancers, several randomized trials as well as meta-analyses demonstrate improved survival and efficacy with preoperative chemoradiation therapy compared to local therapy alone (surgery or radiation).

5 Role of Adjuvant Chemoradiotherapy for Gastroesophageal Tumors

Several trials have evaluated the role of adjuvant chemoradiation in patients with resectable tumors of the GEJ or stomach. The INT 0116 trial investigated patients with AC of the GEJ or stomach and randomized 556 patients to surgery plus postoperative chemoradiation or surgery alone [27]. The adjuvant chemoradiation included 5-FU and 45 Gy. The median overall survival in the chemoradiation group was significantly improved at 36 months compared with 27 months in the surgery alone group. The survival benefit was confirmed in the 10-year follow-up study [28]. The study conducted by Lv et al. [23] mentioned above with only SqCC patients included a postoperative chemoradiation group which had a statistically improved survival compared with the surgery alone group although the study was not powered to detect differences between the pre-operative chemoradiation group and the post-operative chemoradiation group.

6 Role of Neoadjuvant Chemotherapy

Due to the controversy surrounding radiation therapy and its utility in esophageal and gastric cancers, multiple trials have evaluated chemotherapy prior to surgery compared to surgery alone. At least 9 randomized trials have evaluated this question (Table 2). Similar to neoadjuvant chemoradiation, these trials are a mixture of SqCC and EAC and the results are mixed regarding survival benefit. Six trials did not show a benefit [29–34] while four did show a significant survival benefit [35–38]. One of the largest randomized control trials was the MAGIC trial which randomly assigned patients with resectable AC (stage II or higher with no evidence of metastases) of the stomach (74 %), GEJ (11 %), or lower esophagus (15 %) to either perioperative chemotherapy and surgery (250 patients) or surgery alone (253 patients) [36]. Chemotherapy consisted of three cycles each pre- and post-operatively of epirubicin, cisplatin, and 5-FU. The complication rate and 30-day mortality of both groups was similar. The perioperative chemotherapy group had a statistically increased 5-year survival rate of 36 % compared to 23 % in the surgery alone group. One limitation of the treatment strategy is that only 42 % of the perioperative chemotherapy group actually received the postoperative chemotherapy. A similar trial by Ychou et al. [38] again included only patients with resectable AC of the stomach, GEJ, and distal

Table 2 Neoadjuvant chemotherapy versus surgery alone

Trial	N	Histology (%)	Chemotherapy regimen	Perioperative mortality (%)	3 year OS (%)	*p* value
Cunningham et al. [36]	253 S	AC 100	Epirubicin, cisplatin, 5FU (pre-op and post-op)	5.9	23 (5 year)	0.009
	250 C			5.6	36 (5 year)	
Ychou et al. [38]	111 S	AC 100	Cisplatin, 5FU (pre-op and post-op)	4.5	24 (5 year)	0.02
	113 C			4.6	38 (5 year)	
	19 C			12		
Schlag [30]	24 S	SqCC 100	Cisplatin, 5FU	10	10 m (MS)	NS
	22 C			19	10 m (MS)	
Law et al. [32]	73 S	SqCC 100	Cisplatin, 5FU	8.7	13 m (MS)	NS
	74 C			8.3	16.8 m (MS)	
Kelsen et al. [33]	227 S	AC 53	Cisplatin, 5FU	–	26	NS
	216 C			–	23	
Ancona et al. [34]	48 S	SqCC 100	Cisplatin, 5FU	4.2	22 (5 year)	NS
	48 C			4.2	34 (5 year)	
Allum et al. [37] (MRC)	402 S	AC 67	Cisplatin, 5FU	10	17 (5 year)	0.03
	400 C			10	23 (5 year)	
Boonstra et al. [35]	84 S	SqCC 100	Cisplatin, etoposide	4	17 (5 year)	0.03
	85 C			5	26 (5 year)	
Maipang et al. [31]	22 S	SqCC 100	Cisplatin, vinblastine, bleomycin	–	36	NS
	24 C			17	31	

N number, *S* surgery, *C* chemotherapy, *AC* adenocarcinoma, *SqCC* squamous cell carcinoma, *FU* fluorouracil, *OS* overall survival, *NS* not significant

esophagus and randomized 113 patients to the perioperative chemotherapy group and 111 patients to the surgery alone group. A key difference in this trial compared to the MAGIC trial was the patient population. In the MAGIC trial 74 % of the patients had gastric cancer compared to 25 % in this trial, and GEJ/distal esophageal comprised 26 % in the MAGIC trial compared to 75 % in this trial. The chemotherapy regimen in this trial included two or three cycles of cisplatin and 5FU preoperatively and three or four cycles postoperatively. The perioperative chemotherapy group had a significant increase in 5-year survival of 38 % compared to the surgery alone group at 24 %. Perioperative chemotherapy also significantly improved the curative resection rate from 73 to 84 %. Another large trial by the Medical Research Council (MRC) included 802 patients. This patient population included 67 % with EAC although it did not include gastric cancer [39]. Patients were randomized to preoperative chemotherapy consisting of cisplatin and 5FU followed by surgery or surgery alone. Overall survival was significantly improved in the preoperative chemotherapy group compared to surgery alone with a hazard ratio of 0.79. A follow-up study by Allum verified improved survival for the preoperative chemotherapy group with a 5-year survival of 23 % compared to 17 % for the surgery alone group [37]. This survival benefit held true for both EAC and SqCC. A similar trial by

Kelsen did not show a survival benefit [33]. In this randomized trial 216 patients underwent preoperative chemotherapy with cisplatin and 5-FU and 227 patients underwent surgery alone. The histological type was split 50/50 between EAC and SqCC. There was not a significant difference in survival between the neoadjuvant chemotherapy group and the surgery alone group although there was a survival benefit for those patients that responded to chemotherapy. The reason that there was no difference in survival in this study is unclear as similar chemotherapeutic agents were used. One possibility for the difference was the study size of the MRC trial included almost twice as many patients and another is that the percentage of patients with SqCC versus EAC was different.

7 Role of Adjuvant Chemotherapy

Adjuvant chemotherapy is generally only recommended in patients with positive lymph nodes. Studies that have included adjuvant chemotherapy after neoadjuvant chemotherapy and/or surgery include the MAGIC trial and the French trial [36, 38] although in both of these trials only about 50 % of patients intended to receive postoperative chemotherapy actually did. There are a few trials evaluating adjuvant chemotherapy only. Ando randomized 205 patients with esophageal SqCC to either surgery alone or surgery followed by cisplatin and vindesine. The study did not find a statistical significance in 5-year survival between the two groups [40]. A subsequent study by Ando again included patients with esophageal SqCC randomized to surgery alone versus chemotherapy including cisplatin and 5FU. The 5-year survival rates were 52 and 61 % for surgery alone and surgery plus chemotherapy, respectively. This difference was not statistically significant [41]. It is important to realize that both of these studies only included those patients with esophageal cancer and furthermore only SqCC histology.

The question of neoadjuvant chemotherapy compared to adjuvant chemotherapy has been evaluated by a Japanese trial in which patients with esophageal SqCC were randomized to cisplatin and 5FU either pre- or post-operatively. Overall 5-year survival rates were significantly improved in the preoperative chemotherapy group (55 %) compared to the postoperative chemotherapy group (43 %) [42].

8 Summary

In conclusion, the evidence suggests that neoadjuvant chemotherapy or chemoradiotherapy provides better outcomes compared to surgery alone for esophageal cancer, GEJ, and gastric cancers. Meta-analyses indicate a trend towards improved survival in neoadjuvant chemoradiotherapy compared to neoadjuvant chemotherapy. For those patients that have undergone resection for node-positive esophageal cancer without receiving neoadjuvant therapy, some form of adjuvant treatment is generally recommended although there is no evidence supporting chemoradiation versus chemotherapy alone. One of the barriers to using randomized control trials in CER is that to answer certain questions the number of patients needed to enroll would be prohibitive both logistically and financially. Utilization of large databases is often beneficial to examine these questions from a different angle. One important question that must be addressed is how are clinicians using the information from these trials and consensus guidelines to treat their everyday patients?

9 Implementation of Consensus Guidelines for Esophageal Cancer Treatment

It is evident that surgery alone is insufficient for treatment of locally advanced esophageal and GEJ cancers and a plethora of randomized trials indicate that neoadjuvant treatment is superior to surgery alone. Consensus groups such as the National Comprehensive Cancer Network (NCCN) recommend as standard of care neoadjuvant therapy for stage II and III esophageal cancer [43]. Multimodality therapy for esophageal cancer was advocated in the 1980s when it became evident that surgical resection alone resulted in poor outcomes. Neoadjuvant chemotherapy and chemoradiation was implemented into clinical practice after a few large randomized trials demonstrated survival benefits with neoadjuvant treatment in the late 1990s and early 2000s [18, 22]. The ideal treatment regimen including type of chemotherapy, use of radiation, and if so what dose, were largely unknown due to a heterogeneous and unstandardized mix of trials with often conflicting results. Because of this uncertainty Merkow evaluated the national trends for neoadjuvant use in esophageal cancer to determine the effect of these randomized clinical trials on current esophageal cancer treatment. The study evaluated 8,562 patients from the National Cancer Database (NCDB) that were surgically treated for esophageal cancer between 1998 and 2007 [44]. This study demonstrated that for stage I patients neoadjuvant therapy use significantly decreased from 23.5 % in 1998 to 11.2 % in 2007. For stage II and III patients neoadjuvant use significantly increased: from 48 % in 1998 to 72.5 % in 2007 for stage II patients and from 51 % in 1998 to 90 % in 2007 for stage III patients. Factors that were found to be associated with decreased use of neoadjuvant therapy for stage II and III patients were older age, severity of comorbidity, Medicare insurance coverage, clinical stage II disease, and residence in the western United States [44]. An additional factor evaluated using the NCDB was perioperative mortality. In this study evaluating over 1,000 different hospitals, there was no significant difference in perioperative mortality between the patients treated with neoadjuvant therapy compared to those undergoing surgery alone. There was a significant decrease in surgical margin positivity rate as well as lymph node positivity in those patients who underwent neoadjuvant treatment compared to the surgery alone group.

10 Implementation of Consensus Guidelines for Gastric Cancer Treatment

In a similar study to the one mentioned above, Sherman examined the implementation of gastric cancer guidelines into clinical practice using the NCDB [45]. In some clinical trials proximal gastric adenocarcinoma, GEJ, and distal esophageal tumors are treated similarly [27, 36, 38]. As mentioned before, the Cuningham (MAGIC), Macdonald (INT-0116), and Ychou trials demonstrated that adjuvant therapy use in gastric AC resulted in a significantly improved overall survival [27, 36, 38]. These trials were published in the early 2000s and it was unclear how the results of these trials translated into generalized clinical practice outside the auspices of a trial. Based on these studies, the NCCN guidelines recommend preoperative chemoradiation for localized GEJ AC and perioperative chemotherapy or postoperative chemoradiation therapy for localized gastric AC [43]. To determine the impact of the studies and guidelines, Sherman identified 30,448 patients from the NCDB who underwent surgical resection for a diagnosis of stage IB-III gastric adenocarcinoma between 1998 and 2007 [45]. The proportion of patients with stage IB-III gastric adenocarcinoma who received systemic therapy (either pre- or postoperatively) increased by 71 % (from 35.7 to 61 %) between 1998 and 2007 while the proportion of patients who underwent surgery alone significantly decreased. The largest annual increase occurred between 1999 and 2000 which coincides with the release of the INT-0116 trial findings. The use of neoadjuvant therapy was also significantly increased between 1998 and 2007 from 6 to 20 %, with the largest increase between 2005 and 2006 which corresponded with the release of the MAGIC trial results. Multivariate analysis identified several factors for predicting systemic therapy use (pre- or postoperative): young age, male, fewer comorbidities, higher income, and private insurance. The most predictive factor for receiving neoadjuvant therapy was tumor location in the gastric cardia.

11 Summary

These studies indicate that clinical treatment of gastroesophageal cancer in the United States is changing. These changes seem to correlate with the release of large randomized trials and consensus guideline updates. While many physicians are altering their treatment based on current literature and studies, many physicians have not yet implemented these changes.

12 Gastric Cancer Lymph Node Dissection

One of the first clinicians to promote extended lymphadenectomies in gastric cancer was a Polish-Austrian surgeon Mikulicz [46]. He believed that aggressive locoregional control was paramount in controlling the orderly step-wise progression of cancer metastases through the lymph nodes. Even today the debate continues: those surgeons that advocate a D2 or D3 resection echo Mikulicz's beliefs for locoregional control, and opponents argue that extensive surgery only adds perioperative morbidity and mortality without a survival advantage. Most patients who present with gastric cancer in the United States have advanced disease and the majority who undergo resection are found to have nodal disease [47, 48]. Controversy continues as Asian countries have been performing extended lymphadenectomies for decades while Western countries have only recently incorporated extended lymphadenectomies (D2) into their guidelines [43, 49]. Gastric cancer lymphatic drainage generally follows the vasculature. The most common locations for nodal metastases are lesser curvature (29 %), infra-pyloric (23 %), greater curvature (22 %), right cardia (19 %) and left gastric artery (19 %) [50]. Generally gastric lymph node dissections can be divided into D1 through D4 and the lymph node stations are numbered (Fig. 1). A D1 dissection involves removal of the stomach and the perigastric lymph nodes. In a D2 dissection, additional lymph nodes are removed including nodes along the left gastric, common hepatic, splenic, and left hepatoduodenal artery. D3 and D4 dissections include posterior hepatoduodenal and para-aortic lymph nodes [51]. Much of the controversy surrounding lymph node dissections in gastric cancer started in the 1980s when stage-specific 5-year survival in Japan was shown to be superior to that in the United States [52]. It was theorized that this difference was due to the extended lymphadenectomies performed in Japan

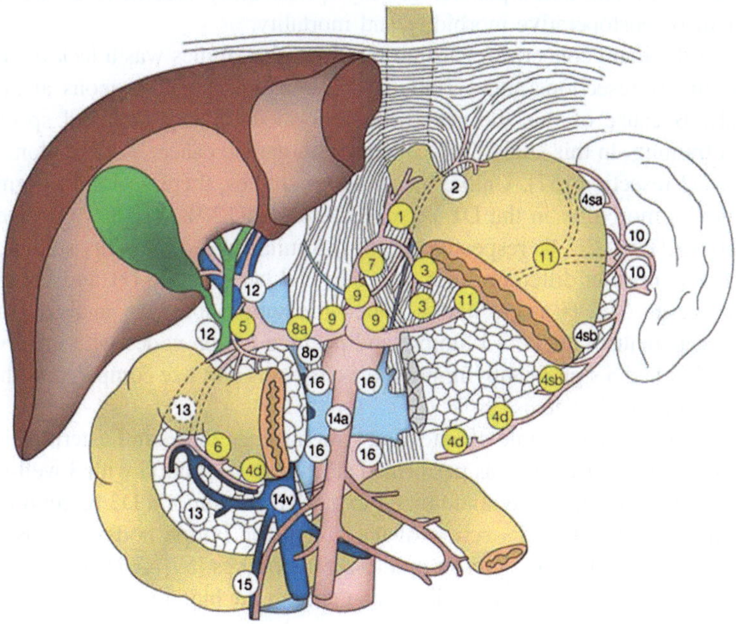

Fig. 1 Gastric lymph node stations [91]

compared to the United States. This stimulated multiple randomized trials comparing the extent of gastric lymphadenectomies.

One of the first trials was performed in South Africa by Dent in the late 1980s. In this study 22 patients were randomized to a D1 resection and 21 patients to the D2 resection group. While the morbidity was found to be higher in the D2 group, the survival at 3 years was similar between the two groups [53]. A larger trial was performed in the United Kingdom with a total of 400 patients who were randomized to a D1 or D2 lymphadenectomy [54]. For tumors in the middle and upper third, a distal pancreaticosplenectomy was performed to obtain the splenic hilar nodes and retropancreatic nodes. There was no significant difference in 5-year survival between the two groups: 35 % compared to 33 % for D1 versus D2 groups respectively. Although there was no overall survival difference, on multivariate analysis, those patients who underwent a D2 resection but did not undergo a distal pancreaticosplenectomy did have an improved survival rate compared to the D1 group. A similar trial performed in the Netherlands accrued patients with gastric cancer from 80 Dutch hospitals and randomized 380 patients to a D1 lymphadenectomy and 331 to a D2 lymphadenectomy [55]. The 5-year survival rates were not significantly different: 45 % for the D1 group and 47 % for the D2 group. There was a significant increase in complications (25 % vs. 43 %) and postoperative deaths (4 % vs. 10 %) in the D2 group compared to the D1 group. When the study was followed out to 11 years the survival for the two groups remained similar: 30 % versus 35 % for the D1 and D2 groups respectively [56]. When subgroups were analyzed, it was determined that a D2 lymphadenectomy may benefit those patients with N2 disease and that a pancreatectomy/splenectomy seemed to be the biggest risk factor of postoperative morbidity and mortality.

One of the main concerns regarding the two prior studies was a lack of surgeon training in D2 resections and variations between individual surgeons at different hospitals. Because of this the next trial performed in Italy included specialized surgeon training. In this study, 267 patients with gastric cancer were randomized to a D1 or D2 resection [57]. Unlike the previous studies, there was not a significant difference in morbidity in the D1 versus D2 groups (12 % vs. 18 %) or operative mortality (3 % vs. 2.2 % respectively) [58]. Similar to the previous studies, there was not a significant difference in 5-year survival between the D1 and D2 groups: 66.5 % versus 64.2 % respectively. When the subgroups were analyzed, it was found that patients with T2-T4 tumors and positive lymph nodes who underwent a D2 resection had a significantly improved 5-year survival rate compared to those in the D1 group: 59 % versus 38 %.

To determine the outcome of extended lymphadenectomies in Eastern patients, a randomized trial in Taiwan was performed at a single institution with 3 well-trained surgeons [59]. Patients were randomized to a D1 resection or a D3 resection. A D1 resection was defined as dissection of the perigastric lymph nodes in close proximity to the tumor along the greater and lesser curvatures [59]. A D3 dissection was defined as additional lymph node dissection around the blood vessels supplying the stomach such as the left gastric, common hepatic, and splenic, as well as lymph nodes in the hepatoduodenal ligament and retropancreatic region. Overall 5-year survival was significantly improved in the D3 resection group at 60 % compared with the D1 group at 53.6 %. Quality control for the surgeons was attempted by having only 3 surgeons perform the operations and each completed at least 25 D3 resections prior to the study. This study implies that in gastric cancer a D3 resection by well-trained surgeons offers a survival benefit compared to a D1 resection. A Japanese study evaluated whether an even more extensive lymphadenectomy known as a para-aortic lymph node dissection (PAND) was superior to the standard D2 lymphadenectomy with gastric resection [60]. The trial was performed in 24 hospitals and 523 patients with curable gastric cancer were randomized to either the standard D2 resection or a D2 resection plus PAND. There was a trend toward increased complications in the D2 plus PAND group with 28 % compared to the D2 group at 21 %. There was no significant difference in 5-year survival between the two groups: 70.3 % for the D2 plus PAND group compared to 69.2 % for the D2 alone group.

13 Gastric and Esophageal Lymph Node Examination in the United States

Regardless of one's opinions about the ideal lymphadenectomy, what has been shown is that lymph node metastases are an important prognostic factor after gastric resection [61–64]. An adequate lymphadenectomy is necessary to allow for accurate pathologic staging. Several studies have investigated this issue and current consensus guidelines recommend a minimum of 15 lymph nodes to allow for reliable staging [43, 65–67]. Similar to esophageal and gastric cancer guidelines, it was unclear how treatment across the United States reflected these recommendations. Bilimoria evaluated how hospital type and volume effected the adequacy of the lymph node resection in gastric cancer [68]. The NCDB was used to identify 3,088 patients who underwent resection for gastric cancer. Of these patients, only 23.2 % had greater than or equal to 15 lymph nodes resected for pathologic evaluation, with an average of 7 lymph nodes [68]. The study also demonstrated that patients were significantly more likely to have greater than 15 lymph nodes examined if they underwent resection at an NCCN-NCI center compared to other academic or community hospitals. Patients were also significantly more likely to have greater than 15 lymph nodes examined if they underwent resection at the highest volume centers compared to high, moderate, or low volume centers.

Like gastric cancer, the NCCN guidelines recommend examining greater than 15 lymph nodes for adequate staging. The adequacy of lymph node resections following esophageal resection in the United States was unknown prior to a study by Merkow which evaluated this question. The study identified 13,995 patients from the NCDB of which 23.5 % had a least 15 lymph nodes examined [69]. During the most recent period of study from 2005 to 2007, greater than 15 lymph nodes were examined in 39 % of academic hospitals compared to 28 % at community hospitals, and in 44.1 % at high-volume centers compared to 29.3 % at low-volume centers.

14 Surgical Treatment for Esophageal and Gastric Tumors

Another source of controversy in esophageal cancer is the surgical management. Esophagectomy is the surgical treatment of esophageal cancer. The type of esophageal resection is dictated by the location of the tumor, the available choices for conduit, and surgeon experience. Surgical therapy remains the mainstay for patients with localized lesions who are fit for major resection, and in the absence of metastatic disease, resection with negative microscopic margins offers the best chance for long-term survival [70, 71]. Appropriate surgical resection depends upon the location and extent of the primary tumor. Surgical strategy should provide the optimal cancer operation with minimal morbidity. For patients with GEJ or proximal gastric lesions, the surgeon will have to make a choice between performing a transabdominal total gastrectomy with esophagojejunal anastomosis versus a combined transthoracic and transabdominal resection of the distal esophagus and proximal stomach with intrathoracic esophagogastric anastomosis (traditional Ivor-Lewis procedure) or transhiatal esophagectomy with cervical esophagogastric anastomosis. In general, if the tumor is limited to the proximal portion of the stomach with minimal extension past the GEJ, a total gastrectomy with intraabdominal esophagojejunal anastomosis is our procedure of choice. We recognize that a longer (>5 cm) negative distal margin will not enhance survival for patients with proximal lesions, but this procedure may minimize post-gastrectomy complications compared to proximal subtotal gastrectomy.

15 Transhiatal Versus Transthoracic Esophagectomy

In an effort to obtain an adequate esophageal margin for more proximal esophageal lesions, an esophagectomy is often required. While there is debate as to whether a transhiatal approach versus a transthroacic approach is preferred, there is no clear evidence indicating the ideal approach [72, 73]. In a meta-analysis by Rindani comparing those two techniques, esophagectomy data from 5,500 patients (44 series) were analyzed [74]. The results demonstrated similar rates of postoperative respiratory and cardiovascular complications. A higher incidence of anastomotic leaks and recurrent laryngeal nerve injuries was found in the transhiatal group [74]. While the 30-day mortality was 6.3 % in the transhiatal group compared to 9.5 % in the transthoracic group, the 5-year survival was similar [74]. In a landmark study, Hulscher et al. [75] assigned 220 patients with adenocarcinoma of the mid-to-distal esophagus or gastric cardia involving the distal esophagus either to transhiatal esophagectomy or to transthoracic esophagectomy with extended en bloc lymphadenectomy. Both operative time and estimated blood loss (EBL) were significantly lower with the transthoracic esophagectomy: 3.5 h versus 6 h and 1 L versus 1.9 L respectively [75]. Although pulmonary complications and chylous leakage were higher after transthoracic esophagectomy (57 % vs. 27 % and 10 % vs. 2 %

respectively) the in-hospital mortality was not significantly different. Duration of mechanical ventilation, ICU and hospital time was shorter in the transhiatal group. Furthermore, there was no significant difference in overall or disease free survival for patients who underwent transhiatal esophagectomy versus those who underwent transthoracic esophagectomy. In 2008, Chang published data from a large population-based study comparing both approaches through the Surveillance, Epidemiology and End Results (SEER) and found a lower operative mortality after transhiatal esophagectomy; 6.7 % versus 13.1 % [76]. Although a higher 5-year survival was noted after transhiatal esophagectomy, after adjusting for other variables, no significant difference was found.

16 Minimally Invasive Approaches of Esophagectomy

16.1 Ivor Lewis Esophagectomy

The minimally invasive Ivor Lewis esophagectomy begins with five-port laparoscopy in supine position. After gastric mobilization and abdominal lymphadenectomy the gastric conduit is created by use of an endoscopic linear stapler. Once the phrenoesophageal ligament is divided, the abdominal part of the procedure is complete and the patient is repositioned in either the left lateral decubitus position or the prone position. The procedure is continued with four-port thoracoscopy. The first thoracic step is the division of the pulmonary ligament followed by circumferential mobilization of the esophagus, division of the azygos vein and dissection of paraesophageal, lower and middle mediastinal, subcarinal and right-sided paratracheal lymph nodes. When the gastric conduit is mobilized into the thorax, the esophagus is divided just superior to the level of the carina and an intrathoracic anastomosis can be accomplished with transoral and transthoracic staplers. Based on a recent review comparing open and minimally invasive esophagectomy in terms of anastomotic leakage and stenosis rates, both techniques can be considered equally safe and effective [77, 78]. However, a hybrid minimally invasive technique combining the open and endoscopic techniques for transthoracic resection has also been described.

17 McKeown Esophagectomy

The 3-incisional McKeown esophagectomy combines features of the transhiatal and the Ivor-Lewis transthoracic technique. The abdominal and thoracic stages of the procedure are comparable to the previously described Ivor-Lewis technique and allow the surgeon to perform the same two-field (upper abdominal and mediastinal) lymphadenectomy under direct vision. The main difference however, is the addition of a left cervical incision to allow a cervical anastomosis. Although robust scientific evidence is lacking, cervical reconstruction is considered to have clinical advantages compared to an intrathoracic anastomosis. The advantages include improved leak management in the event of an anastomotic breakdown, and wider proximal resection margins. A high rate of anastomotic leakage and stenosis are the disadvantages of this technique [79, 80]. The thoracoscopic and laparoscopic portion of the minimally invasive McKeown technique are comparable to the descriptions above. However, the procedure usually begins with a thoracic stage to avoid the need for extra repositioning. Removal of the resection specimen and construction of the gastric conduit usually occurs through an accessory upper midline incision of 5 cm. Subsequently the gastric conduit is delivered to the cervical region where again a hand-sewn or stapled anastomosis can be performed. Similar to the minimally invasive Ivor Lewis approach, hybrid minimally invasive McKeown procedures can be performed.

18 Robotic Esophagectomy

A robot-assisted esophagectomy has also been described, allowing three-dimensional visualization, improved magnification, and a greater range of instrument motion. Robotic assistance has been described for gastric mobilization (in both transhiatal and transthoracic resections), mediastinal lymphadenectomy, dissection of the esophagus and generation of an intrathoracic anastomosis. The need for single-lung ventilation is a potential limitation. However, preliminary studies showing equality with above-mentioned techniques in terms of safety and efficacy have led to the ROBOT trial, comparing open and robot assisted esophagectomy [81, 82]. A combination of randomized controlled trials (RCT) and meta-analyses have compared open versus minimally invasive esophagectomy with the goal of determining the most effective approach for esophageal cancer [77, 83, 84]. The following section will compare open versus minimally invasive esophagectomy in terms of their respective outcomes.

19 Outcomes

Nagpal et al. [85] addressed intraoperative outcomes based on five comparative studies and found that blood loss was significantly lower in the minimally invasive group. This beneficial effect of minimally invasive surgery was confirmed by the recent TIME trial by Biere, comparing minimally invasive versus open esophagectomy for patients with esophageal cancer. There was a significant decrease in blood loss in the minimally invasive group (200 mL) versus the open esophagectomy group (475 mL) [77]. Comparative studies evaluating operative time have demonstrated decreased operative times in the laparoscopic group compared to the open transhiatal esophagectomy group [85]. In a recent systematic review, seven out of nine included studies (including the TIME trial) showed a significantly increased operative time in case of thoracoscopic resection [77]. Additional studies comparing a minimally invasive approach to an open approach are listed in Table 3.

Table 3 Minimally invasive esophagectomy versus open esophagectomy

Authors	Study design	Sample size/ number of study	MIE	Open techniques	EBL (ml)	Pulmonary complications/ nerve injury	Oncologic adequacy (R0) MIE versus open	30 day mortality MIE versus open
Nagpal et al. [85]	Meta-analysis	216/5	TTE	TTE	**268.5	*OR 0.58 $P = 0.04$/OR 0.76 $P = 0.71$	NR	OR = 0.55 $P = 0.26$
Biere et al. [77]	Randomized control trials	115/NA	TTE (59)	TTE (56)	200 versus 475	9 % versus 29 % $P = 0.005$/2 % versus 14 % $P = 0.012$	NS	NS
Sgourakis et al. [83]	Meta-analysis	163/5	TTE	TTE	NR	OR 1.31 $P = 0.73$/OR 0.57 $P = 0.52$	NR	RR = 1.45 $P = 0.47$
Schoppman et al. [86]	Cohort	62	TTE (31)	TTE (31)	NR	OR 0.15 $P = 0.001$/OR 0.0095 $P = 0.005$	NS	NS
Sihag et al. [87]	Prospective	114	TTE (38)	TTE (76)	200 versus 250	NR/NR	NS	0 % versus 2 %
Braghetto et al. [90]	Prospective	166	TTE (47)	TTE (60) THE (59)	NR	NR/NS	NR	6.3 % versus 10.9 %

TTE transthoracic esophagectomy, *THE* transhiatal esophagectomy, *MIE* minimally invasive esophagectomy, *OR* odds ratio, *EBL* estimated blood loss, *NR* not recorded, *RR* relative risk, *NS* not significant, *OR in favor of MIE, **EBL in favor of MIE

The most significant factor for the decreased overall morbidity after minimally invasive esophagectomy is the reduction in pulmonary complications. This is reflected by significant differences demonstrated in the meta-analyses of Nagpal, the TIME trial, and to a lesser extent by an observed trend in the meta-analysis by Sgourakis et al. [83]. The evidence about laryngeal nerve palsy is contradictory. The TIME trail showed a significantly lower rate of recurrent laryngeal nerve palsy after minimally invasive resection, which is in accordance with the study by Schoppmann although this contradicts the findings in a meta-analysis [77, 86]. Patients treated in the minimally invasive arm of the TIME trial reported a significantly higher short-term quality of life in terms of physical status, global health and in relation to common postoperative symptoms like pain and speech impediment [77]. Based on the discussed literature, minimally invasive esophagectomy should be regarded as a safe alternative to open resection with proven short-term advantages with respect to pulmonary status, vocal cord function and quality of life.

One of the most controversial issues in the surgical treatment of esophageal cancer is the oncological adequacy of a minimally invasive resection. A major factor in oncologic adequacy is the proportion of R0 resections. Unfortunately, comparisons of R0 resection rates between open- and minimally invasive esophagectomy are rarely reported. In three recent comparative studies R0 resection rates were reported [77, 87, 88]. In the TIME trial an insignificant difference of 8 % (92 % vs. 84 %) in favor of minimally invasive esophagectomy was observed [77]. Two similar studies by Sihag and Sundaram, comparing perioperative outcomes following open versus minimally invasive Ivor Lewis esophagectomy, found no significant differences in R0 resection: (100 % vs. 93.4 %) and (93.6 % vs. 92.3 %) respectively [87, 88]. Contrary to R0 resection rates, the total number of retrieved lymph nodes is a commonly reported outcome measure. One of the three meta-analyses on this topic reported a significant increase in median number of nodes, 16 versus 10, in favor of minimally invasive esophagectomy [84]. In the same review the described increase in lymph node retrieval did not seem to translate to a survival benefit as no significant differences were found in one-, two-, three- and five-year survival [84]. Currently available data imply that oncologic outcomes of minimally invasive esophagectomy are not inferior to those of open esophagectomy.

References

1. Siegel R, Naishadham D, Jemal A (2013) Cancer statistics, 2013. CA Cancer J Clin 63(1):11–30
2. Devesa SS, Blot WJ, Fraumeni JF Jr (1998) Changing patterns in the incidence of esophageal and gastric carcinoma in the United States. Cancer 83(10):2049–2053
3. Siegel R, Naishadham D, Jemal A (2012) Cancer statistics, 2012. CA Cancer J Clin 62(1):10–29
4. Sox HC, Greenfield S (2009) Comparative effectiveness research: a report from the institute of medicine. Ann Intern Med 151(3):203–205
5. Shridhar R et al (2013) Curative treatment of esophageal cancer; an evidenced based review. J Gastrointest Cancer 44(4):375–384

6. Cooper JS et al (1999) Chemoradiotherapy of locally advanced esophageal cancer: long-term follow-up of a prospective randomized trial (RTOG 85-01). Radiation therapy oncology group. JAMA 281(17):1623–1627
7. Herskovic A et al (1992) Combined chemotherapy and radiotherapy compared with radiotherapy alone in patients with cancer of the esophagus. N Engl J Med 326(24):1593–1598
8. Raman NV, Small W Jr (1999) The role of radiation therapy in the management of esophageal cancer. Cancer Control 6(1):53–62
9. Newaishy GA et al (1982) Results of radical radiotherapy of squamous cell carcinoma of the oesophagus. Clin Radiol 33(3):347–352
10. Petrovich Z et al (1991) Management of carcinoma of the esophagus: the role of radiotherapy. Am J Clin Oncol 14(1):80–86
11. Van Houtte P (1977) Radiotherapy of oesophagus cancer. A review of 136 cases treated at the Institut Bordet (author's transl). Acta Gastroenterol Belg 40(3–4):121–128
12. Arnott SJ et al (2005) Preoperative radiotherapy for esophageal carcinoma. Cochrane Database Syst Rev 4:CD001799
13. Fok M et al (1993) Postoperative radiotherapy for carcinoma of the esophagus: a prospective, randomized controlled study. Surgery 113(2):138–147
14. Teniere P et al (1991) Postoperative radiation therapy does not increase survival after curative resection for squamous cell carcinoma of the middle and lower esophagus as shown by a multicenter controlled trial. French university association for surgical research. Surg Gynecol Obstet 173(2):123–130
15. Wong R, Malthaner R (2006) Combined chemotherapy and radiotherapy (without surgery) compared with radiotherapy alone in localized carcinoma of the esophagus. Cochrane Database Syst Rev 1:CD002092
16. Smith TJ et al (1998) Combined chemoradiotherapy versus radiotherapy alone for early stage squamous cell carcinoma of the esophagus: a study of the Eastern cooperative oncology group. Int J Radiat Oncol Biol Phys 42(2):269–276
17. Minsky BD et al (2002) INT 0123 (radiation therapy oncology group 94-05) phase III trial of combined-modality therapy for esophageal cancer: high-dose versus standard-dose radiation therapy. J Clin Oncol 20(5):1167–1174
18. Walsh TN et al (1996) A comparison of multimodal therapy and surgery for esophageal adenocarcinoma. N Engl J Med 335(7):462–467
19. Urba SG et al (2001) Randomized trial of preoperative chemoradiation versus surgery alone in patients with locoregional esophageal carcinoma. J Clin Oncol 19(2):305–313
20. Lee JL et al (2004) A single institutional phase III trial of preoperative chemotherapy with hyperfractionation radiotherapy plus surgery versus surgery alone for resectable esophageal squamous cell carcinoma. Ann Oncol 15(6):947–954
21. Burmeister BH et al (2005) Surgery alone versus chemoradiotherapy followed by surgery for resectable cancer of the oesophagus: a randomised controlled phase III trial. Lancet Oncol 6 (9):659–668
22. Tepper J et al (2008) Phase III trial of trimodality therapy with cisplatin, fluorouracil, radiotherapy, and surgery compared with surgery alone for esophageal cancer: CALGB 9781. J Clin Oncol 26(7):1086–1092
23. Lv J et al (2010) Long-term efficacy of perioperative chemoradiotherapy on esophageal squamous cell carcinoma. World J Gastroenterol 16(13):1649–1654
24. Mariette C, Piessen G, Triboulet JP (2007) Therapeutic strategies in oesophageal carcinoma: role of surgery and other modalities. Lancet Oncol 8(6):545–553
25. van Hagen P et al (2012) Preoperative chemoradiotherapy for esophageal or junctional cancer. N Engl J Med 366(22):2074–2084
26. Sjoquist KM et al (2011) Survival after neoadjuvant chemotherapy or chemoradiotherapy for resectable oesophageal carcinoma: an updated meta-analysis. Lancet Oncol 12(7):681–692
27. Macdonald JS et al (2001) Chemoradiotherapy after surgery compared with surgery alone for adenocarcinoma of the stomach or gastroesophageal junction. N Engl J Med 345(10):725–730

28. Smalley SR et al (2012) Updated analysis of SWOG-directed intergroup study 0116: a phase III trial of adjuvant radiochemotherapy versus observation after curative gastric cancer resection. J Clin Oncol 30(19):2327–2333
29. Roth JA et al (1988) Randomized clinical trial of preoperative and postoperative adjuvant chemotherapy with cisplatin, vindesine, and bleomycin for carcinoma of the esophagus. J Thorac Cardiovasc Surg 96(2):242–248
30. Schlag PM (1992) Randomized trial of preoperative chemotherapy for squamous cell cancer of the esophagus. The Chirurgische Arbeitsgemeinschaft Fuer Onkologie der Deutschen Gesellschaft Fuer Chirurgie Study Group. Arch Surg 127(12):1446–1450
31. Maipang T et al (1994) Induction chemotherapy in the treatment of patients with carcinoma of the esophagus. J Surg Oncol 56(3):191–197
32. Law S et al (1997) Preoperative chemotherapy versus surgical therapy alone for squamous cell carcinoma of the esophagus: a prospective randomized trial. J Thorac Cardiovasc Surg 114 (2):210–217
33. Kelsen DP et al (2007) Long-term results of RTOG trial 8911 (USA Intergroup 113): a random assignment trial comparison of chemotherapy followed by surgery compared with surgery alone for esophageal cancer. J Clin Oncol 25(24):3719–3725
34. Ancona E et al (2001) Only pathologic complete response to neoadjuvant chemotherapy improves significantly the long term survival of patients with resectable esophageal squamous cell carcinoma: final report of a randomized, controlled trial of preoperative chemotherapy versus surgery alone. Cancer 91(11):2165–2174
35. Boonstra JJ et al (2011) Chemotherapy followed by surgery versus surgery alone in patients with resectable oesophageal squamous cell carcinoma: long-term results of a randomized controlled trial. BMC Cancer 11:181
36. Cunningham D et al (2006) Perioperative chemotherapy versus surgery alone for resectable gastroesophageal cancer. N Engl J Med 355(1):11–20
37. Allum WH et al (2009) Long-term results of a randomized trial of surgery with or without preoperative chemotherapy in esophageal cancer. J Clin Oncol 27(30):5062–5067
38. Ychou M et al (2011) Perioperative chemotherapy compared with surgery alone for resectable gastroesophageal adenocarcinoma: an FNCLCC and FFCD multicenter phase III trial. J Clin Oncol 29(13):1715–1721
39. Medical Research Council Oesophageal Cancer Working, G (2002) Surgical resection with or without preoperative chemotherapy in oesophageal cancer: a randomised controlled trial. Lancet 359(9319):1727–1733
40. Ando N et al (1997) A randomized trial of surgery with and without chemotherapy for localized squamous carcinoma of the thoracic esophagus: the Japan clinical oncology group study. J Thorac Cardiovasc Surg 114(2):205–209
41. Ando N et al (2003) Surgery plus chemotherapy compared with surgery alone for localized squamous cell carcinoma of the thoracic esophagus: a Japan clinical oncology group study (JCOG9204). J Clin Oncol 21(24):4592–4596
42. Ando N et al (2012) A randomized trial comparing postoperative adjuvant chemotherapy with cisplatin and 5-fluorouracil versus preoperative chemotherapy for localized advanced squamous cell carcinoma of the thoracic esophagus (JCOG9907). Ann Surg Oncol 19 (1):68–74
43. The National Comprehensive Cancer Network Guidelines in Oncology (cited 2014 Feb 6). Available from. http://www.nccn.org
44. Merkow RP et al (2012) Use of multimodality neoadjuvant therapy for esophageal cancer in the United States: assessment of 987 hospitals. Ann Surg Oncol 19(2):357–364
45. Sherman KL et al (2013) Treatment trends and predictors of adjuvant and neoadjuvant therapy for gastric adenocarcinoma in the United States. Ann Surg Oncol 20(2):362–370
46. Olch PD (1960) Johann von Mikulicz-Radecki. Ann Surg 152:923–926
47. Wanebo HJ et al (1993) Cancer of the stomach. A patient care study by the American college of surgeons. Ann Surg 218(5):583–592

48. Hundahl SA et al (1997) The national cancer data base report on gastric carcinoma. Cancer 80 (12):2333–2341
49. Okines A et al (2010) Gastric cancer: ESMO clinical practice guidelines for diagnosis, treatment and follow-up. Ann Oncol 21(Suppl 5):v50–v54
50. Maruyama K et al (1989) Lymph node metastases of gastric cancer. General pattern in 1931 patients. Ann Surg 210(5):596–602
51. Kajitani T (1981) The general rules for the gastric cancer study in surgery and pathology. Part I. Clinical classification. Jpn J Surg 11(2):127–139
52. Maruyama K, Okabayashi K, Kinoshita T (1987) Progress in gastric cancer surgery in Japan and its limits of radicality. World J Surg 11(4):418–425
53. Dent DM, Madden MV, Price SK (1988) Randomized comparison of R1 and R2 gastrectomy for gastric carcinoma. Br J Surg 75(2):110–112
54. Cuschieri A et al (1999) Patient survival after D1 and D2 resections for gastric cancer: long-term results of the MRC randomized surgical trial. Surgical co-operative group. Br J Cancer 79 (9–10):1522–1530
55. Bonenkamp JJ et al (1999) Extended lymph-node dissection for gastric cancer. N Engl J Med 340(12):908–914
56. Hartgrink HH et al (2004) Extended lymph node dissection for gastric cancer: who may benefit? Final results of the randomized Dutch gastric cancer group trial. J Clin Oncol 22(11):2069–2077
57. Degiuli M et al (2010) Morbidity and mortality in the Italian gastric cancer study group randomized clinical trial of D1 versus D2 resection for gastric cancer. Br J Surg 97(5):643–649
58. Degiuli M et al (2014) Randomized clinical trial comparing survival after D1 or D2 gastrectomy for gastric cancer. Br J Surg 101(2):23–31
59. Wu CW et al (2006) Nodal dissection for patients with gastric cancer: a randomised controlled trial. Lancet Oncol 7(4):309–315
60. Sasako M et al (2008) D2 lymphadenectomy alone or with para-aortic nodal dissection for gastric cancer. N Engl J Med 359(5):453–462
61. Peeters KC et al (2005) Validation of a nomogram for predicting disease-specific survival after an R0 resection for gastric carcinoma. Cancer 103(4):702–707
62. Siewert JR et al (1998) Relevant prognostic factors in gastric cancer: ten-year results of the German gastric cancer study. Ann Surg 228(4):449–461
63. Kodera Y et al (1998) The number of metastatic lymph nodes: a promising prognostic determinant for gastric carcinoma in the latest edition of the TNM classification. J Am Coll Surg 187(6):597–603
64. Kim JP et al (1998) Clinicopathologic characteristics and prognostic factors in 10 783 patients with gastric cancer. Gastric Cancer 1(2):125–133
65. Karpeh MS et al (2000) Lymph node staging in gastric cancer: is location more important than number? An analysis of 1,038 patients. Ann Surg 232(3):362–371
66. Lee HK et al (2001) Influence of the number of lymph nodes examined on staging of gastric cancer. Br J Surg 88(10):1408–1412
67. Bouvier AM et al (2002) How many nodes must be examined to accurately stage gastric carcinomas? Results from a population based study. Cancer 94(11):2862–2866
68. Bilimoria KY et al (2008) Effect of hospital type and volume on lymph node evaluation for gastric and pancreatic cancer. Arch Surg 143(7):671–678; discussion 678
69. Merkow RP et al (2012) Variation in lymph node examination after esophagectomy for cancer in the United States. Arch Surg 147(6):505–511
70. Brennan MF (1995) Benefit of aggressive multimodality treatment for gastric cancer. Ann Surg Oncol 2(4):286–287
71. Brennan MF, Karpeh MS Jr (1996) Surgery for gastric cancer: the American view. Semin Oncol 23(3):352–359

72. Griffin SM, Shaw IH, Dresner SM (2002) Early complications after Ivor Lewis subtotal esophagectomy with two-field lymphadenectomy: risk factors and management. J Am Coll Surg 194(3):285–297
73. Hulscher JB et al (2001) Transthoracic versus transhiatal resection for carcinoma of the esophagus: a meta-analysis. Ann Thorac Surg 72(1):306–313
74. Rindani R, Martin CJ, Cox MR (1999) Transhiatal versus Ivor-Lewis oesophagectomy: is there a difference? Aust NZ J Surg 69(3):187–194
75. Hulscher JB et al (2002) Extended transthoracic resection compared with limited transhiatal resection for adenocarcinoma of the esophagus. N Engl J Med 347(21):1662–1669
76. Chang AC et al (2008) Outcomes after transhiatal and transthoracic esophagectomy for cancer. Ann Thorac Surg 85(2):424–429
77. Biere SS et al (2012) Minimally invasive versus open oesophagectomy for patients with oesophageal cancer: a multicentre, open-label, randomised controlled trial. Lancet 379 (9829):1887–1892
78. Watanabe M et al (2013) Minimally invasive esophagectomy for esophageal cancer: an updated review. Surg Today 43(3):237–244
79. Pennathur A et al (2010) The "best operation" for esophageal cancer? Ann Thorac Surg 89(6): S2163–S2167
80. Yamamoto M et al (2013) Minimally invasive surgery for esophageal cancer: review of the literature and institutional experience. Cancer Control 20(2):130–137
81. Verhage RJ et al (2009) Minimally invasive surgery compared to open procedures in esophagectomy for cancer: a systematic review of the literature. Minerva Chir 64(2):135–146
82. van der Sluis PC et al (2012) Robot-assisted minimally invasive thoraco-laparoscopic esophagectomy versus open transthoracic esophagectomy for resectable esophageal cancer, a randomized controlled trial (ROBOT trial). Trials 13:230
83. Sgourakis G et al (2010) Minimally invasive versus open esophagectomy: meta-analysis of outcomes. Dig Dis Sci 55(11):3031–3040
84. Dantoc M, Cox MR, Eslick GD (2012) Evidence to support the use of minimally invasive esophagectomy for esophageal cancer: a meta-analysis. Arch Surg 147(8):768–776
85. Nagpal K et al (2010) Is minimally invasive surgery beneficial in the management of esophageal cancer? A meta-analysis. Surg Endosc 24(7):1621–1629
86. Schoppmann SF et al (2010) Open versus minimally invasive esophagectomy: a single-center case controlled study. Surg Endosc 24(12):3044–3053
87. Sihag S et al (2012) Comparison of perioperative outcomes following open versus minimally invasive Ivor Lewis oesophagectomy at a single, high-volume centre. Eur J Cardiothorac Surg 42(3):430–437
88. Sundaram A et al (2012) Survival and quality of life after minimally invasive esophagectomy: a single-surgeon experience. Surg Endosc 26(1):168–176
89. Mariette C, Seitz JF, Maillard E et al (2010) Surgery alone versus chemoradiotherapy followed by surgery for localized esophageal cancer: analysis of a randomized controlled phase III trial FFCD 9901. J Clin Oncol 28(15 supplement):4005
90. Braghetto I et al (2006) Open transthoracic or transhiatal esophagectomy versus minimally invasive esophagectomy in terms of morbidity, mortality and survival. Surg Endosc 20 (11):1681–1686
91. Roukos DH, Kappas AM (2005) Perspectives in the treatment of gastric cancer. Nat Clin Pract Oncol 2:98–107. doi:10.1038/ncponc0099

Comparative Effectiveness in Colon and Rectal Cancer

Christine C. Jensen and Robert D. Madoff

Abstract

Treatment of colorectal cancer is becoming more uniform, with wider acceptance of standardized guidelines. However, areas of controversy exist where the appropriate treatment is not clear, including:

- should a segmental colectomy or a more extensive resection be performed in hereditary nonpolyposis colorectal cancer?
- should an asymptomatic primary cancer be resected in the presence of unresectable metastatic disease?
- what is the role of extended lymph node resection in colon and rectal cancer?
- are there clinically significant benefits for a robotic approach to colorectal resection versus a laparoscopic approach?

This chapter will examine these issues and discuss how they may be resolved.

Keywords

Hereditary nonpolyposis colorectal cancer · Complete mesocolic excision · Metastatic colon cancer · Robotic surgery

Contents

C.C. Jensen (✉) · R.D. Madoff
University of Minnesota, Minneapolis, MN, USA
e-mail: cjensen@crsal.org

C.C. Jensen
Colon and Rectal Surgery Associates, Minneapolis, MN, USA

K.Y. Bilimoria et al. (eds.), *Comparative Effectiveness in Surgical Oncology*,
Cancer Treatment and Research 164, DOI 10.1007/978-3-319-12553-4_9

1 Extended Versus Segmental Resection for Hereditary Nonpolyposis Colorectal Cancer

Persons with hereditary nonpolyposis colorectal cancer (HNPCC) are at increased risk for metachronous cancers compared to the general population. This risk has been estimated to be 40 % by 10 years [1]. In addition, the adenoma-carcinoma sequence appears to be accelerated in HNPCC, so that persons with HNPCC can progress from a normal colonoscopy to carcinoma within 2–3 years, [2, 3] mandating colonoscopy every 1–2 years. Such surveillance has been shown to decrease the risk of subsequent cancer by more than 63 %, even when conducted only every 3 years, and also decreases the risk of death related to colorectal cancer [4]. However, some studies have shown a significant risk for development of cancer despite intensive surveillance, ranging from 6 to 25 % [2, 5, 6]. In addition, the rate of missed adenomas on colonoscopy has been found to be as high as 55 % in HNPCC, [7] suggesting that there continues to be significant risk of subsequent cancer even with intensive surveillance. Because of this uncertainty, the NCCN guidelines recommend the surgeon "consider more extensive colectomy for patients with a strong family history of colon cancer or young age (<50)," but stop short of recommending this [8].

The ability to detect microsatellite instability and defective mismatch repair genes preoperatively has blossomed over the last several years. Patients with likely HNPCC can be diagnosed preoperatively using germline testing when there is an established family history of HNPCC. The diagnosis can also be suggested when immunohistochemistry testing fails to show intact mismatch repair enzymes or when there is microsatellite instability in a biopsy specimen, even if there is no suggestive family history. Now much more frequently than before, an individual is known to be an HNPCC carrier prior to surgery. Thus, the question arises whether patients with a colorectal cancer in the setting of HNPCC should have a more extensive resection, such as a subtotal or total colectomy or an ileoanal pouch. This may reduce their risk of a subsequent cancer more than having a segmental resection but is associated with functional consequences. Also undetermined is whether a known HNPCC carrier should have a prophylactic colectomy, and if so which procedure should be performed.

Several attempts have been made to compare these operative strategies. In a study of colorectal cancer patients in known HNPCC families, Mecklin and Jarvinen [9] found metachronous cancers in 41 % of patients who had undergone segmental resection versus 24 % who had subtotal colectomy during 7 years of follow up. Similarly, Van Dalen [10] found no metachronous cancer among patients who had total colectomies versus 16 cancers in 70 patients who had segmental resections (although the rate of metachronous cancer in this group was quite different depending on whether the patients had been followed up at the original institution or another institution). These results would suggest that patients with HNPCC may benefit from a more extensive resection.

Decision analysis has also been used as a tool to model outcomes between the two strategies. Maeda et al. [11] performed a decision analysis of segmental versus total abdominal colectomy for a hypothetical cohort of 30-year-old patients with HNPCC. For this population, total abdominal colectomy led to an improvement in survival of 0.7 years and no appreciable difference in quality-adjusted life years. Which operation was preferred was dependent on the quality of life associated with each operation, the patient's age and the hypothesized risk of metachronous cancer, so the authors recommended the procedure to be performed should be chosen on a case-by-case basis taking these factors into account. Cappel et al. [12] in a study that did not examine quality of life, found a predicted 2.3-year survival benefit among a cohort of 27-year-old patients with cancer undergoing total abdominal colectomy as compared to segmental resection, although this survival benefit decreased with age.

Despite the predominance of right-sided cancers in HNPCC, approximately 15 % of initial cancers in HNPCC patients will be rectal cancers [13]. For a patient with rectal cancer in the setting of HNPCC, the functional difference between a segmental and extended resection becomes more stark, as extended resection would require an ileoanal pouch, as has been recommended by some [14]. There are few studies examining this specific area, other than the case series by Kalady et al. [2] demonstrating a greater than 50 % risk of high-risk adenoma or carcinoma after proctectomy, despite colonoscopic surveillance. In that series, one patient developed a metachronous cancer within 2 years of a normal colonoscopy.

For a patient known to have HNPCC who has not yet been diagnosed with a colorectal cancer, there is little data on whether they should be offered a prophylactic colectomy. Some authors have suggested prophylactic colectomies for known gene carriers may be appropriate in certain situations [14, 15]. A decision analysis study by Syngal et al. [16] found that for a hypothetical 25-year-old HNPCC carrier, prophylactic proctocolectomy was associated with an increase in survival of 15.6 years versus no intervention, whereas intensive surveillance was associated with an increase of 13.5 years. With increasing age prophylactic proctocolectomy became less beneficial, and when health-related quality of life was considered, surveillance led to greater benefit than prophylactic proctocolectomy. However, there is no retrospective or prospective data to guide this decision making.

There are several barriers that have prohibited more conclusive research in this area. First, HNPCC represents approximately only 3 % of colorectal cancers, so obtaining adequate numbers of patients would require a multi-institutional study or a study spanning many years at a single institution. Second, the functional consequences of a segmental resection versus a more extensive resection mean that patients may have a strong preference for one option versus another, and some patients may not be a candidate for a more extensive resection due to pre-existing incontinence or diarrhea. Third, the diagnosis of HNPCC has historically been based on the Amsterdam criteria rather than genetic testing, leading to exclusion of patients from studies if their family history was not strongly suggestive of HNPCC due to a small family size or de novo genetic mutation. Patients may also have been incorrectly classified as having HNPCC based on the Amsterdam criteria even when their genetic predisposition was instead due to another cause such as Familial Colorectal Cancer Type X.

The time may be right for a randomized controlled trial of extended versus segmental resection for established colorectal cancer, which would clearly provide the best quality evidence regarding the optimal surgical procedure. The ability to diagnose HNPCC prior to surgery, even in persons who may not have been suspected to have HNPCC based on family history, and the ability for institutions to collaborate through the use of registries may lead to a sufficient number of patients being available for enrollment in a study. The risks and benefits of a segmental versus extended resection do not currently show one of these strategies to be clearly superior and therefore it is acceptable from an ethical standpoint to enroll patients in a randomized trial on this subject. With metachronous cancer rates being as high as 40 % at 10 years, [1] the randomized trial may not require an extensive period of time to show whether there is an effect on the rate of metachronous cancer, provided enough patients can be enrolled. At a minimum, the use of a centralized registry of HNPCC patients would allow for a case series to be conducted with larger number of patients than the studies already in existence, thus providing more reliable information regarding the risk of subsequent cancer.

It would be difficult to use a randomized controlled trial to evaluate surgical options for HNPCC patients presenting with rectal cancer or persons known to carry a mismatch repair gene defect who have not yet developed cancer. In these patients, the functional differences between standard resection and total proctocolectomy for the rectal cancer patients, and no surgery and total proctocolectomy for the mismatch repair gene defect patients, are disparate enough that it would likely be difficult to recruit patients to this sort of trial. Since both of these situations represent a very small minority of the colorectal cancer patients seen by the typical surgeon, this is a case where a centralized registry may help with compiling such cases and allow analysis of outcomes through a case series. Ideally, quality of life data would also be gathered, but this would be difficult given the likely large number of contributors to the registry.

Thus, there are no compelling data that mandate the appropriate surgery for a patient with HNPCC and colon cancer. At present, the decision must be individualized based upon the patient's age, disease status, bowel function and individual preference. Even less clear is what should be done for the patient with an HNPCC-associated rectal cancer, or a mismatch repair gene defect carrier who has not yet developed a colorectal cancer. However, due to an increased ability to identify mismatch repair gene carriers, there is great promise for future research in this area.

2 Resection of an Asymptomatic Primary Tumor in Unresectable Metastatic Disease

As many as 20–25 % of patients will have metastatic disease at the time of presentation with colorectal cancer [17]. Even within this group, presentations can vary, from the patient with a symptomatic primary and minimal metastatic disease, to the patient with no symptoms from the primary and extensive metastatic disease, to the patient with both primary and metastatic disease that may become resectable after chemotherapy. The patient with an asymptomatic primary tumor and unresectable metastatic disease represents a special case. In this situation, the NCCN guidelines recommend chemotherapy with monitoring of response every 2 months. Surgery is recommended only if both the primary and the metastases become completely resectable [8].

In reality, the situation may not be so straightforward. Resection of the asymptomatic primary may be advisable for two reasons. First, it may prevent complications from the tumor during chemotherapy, such as perforation or obstruction, or allow use of additional chemotherapeutic agents such as bevacizumab. Second, and more controversially, it may prolong survival even in the presence of unresectable metastatic disease.

The risk of tumor complications from an unresected primary tumor during chemotherapy has been widely variable in the literature (Table 1). Complications can include perforation, bleeding and obstruction. There have been particular concerns about the use of bevacizumab contributing to an increased risk of tumor perforation, leading some oncologists to avoid use of bevacizumab when there is an intact primary tumor. Other authors have not found this to be the case and have recommended use of bevacizumab with an intact primary tumor [18].

Resection of the primary has its own risks. The risk of mortality with resection of the primary has been found to be between 1.6 and 4.6 % [19, 20]. Resection of the primary tumor delays initiation of systemic therapy, particularly if postoperative complications occur, potentially allowing progression of metastases. Rarely, patients may still be at risk for complications from the primary tumor, such as

Table 1 Risk of complications from primary tumor during chemotherapy with unresectable metastatic disease

Author, year	Complications due to primary (%)
Benoist, 2005	15
Cellini, 2010	67
Galizia, 2008	30
Karoui, 2011	19
McCahill, 2012	14
Muratore, 2007	8.6
Ruo, 2003	29
Scoggins, 1999	8.7
Seo, 2010	19.9
Tebutt, 2003	9.8

obstruction or perforation, if there is recurrence of the tumor either at an anastomosis or at another site in the bowel. In fact, a recent Cochrane review concluded there was no significant reduction in the risk of complications when surgery as the initial therapy was compared to chemotherapy and/or radiation as the initial therapy [21]. These findings have lead several authors to recommend avoidance of resection for asymptomatic primary tumors, [18, 20, 22, 23] while others recommend resection, particularly for patients who are low-risk for surgery from a medical standpoint [24, 25].

Resection of the primary could also theoretically slow the progression of the disease by debulking the tumor, allowing chemotherapy to work more effectively on the remaining disease. Many studies have examined the possibility of a survival benefit with resection of the primary tumor, but these have been hampered by the strong influence of patient selection since these were retrospective studies. Often patients who were in better medical condition or those who were thought to have a possibility of cure with from a combination of resection and chemotherapy were chosen for resection, leading to a bias toward much more advanced disease in the nonresected subjects. Results of such studies have varied widely. For studies limited to patients with asymptomatic primary tumors and unresectable metastatic disease, some studies have shown a survival benefit while the majority have not (Table 2). The authors of these studies have been split on whether resection of the primary is beneficial. Some have advocated for this approach [26] whereas others have not [20, 27–29]. If the criteria are expanded so that studies that include symptomatic primaries or resectable metastatic disease are included (Table 3), the picture becomes even more clouded. In these studies, it is difficult to determine how much of the improvement in survival, if demonstrated, could be due to patients who are curable. Some multivariate analyses have found tumor resection to be an independent predictor of survival [30–32] while others have not [33]. A Cochrane review on the subject concluded there is no consistent improvement in overall survival with resection of the primary tumor [21].

Thus, retrospective data have been very limited in their ability to allow reliable conclusions about the role of resection of the primary due to issues with patient selection. Ideally, a randomized controlled trial could be done among patients with asymptomatic primaries and unresectable metastatic disease who are medically fit to undergo resection, thus eliminating these patient selection factors that have plagued retrospective studies. However, recruitment for such studies has been difficult, with at least two studies being closed due to lack of recruitment [34, 35]. This difficulty with recruitment likely relates to patients being unwilling to undergo surgery for unclear benefit, or care providers encouraging them to have resection due to the perceived risk of complications from the primary. There is currently another randomized controlled trial on this subject underway, [36] which one hopes will provide definitive data as to whether primary tumor resection is associated with decreased complications or lengthened survival.

Other important issues in these cases are quality of life and patient preferences. Since surgery can be associated with short-term decreases in quality of life, this could be a major consideration in patients who likely have a limited life expectancy.

Table 2 Case series evaluating resection of primary in unresectable metastatic colon and rectal cancer with asymptomatic primary tumors

Author, year	Number of patients	Follow up, months	Survival, months	Comments
Benoist, 2005				Difference in survival not significant
Resection of primary	32	Not stated	2-year OS: 44 %	
No resection	27		2-year OS: 41 %	
Galizia, 2008				$p = 0.03$ for difference in survival
Resection of primary	42	16	15	
No resection	23	12	12	
Ruo, 2003				$p < 0.001$ for difference in survival
Resection of primary	127	>80 % followed until death	16	
No resection	103		9	
Scoggins, 1999				Difference in survival not significant
Resection of primary	66	Not stated	14.5	
No resection	23		16.6	
Seo, 2010				Survival different in univariate but not multivariate analysis
Resection of primary	144	49	22.0	
No resection	83		14.0	
Tebutt, 2003				Difference in survival not significant in multivariate analysis
Resection of primary	280	30	14.0	
No resection	82	19	8.2	

Unless otherwise noted, follow up and survival numbers are reported as medians
OS overall survival

Patient preferences in this area could be examined with the time-trade-off method, where patients are given a hypothetical scenario where the typical postoperative course for surgery is described in detail and patients are asked if an increased survival of 6 months, for example, would lead them to choose surgery and its associated recovery in order to gain this survival benefit. The anticipated increase in survival is then lessened and the same question asked again, with the process repeated until the patient no longer reports they would be willing to have surgery for the anticipated survival benefit. Such a study could provide information as to whether most patients would consider resection of the primary, even if it were proven to be associated with some definite increase in survival.

Thus, it remains unclear whether resection of the primary tumor is associated with a decrease in complications from the primary tumor or an increase in survival. Patient preferences in this area have not been well studied and are likely to play a significant role in whether surgical intervention for the primary tumor is pursued.

Table 3 Studies evaluating resection of primary in metastatic colon and rectal cancer, resectable metastatic disease and symptomatic primaries included

Author, year	Number of patients	Follow up, months	Survival, months	Comments
Cellini, 2010				Difference in survival not significant
Staged primary and liver	13	23	50	
Synchronous primary and liver	30		54	
Primary only	22		32	
No resection	9		37	
Chan, 2010				
Resection of primary	286	Variable	14	
No resection	125		6	
Chew, 2012				Patients routinely received primary resection unless contraindication
Resection of primary	696	9	1-year cancer-spec.: 48.7 %	
No resection	22		1-year cancer-spec.: 9 %	
Cook, 2005				Analysis of the SEER database
Resection of primary	17,658	Not stated	11 colon, 16 rectal	
No resection	9,097		2 colon, 6 rectal	
Karoui, 2011				Resection independent predictor of survival in multivariate analysis
Resection of primary	85	19.7	30.7	
No resection	123		21.9	
Konyalian, 2007				Resection independent predictor of survival in multivariate analysis
Resection of primary	62	Not stated	12.3	
No resection	47		4.5	

Unless otherwise noted, follow up and survival numbers are reported as medians
SEER Surveillance, Epidemiology and End Results

3 Standard Versus Extended Lymph Node Resection for Colon and Rectal Cancer

Great emphasis has been placed on ensuring appropriate oncologic resection for colon and rectal cancer, with 12 nodes in the specimen being a generally accepted standard to ensure an adequate resection and accurate staging. This standard does not take into account factors that are associated with decreased lymph node number (such as radiation, left-sided resections or variations in pathology practice), [37] or whether an increased number of lymph nodes was obtained by resecting a greater length of bowel, a longer segment of the feeding vessel, or a more complete mesocolic/mesorectal excision. Some have advocated a more aggressive resection of the lymph nodes, beyond this numerical standard, for both colon cancer and for rectal cancer. It remains unclear whether this results in better oncologic outcomes.

3.1 Colon Cancer

For colon cancer, more aggressive resection is termed complete mesocolic excision (CME). For the right colon, this entails a Kocher maneuver with mobilization of the mesenteric root up to the base of the superior mesenteric artery, including dissection of the mesentery off of the uncinate process of the pancreas and duodenum. For the left colon, this involves takedown of the splenic flexure and resection of the transverse mesocolon at the lower edge of the pancreas [38]. In both cases, close attention is paid to maintaining an intact mesocolic fascia. Some authors also resect a greater length of colon as part of this approach [39, 40]. Similar to total mesorectal excision in rectal cancer, the theory is that maintaining intact embryologic planes and ensuring complete resection of the mesentery will improve oncologic outcomes.

Results of this approach have generally shown acceptable operative times, blood loss and postoperative complications [38, 41, 42]. CME has also been demonstrated to result in a greater incidence of an intact mesocolon and a greater number of lymph nodes resected [39, 40]. Attempts have been made to determine whether this results in improved oncologic outcomes. Hohenberger et al. [38] showed that among node-negative patients, those with resection of 28 or more lymph nodes had 96.3 % cancer-related 5-year survival versus 90.7 % if less than 28 lymph nodes were resected, but a similar analysis among node-positive patients was not significant. CME was the standard practice at that institution, so the differences in survival were not associated with whether CME was attempted. Other studies have shown improved outcomes with preservation of anatomic planes [43, 44] or more extensive resection [45]. However, it remains unclear whether there is a benefit in terms of survival or local recurrence. The primary problem is that individual centers tend to pursue either CME or standard resection exclusively, and there are therefore no appropriate patients to serve as comparators. Comparing outcomes from patients operated on at different centers introduces an increased risk that any differences observed are due to factors other than the surgical approach.

Conclusive evidence demonstrating whether there is a benefit to CME would require a randomized clinical trial of CME versus more standard resection. However, the number of patients required to demonstrate this difference could be prohibitive, depending on the endpoints chosen for the study. As an example, power calculations can be estimated using the local recurrence rate (4.8 %) and cancer-specific survival rate (85.2 %) from Weber et al.'s [42] study of 1,452 patients undergoing CME who were followed for at least 5 years. Assuming an 80 % power and a significance level of 0.05, 11,136 patients would be required to demonstrate a 25 % difference in local recurrence. In contrast, 792 patients would be required to demonstrate a 10 % difference in cancer-specific survival. While this latter example may represent a feasible number of patients to recruit to such a study, the number of patients required is exquisitely sensitive to the estimated difference in cancer-specific survival, and the 10 % difference estimate may be too high. Changing the estimated difference in cancer-specific survival to 5 % rather than 10 % increases the number of patients required to 2,614.

A more feasible approach may be a pathology-based study. CME could be performed in patients, and the surgeon could delineate which areas of the specimen they believe would have been removed in a standard resection and which areas were resected only as a result of the CME. It may be best to have two surgeons come to an agreement regarding these boundaries, to prevent the surgeon from under- or overestimating the amount of tissue that would have been removed with a standard resection, as Spasojevic et al. [46] found surprising lengths of artery remaining after what were reportedly standard resections with high ligation. The two areas of the specimen could then be dissected apart and processed separately. If additional nodal metastases or tumor deposits are found frequently in the additional tissue, this would lend more credence to the argument to perform a more extensive resection. If, however, metastasis is infrequent in the additional tissue, this would make it unlikely that CME contributes to a clinically significant difference in outcomes. A similar study, looking at the location of lymph node metastases in right-sided colon cancers, found less than 1 % of lymph node metastases were located more than 10 cm from the primary tumor (Fig. 1) [47].

3.2 Rectal Cancer

In contrast to colon cancer, in rectal cancer dissection along embryologic planes is accepted practice. However, controversy remains about whether more extensive lymph node dissection is of benefit. Particularly in Japan, a more aggressive

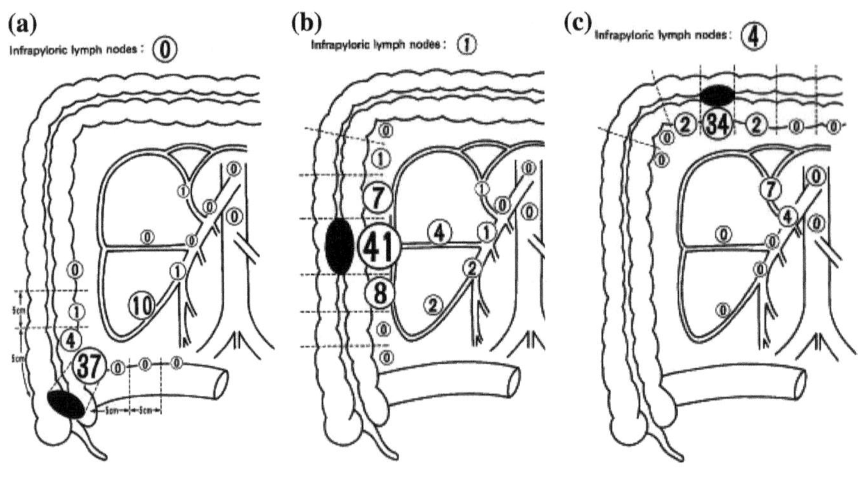

Fig. 1 Rates of lymph node metastases for cecal (**a**), ascending (**b**) and transverse colon cancers (**c**). From Toyota et al. [47]

resection is often used, including dissection of the lateral pelvic lymph nodes. This has been shown to result in increased survival [48, 49] in some studies, although other studies have shown no difference [50, 51]. A recent meta-analysis showed no difference in overall or disease-free survival (Fig. 2) [52].

There are a few issues that make it difficult to determine whether extended lymph node resection for rectal cancer is associated with a benefit. For the studies demonstrating a survival advantage with more aggressive lymph node resection, stage migration could be a confounding issue. More accurate staging due to a larger number of lymph nodes being resected could theoretically correctly classify some early stage III cancers that would have been erroneously classified as stage II, thus improving the survival of both stage II and stage III cancers as a whole, even if there is no actual survival benefit for extended lymph node resection. Another pertinent issue is the use of radiation. Many of these patients do not receive pre-operative chemotherapy and radiation. However, in other countries where preoperative radiation for node-positive rectal cancer is more common, such as the United States, extended node dissection is not standard practice. There is some evidence that these two approaches have similar effectiveness [53]. However, it is unclear whether adding extended node dissection to radiation may further improve outcomes. Finally, the average body mass index is generally much lower in countries which practice extended lymph node resection, raising the question of whether this technique can be generalized while maintaining the same results.

Whether lateral node dissection should be undertaken is particularly important because there can be significant adverse effects. In this dissection, the pelvic nerves

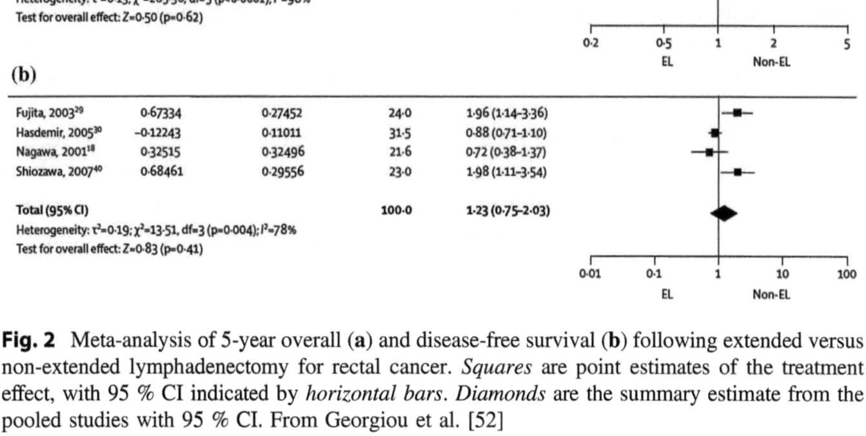

Fig. 2 Meta-analysis of 5-year overall (**a**) and disease-free survival (**b**) following extended versus non-extended lymphadenectomy for rectal cancer. *Squares* are point estimates of the treatment effect, with 95 % CI indicated by *horizontal bars*. *Diamonds* are the summary estimate from the pooled studies with 95 % CI. From Georgiou et al. [52]

are often damaged or even intentionally sacrificed, and this results in a very high incidence of urinary and sexual dysfunction [50, 54, 55]. For example, Akasu et al. [54] found that with unilateral or bilateral pelvis plexus sacrifice, rates of inability to have sexual intercourse at 1 year were 55 and 100 %, respectively. Urinary symptoms were present in 100 % of male and 90 % of female patients in one study, and 1 year after surgery 44 % of men and 17 % of women still required self-catheterization [55]. Lateral node dissection has also been associated with increased operative time [50, 52, 56] and blood loss [52, 56].

Ideally, a randomized controlled trial would determine whether extended lymph node resection contributes any additional benefit among patients who have undergone preoperative chemotherapy and radiation. Indeed, this study has already been performed by Nagawa et al. [57]. They found no difference in survival between patients undergoing a standard resection versus an extended lymph node resection after preoperative chemotherapy and radiation. However, only 45 patients were enrolled in this study, severely limiting its ability to detect a difference in survival. In addition, patients with evidence of lateral pelvic or para-aortic lymph node metastasis were excluded, although it seems this staging may have been done after chemotherapy and radiation were completed.

A more informative study may be obtained by selecting only patients who have evidence of lateral pelvic or para-aortic lymph node metastasis before chemotherapy and radiation, then randomizing them to standard versus extended lymph node resection after neoadjuvant therapy. Limiting this analysis to patients who are preoperatively known to have advanced nodal metastasis achieves two ends. One, it increases the likelihood of local recurrence [49] and therefore decreases the sample size needed to demonstrate a difference related to extended node dissection, similar to the discussion of CME for colon cancer. Second, it could help resolve the ethical dilemma of exposing patients to the high risk of urinary and sexual dysfunction associated with lateral node dissection; if patients are strongly suspected to have lateral node metastasis prior to radiation these risks may be more acceptable in light of an increased risk of poor outcome. Thus, the pertinent question seems to be not whether radiation or extended lymph node resection is preferable, but if extended resection can improve upon the outcomes already obtained with preoperative chemotherapy and radiation in cases of known lateral pelvic or para-aortic lymph node metastasis, and whether the combination of radiation and extended lymph node resection would lead to prohibitively severe morbidity.

While extended lymph node resection for colon and rectal cancer seems as if it would be preferable, current data do not allow conclusions to be drawn about whether this approach has benefits that would justify any increase in operative time or complications. A variety of methods may be used to provide additional data in this area.

4 Robotic Versus Laparoscopic Resection for Colorectal Cancer

When reports of laparoscopic colon and rectal resection first appeared, the relative merits of laparoscopic and open surgery were hotly debated. Many surgeons now believe that laparoscopic resection is associated with improved postoperative recovery and similar oncologic outcomes, but even so both open and laparoscopic surgery continue to have their proponents, and only 10.5 % of elective colon resections in the United States were performed laparoscopically as recently as 2007 [58]. The appearance of robotic surgery has renewed the debate regarding the optimal approach to colorectal cancer resections.

Potential benefits of the robotic approach center around the ability to have seven degrees of freedom in movement, and the increased visibility resulting from a three-dimensional view and greater magnification (Table 4). Particularly in the pelvis, where dissection can be quite difficult due to the bony pelvis, patient obesity and a bulky tumor, these may be significant advantages. Laparoscopic resections in this area can be difficult due to the fulcrum effect of the laparoscopic instruments on the sacral promontory. The robot also stabilizes physiologic tremor. Robotic surgery has thus been hypothesized to result in a better surgical specimen, with some evidence to support this [59].

Potential drawbacks of the robotic approach include operative time and cost. The majority of studies have found that robotic surgery is associated with increased operative times, which can range from a difference of 42–64 min for a low anterior or abdominoperineal resection [60–67]. Only a few studies have shown operative times to be similar, [68–71] and one showed a decreased operative time for robotic compared to laparoscopic low anterior resections [72]. Increased operative time exposes patients to increased risk of certain complications, in particular venous thromboembolism [73]. In addition, there are some technical drawbacks of the robot. Colorectal resections often encompass dissection over a large area of the abdomen, such as from the splenic flexure to the pelvis, which can result in the need to re-dock the robot several times to perform the dissection robotically. More

Table 4 Potential advantages of robotic colorectal surgery as compared to laparoscopic surgery

Potential advantages of robotic surgery
Increased degrees of freedom and "wristed" movements
Improved visualization due to magnification and steady camera
Stabilization of physiologic tremor
Absence of fulcrum effect during mesorectal dissection
Potential advantages of laparoscopic surgery
Decreased operative time
Decreased expense
Greater familiarity with technique among surgeons
Haptic feedback

instruments may be needed than there are available robotic arms, leading some surgeons to use a laparoscopic port and an assistant during the robotic dissection. Because of these factors, surgeons often approach a portion of the operation laparoscopically or through an open incision, and there is great variation in how individual steps of the operation are completed (Table 5).

Four studies have addressed the cost of the robot in comparison to laparoscopy, and all have found the robotic approach to be more expensive. Delaney et al. [60] found that equipment cost was $350 greater in robotic resections (in 2003 dollars) and did not account for the costs of maintenance or depreciation; robot maintenance can be approximately $100,000 per year. DeSouza et al. [61] compared 40 robotic and 135 laparoscopic right colectomies and found total cost was $15,192.00 for robotic cases versus $12,361.50 for laparoscopic cases. Similarly, a randomized controlled trial of right colectomies by Park et al. [65] found the cost to be higher with robotic resections versus laparoscopy ($12,235 vs. $10,320). Tyler et al. [73] reviewed the Nationwide Inpatient Sample and found robotic colon resections cost an average of $3,424 more than laparoscopic resections.

Perioperative results are similar in laparoscopic and robotic cases. Most studies have found no difference in intraoperative complications, [62, 66, 73] estimated blood loss, [60, 61, 65, 66, 68, 70, 72] postoperative complications, [61, 62, 64–66, 68–70, 72–74] anastomotic leak rate, [64, 72] conversion rate, [61, 62, 64–66, 69] readmission [66, 68] and length of stay [60–62, 65, 68, 70, 73, 74]. However, a few studies have found differences in these outcomes, including decreased conversion rates with the robot, [68, 74] decreased blood loss in robotic cases [62] and decreased length of stay for robotic compared to laparoscopic but not hand-assisted laparoscopic cases [66].

Oncologic results have generally been found to be equivalent between the laparoscopic and robotic approaches (Table 6). Both approaches result in a similar number of lymph nodes resected, rates of positive margins and survival data. Although the robotic approach has been promoted as ensuring a more complete mesocolic excision, there is little data to support this claim nor any impact of a more complete excision on survival or local recurrence.

Obtaining high-quality data in this area has been difficult. Many of the currently published studies are case series or case-matched studies that document the early experience with robotic colorectal resections and therefore may not be representative of current results. Few have long-term follow up to assess oncologic outcomes, and most of these do not go beyond two- to three-year follow up. Therefore, even in the absence of a more rigorous study such as a randomized controlled trial, more current case-matched studies with longer follow up could provide valuable information on the results of robotic colon and rectal surgery now that some of the initial learning curve has passed. Prior to embarking on additional prospective studies, a few considerations should be taken into account. First, any potential study should split resections that include a rectal dissection from those that do not, as rectal dissection is where the majority of the potential benefit from the robotic approach appears to lie. It would also be useful if a consensus approach to dissection, resection and anastomosis on the left side could be developed, given the

Table 5 Differences in robotic technique for left-sided resections

Author, year	Stage of operation					Comments
	Transection of vessels	Flexure mobilization	Rectal dissection	Rectal transection	Anastomosis	
Baek, 2013	R	R	R	R	R or TA	
Bianchi, 2010	R	25 % L 75 % R	R	R	L	
Choi, 2009	R	R	R	L	L	Laparoscopy for initial exposure
D'Annibale, 2004	R	R	R	R	L or TA	
Delaney, 2003	R	R	R	O	O	Laparoscopy for takedown of adhesions
DeSouza, 2011	L (R if APR)	L (R if APR)	R	R or TA	R or TA	
Kwak, 2011	R	R	R	L	L	Laparoscopy for initial exposure
Luca, 2009	R	R	R	R	R	
Patriti, 2009	L	L	R	R	R? or TA	Unclear whether anastomosis was R or L
Pigazzi, 2010	L	L	R	L	R?	
Ragupathi, 2011	R	L	R	R	R	

R robotic, *L* laparoscopic, *O* open, *TA* transanal

Table 6 Oncologic outcomes in robotic and laparoscopic colorectal cancer resections

Author, year	Lymph nodes, mean		Positive circumferential margin (%)		Survival	
	Robotic	Laparoscopic	Robotic	Laparoscopic	Robotic	Laparoscopic
Baek, 2013	10.6	14.1	2.1	8.1	3-year OS 86.5 %	3-year OS 90.7 %
Baik, 2013 [76]	15.6	n/a	5.7	n/a	3-year OS 93.1 %	n/a
Bianchi, 2010	18	17	0	4.0		
Choi, 2009 [77]	20.6	n/a	2.0	n/a		
D'Annibale, 2004	17	16	0	0		
deSouza, 2011	15.0	16.8	0	5.9		
deSouza, 2010	14	n/a	0	n/a		
Kwak, 2011	20	21	0.9	0	Recurrence 5.5 % over median 17 months	Recurrence 5.6 % over median 13 months
Luca, 2009	18.5	n/a	0	n/a		
Patel, 2011	17.3	20.9	0	0		
Patriti, 2009	10.3	11.2	0	0	No difference in OS or DS over mean follow up of 29 (robotic) and 19 months (laparoscopic)	
Pigazzi, 2010 [78]	14.1	n/a	0.7	n/a	Robotic only; 3-year overall survival 97 % with no local recurrence at mean follow up of 17 months	

No differences in this table were significant at $p < 0.05$ or less
OS overall survival

variation in technique detailed in Table 5. Even if a study were to examine robotic versus laparoscopic left-sided resections, it would be difficult to generalize the data to robotic resections performed by other surgeons, given the variations in technique. A difference in the number of re-dockings required, the technique of anastomosis, or the use of laparoscopy for a portion of the procedure can greatly affect the operative times, cost and complications associated with robotic surgery. Of course, a randomized controlled trial would provide even more reliable information on the outcomes of these two approaches. There is currently a randomized controlled trial entitled "Robotic versus Laparoscopic Resection for Rectal Cancer" (ROLARR) which will attempt to answer these questions for rectal cancer [75]. This study will include quality of life and cost data to allow a cost-effectiveness analysis to be performed. Cost-effectiveness analysis lends itself particularly well toward comparing robotic and laparoscopic colorectal resections for cancer. Since most studies have found similar outcomes, the question becomes whether the difference in cost between laparoscopic and robotic resections is justified by an improvement in quality of life.

Robotic and laparoscopic surgery in colorectal resections thus have much more similar results than a similar comparison between laparoscopic and open resection, but a much greater difference in cost and operative times. Areas of future research should therefore focus on quality of life and cost in addition to surgical and oncologic outcomes to provide information on whether robotic surgery is the preferred approach in colon and rectal cancer.

5 Conclusion

Surgical treatment in colon and rectal cancer has become more standardized, but there remain a number of areas of controversy, ranging from surgical treatment of HNPCC to the role of robotic surgery, where the appropriate choices are not clear. Further study in these areas can be accomplished by a variety of approaches, with certain methods being more likely than others to provide a solid evidence base for future surgical practice.

References

1. Fitzgibbons RJ Jr, Lynch HT, Stanislav GV, Watson PA, Lanspa SJ, Marcus JN et al (1987) Recognition and treatment of patients with hereditary nonpolyposis colon cancer (lynch syndromes i and ii). Ann Surg 206:289–295
2. Kalady MF, Lipman J, McGannon E, Church JM (2012) Risk of colonic neoplasia after proctectomy for rectal cancer in hereditary nonpolyposis colorectal cancer. Ann Surg 255:1121–1125
3. Rijcken FE, Hollema H, Kleibeuker JH (2002) Proximal adenomas in hereditary non-polyposis colorectal cancer are prone to rapid malignant transformation. Gut 50:382–386

4. Jarvinen HJ, Aarnio M, Mustonen H, Aktan-Collan K, Aaltonen LA, Peltomaki P et al (2000) Controlled 15-year trial on screening for colorectal cancer in families with hereditary nonpolyposis colorectal cancer. Gastroenterology 118:829–834
5. Kalady MF, McGannon E, Vogel JD, Manilich E, Fazio VW, Church JM (2010) Risk of colorectal adenoma and carcinoma after colectomy for colorectal cancer in patients meeting Amsterdam criteria. Ann Surg 252:507–511 discussion 511–503
6. Vasen HF, Abdirahman M, Brohet R, Langers AM, Kleibeuker JH, van Kouwen M et al (2010) One to 2-year surveillance intervals reduce risk of colorectal cancer in families with lynch syndrome. Gastroenterology 138:2300–2306
7. Stoffel EM, Turgeon DK, Stockwell DH, Zhao L, Normolle DP, Tuck MK et al (2008) Missed adenomas during colonoscopic surveillance in individuals with lynch syndrome (hereditary nonpolyposis colorectal cancer). Cancer Prev Res 1:470–475
8. Network NCC (2014) Nccn clinical practice guidlines in oncology: colon cancer
9. Mecklin JP, Jarvinen H (1993) Treatment and follow-up strategies in hereditary nonpolyposis colorectal carcinoma. Dis Colon Rectum 36:927–929
10. Van Dalen R, Church J, McGannon E, Fay S, Burke C, Clark B (2003) Patterns of surgery in patients belonging to amsterdam-positive families. Dis Colon Rectum 46:617–620
11. Maeda T, Cannom RR, Beart RW Jr, Etzioni DA (2010) Decision model of segmental compared with total abdominal colectomy for colon cancer in hereditary nonpolyposis colorectal cancer. J Clin Oncol (official journal of the American Society of Clinical Oncology) 28:1175–1180
12. de Vos tot Nederveen Cappel WH, Buskens E, van Duijvendijk P, Cats A, Menko FH, Griffioen G, et al (2003) Decision analysis in the surgical treatment of colorectal cancer due to a mismatch repair gene defect. Gut 52:1752–1755
13. Lee JS, Petrelli NJ, Rodriguez-Bigas MA (2001) Rectal cancer in hereditary nonpolyposis colorectal cancer. Am J Surg 181:207–210
14. Kalady MF (2011) Surgical management of hereditary nonpolyposis colorectal cancer. Adv Surg 45:265–274
15. Thorson AG, Faria J (2000) Familial adenomatous polyposis, hereditary nonpolyposis colon cancer, and familial risk: what are the implications for the surgeon? Surg Oncol Clin N Am 9:683–697 discussion 699–701
16. Syngal S, Weeks JC, Schrag D, Garber JE, Kuntz KM (1998) Benefits of colonoscopic surveillance and prophylactic colectomy in patients with hereditary nonpolyposis colorectal cancer mutations. Ann Intern Med 129:787–796
17. Manfredi S, Lepage C, Hatem C, Coatmeur O, Faivre J, Bouvier AM (2006) Epidemiology and management of liver metastases from colorectal cancer. Ann Surg 244:254–259
18. McCahill LE, Yothers G, Sharif S, Petrelli NJ, Lai LL, Bechar N et al (2012) Primary mfolfox6 plus bevacizumab without resection of the primary tumor for patients presenting with surgically unresectable metastatic colon cancer and an intact asymptomatic colon cancer: definitive analysis of nsabp trial c-10. Journal Clin Oncol (official journal of the American Society of Clinical Oncology) 30:3223–3228
19. Ruo L, Gougoutas C, Paty PB, Guillem JG, Cohen AM, Wong WD (2003) Elective bowel resection for incurable stage iv colorectal cancer: Prognostic variables for asymptomatic patients. J Am Coll Surg 196:722–728
20. Scoggins CR, Meszoely IM, Blanke CD, Beauchamp RD, Leach SD (1999) Nonoperative management of primary colorectal cancer in patients with stage iv disease. Ann Surg Oncol 6:651–657
21. Cirocchi R, Trastulli S, Abraha I, Vettoretto N, Boselli C, Montedori A et al (2012) Non-resection versus resection for an asymptomatic primary tumour in patients with unresectable stage iv colorectal cancer. Cochrane Database Syst Rev 8:CD008997
22. Muratore A, Zorzi D, Bouzari H, Amisano M, Massucco P, Sperti E et al (2007) Asymptomatic colorectal cancer with un-resectable liver metastases: immediate colorectal resection or up-front systemic chemotherapy? Ann Surg Oncol 14:766–770

23. Stelzner S, Hellmich G, Koch R, Ludwig K (2005) Factors predicting survival in stage iv colorectal carcinoma patients after palliative treatment: a multivariate analysis. J Surg Oncol 89:211–217
24. Cellini C, Hunt SR, Fleshman JW, Birnbaum EH, Bierhals AJ, Mutch MG (2010) Stage iv rectal cancer with liver metastases: is there a benefit to resection of the primary tumor? World J Surg 34:1102–1108
25. Vibert E, Bretagnol F, Alves A, Pocard M, Valleur P, Panis Y (2007) Multivariate analysis of predictive factors for early postoperative death after colorectal surgery in patients with colorectal cancer and synchronous unresectable liver metastases. Dis Colon Rectum 50:1776–1782
26. Galizia G, Lieto E, Orditura M, Castellano P, Imperatore V, Pinto M et al (2008) First-line chemotherapy vs bowel tumor resection plus chemotherapy for patients with unresectable synchronous colorectal hepatic metastases. Arch Surg 143:352–358 discussion 358
27. Benoist S, Pautrat K, Mitry E, Rougier P, Penna C, Nordlinger B (2005) Treatment strategy for patients with colorectal cancer and synchronous irresectable liver metastases. Br J Sur 92:1155–1160
28. Seo GJ, Park JW, Yoo SB, Kim SY, Choi HS, Chang HJ et al (2010) Intestinal complications after palliative treatment for asymptomatic patients with unresectable stage iv colorectal cancer. J Surg Oncol 102:94–99
29. Tebbutt NC, Norman AR, Cunningham D, Hill ME, Tait D, Oates J et al (2003) Intestinal complications after chemotherapy for patients with unresected primary colorectal cancer and synchronous metastases. Gut 52:568–573
30. Platell C, Ng S, O'Bichere A, Tebbutt N (2011) Changing management and survival in patients with stage iv colorectal cancer. Dis Colon Rectum 54:214–219
31. Karoui M, Roudot-Thoraval F, Mesli F, Mitry E, Aparicio T, Des Guetz G et al (2011) Primary colectomy in patients with stage iv colon cancer and unresectable distant metastases improves overall survival: results of a multicentric study. Dis Colon Rectum 54:930–938
32. Konyalian VR, Rosing DK, Haukoos JS, Dixon MR, Sinow R, Bhaheetharan S et al (2007) The role of primary tumour resection in patients with stage iv colorectal cancer. Colorectal Dis Official J Assoc Coloproctol Great Br Irel 9:430–437
33. Zhang S, Gao F, Luo J, Yang J (2010) Prognostic factors in survival of colorectal cancer patients with synchronous liver metastasis. Colorectal Dis Official J Assoc Coloproctol Great Br Irel 12:754–761
34. Obichere A (2012) Chemotherapy with or without surgery in treating patients with metastatic colorectal cancer that cannot be removed by surgery. Clinicaltrials. Gov study number nct01086618
35. Platell C (2012) A randomised phase iii multicenter trial evaluating the role of palliative surgical resection of the primary tumour in patients with metastatic colorectal cancer. Actrn12609000680268
36. Rahbari NN, Lordick F, Fink C, Bork U, Stange A, Jager D et al (2012) Resection of the primary tumour versus no resection prior to systemic therapy in patients with colon cancer and synchronous unresectable metastases (uicc stage iv): synchronous–a randomised controlled multicentre trial (isrctn30964555). BMC Cancer 12:142
37. Baxter NN, Virnig DJ, Rothenberger DA, Morris AM, Jessurun J, Virnig BA (2005) Lymph node evaluation in colorectal cancer patients: a population-based study. J Natl Cancer Inst 97:219–225
38. Hohenberger W, Weber K, Matzel K, Papadopoulos T, Merkel S (2009) Standardized surgery for colonic cancer: complete mesocolic excision and central ligation–technical notes and outcome. Colorectal Dis Official J Assoc Coloproctol Great Br Irel 11:354–364 discussion 364–355
39. West NP, Kobayashi H, Takahashi K, Perrakis A, Weber K, Hohenberger W et al (2012) Understanding optimal colonic cancer surgery: comparison of japanese d3 resection and european complete mesocolic excision with central vascular ligation. J Clin Oncol (official journal of the American Society of Clinical Oncology) 30:1763–1769

40. West NP, Hohenberger W, Weber K, Perrakis A, Finan PJ, Quirke P (2010) Complete mesocolic excision with central vascular ligation produces an oncologically superior specimen compared with standard surgery for carcinoma of the colon. J Clin Oncol (official journal of the American Society of Clinical Oncology) 28:272–278
41. Adamina M, Manwaring ML, Park KJ, Delaney CP (2012) Laparoscopic complete mesocolic excision for right colon cancer. Surg Endosc 26:2976–2980
42. Weber K, Merkel S, Perrakis A, Hohenberger W (2013) Is there a disadvantage to radical lymph node dissection in colon cancer? Int J Colorectal Dis 28:217–226
43. Bokey EL, Chapuis PH, Dent OF, Mander BJ, Bissett IP, Newland RC (2003) Surgical technique and survival in patients having a curative resection for colon cancer. Dis Colon Rectum 46:860–866
44. West NP, Morris EJ, Rotimi O, Cairns A, Finan PJ, Quirke P (2008) Pathology grading of colon cancer surgical resection and its association with survival: a retrospective observational study. Lancet Oncol 9:857–865
45. Jagoditsch M, Lisborg PH, Jatzko GR, Wette V, Kropfitsch G, Denk H et al (2000) Long-term prognosis for colon cancer related to consistent radical surgery: multivariate analysis of clinical, surgical, and pathologic variables. World J Surg 24:1264–1270
46. Spasojevic M, Stimec BV, Gronvold LB, Nesgaard JM, Edwin B, Ignjatovic D (2011) The anatomical and surgical consequences of right colectomy for cancer. Dis Colon Rectum 54:1503–1509
47. Toyota S, Ohta H, Anazawa S (1995) Rationale for extent of lymph node dissection for right colon cancer. Dis Colon Rectum 38:705–711
48. Dong XS, Xu HT, Yu ZW, Liu M, Cu BB, Zhao P et al (2003) Effect of extended radical resection for rectal cancer. World J Gastroenterol WJG 9:970–973
49. Shiozawa M, Akaike M, Yamada R, Godai T, Yamamoto N, Saito H et al (2007) Lateral lymph node dissection for lower rectal cancer. Hepatogastroenterology 54:1066–1070
50. Col C, Hasdemir O, Yalcin E, Guzel H, Tunc G, Bilgen K et al (2005) The assessment of urinary function following extended lymph node dissection for colorectal cancer. Eur J Surg Oncolo Journal Eur Soc Sur Oncol Br Assoc Sur Oncol 31:237–241
51. Hasdemir O, Col C, Yalcin E, Tunc G, Bilgen K, Kucukpinar T (2005) Local recurrence and survival rates after extended systematic lymph-node dissection for surgical treatment of rectal cancer. Hepatogastroenterology 52:455–459
52. Georgiou P, Tan E, Gouvas N, Antoniou A, Brown G, Nicholls RJ et al (2009) Extended lymphadenectomy versus conventional surgery for rectal cancer: a meta-analysis. Lancet Oncol 10:1053–1062
53. Watanabe T, Tsurita G, Muto T, Sawada T, Sunouchi K, Higuchi Y et al (2002) Extended lymphadenectomy and preoperative radiotherapy for lower rectal cancers. Surgery 132:27–33
54. Akasu T, Sugihara K, Moriya Y (2009) Male urinary and sexual functions after mesorectal excision alone or in combination with extended lateral pelvic lymph node dissection for rectal cancer. Ann Surg Oncol 16:2779–2786
55. Matsuoka N, Moriya Y, Akasu T, Fujita S (2001) Long-term outcome of urinary function after extended lymphadenectomy in patients with distal rectal cancer. Eur J Sur Oncol J Eur Soc Sur Oncol Br Assoc Sur Oncol 27:165–169
56. Moriya Y, Sugihara K, Akasu T, Fujita S (1997) Importance of extended lymphadenectomy with lateral node dissection for advanced lower rectal cancer. World J Surg 21:728–732
57. Nagawa H, Muto T, Sunouchi K, Higuchi Y, Tsurita G, Watanabe T et al (2001) Randomized, controlled trial of lateral node dissectionvs. nerve-preserving resection in patients with rectal cancer after preoperative radiotherapy. Dis Colon Rectum 44:1274–1280
58. Rea JD, Cone MM, Diggs BS, Deveney KE, Lu KC, Herzig DO (2011) Utilization of laparoscopic colectomy in the United States before and after the clinical outcomes of surgical therapy study group trial. Ann Surg 254:281–288
59. Luca F, Cenciarelli S, Valvo M, Pozzi S, Faso FL, Ravizza D et al (2009) Full robotic left colon and rectal cancer resection: technique and early outcome. Ann Surg Oncol 16:1274–1278

60. Delaney CP, Lynch AC, Senagore AJ, Fazio VW (2003) Comparison of robotically performed and traditional laparoscopic colorectal surgery. Dis Colon Rectum 46:1633–1639
61. deSouza AL, Prasad LM, Park JJ, Marecik SJ, Blumetti J, Abcarian H (2010) Robotic assistance in right hemicolectomy: is there a role? Dis Colon Rectum 53:1000–1006
62. deSouza AL, Prasad LM, Ricci J, Park JJ, Marecik SJ, Zimmern A et al (2011) A comparison of open and robotic total mesorectal excision for rectal adenocarcinoma. Dis Colon Rectum 54:275–282
63. Fung AK, Aly EH (2013) Robotic colonic surgery: is it advisable to commence a new learning curve? Dis Colon Rectum 56:786–796
64. Kwak JM, Kim SH, Kim J, Son DN, Baek SJ, Cho JS (2011) Robotic versus laparoscopic resection of rectal cancer: short-term outcomes of a case-control study. Dis Colon Rectum 54:151–156
65. Park JS, Choi GS, Park SY, Kim HJ, Ryuk JP (2012) Randomized clinical trial of robot-assisted versus standard laparoscopic right colectomy. The British journal of surgery. 99:1219–1226
66. Patel CB, Ragupathi M, Ramos-Valadez DI, Haas EM (2011) A three-arm (laparoscopic, hand-assisted, and robotic) matched-case analysis of intraoperative and postoperative outcomes in minimally invasive colorectal surgery. Dis Colon Rectum 54:144–150
67. Scarpinata R, Aly EH (2013) Does robotic rectal cancer surgery offer improved early postoperative outcomes? Dis Colon Rectum 56:253–262
68. Baek SJ, Al-Asari S, Jeong DH, Hur H, Min BS, Baik SH et al (2013) Robotic versus laparoscopic coloanal anastomosis with or without intersphincteric resection for rectal cancer. Surg Endosc 27:4157–4163
69. Bianchi PP, Ceriani C, Locatelli A, Spinoglio G, Zampino MG, Sonzogni A et al (2010) Robotic versus laparoscopic total mesorectal excision for rectal cancer: a comparative analysis of oncological safety and short-term outcomes. Surg Endosc 24:2888–2894
70. D'Annibale A, Morpurgo E, Fiscon V, Trevisan P, Sovernigo G, Orsini C et al (2004) Robotic and laparoscopic surgery for treatment of colorectal diseases. Dis Colon Rectum 47:2162–2168
71. Trastulli S, Desiderio J, Farinacci F, Ricci F, Listorti C, Cirocchi R et al (2013) Robotic right colectomy for cancer with intracorporeal anastomosis: short-term outcomes from a single institution. Int J Colorectal Dis 28:807–814
72. Patriti A, Ceccarelli G, Bartoli A, Spaziani A, Biancafarina A, Casciola L (2009) Short- and medium-term outcome of robot-assisted and traditional laparoscopic rectal resection. JSLS J Soc Laparoendosc Surg/Soc Laparoendosc Surg 13:176–183
73. Tyler JA, Fox JP, Desai MM, Perry WB, Glasgow SC (2013) Outcomes and costs associated with robotic colectomy in the minimally invasive era. Dis Colon Rectum 56:458–466
74. Trastulli S, Farinella E, Cirocchi R, Cavaliere D, Avenia N, Sciannameo F et al (2012) Robotic resection compared with laparoscopic rectal resection for cancer: systematic review and meta-analysis of short-term outcome. Colorectal Dis Official J Assoc Coloproctol Great Br Irel 14: e134–e156
75. Robotic versus laparoscopic resection for rectal cancer (rolarr) trial. Online at http://ctru.Leeds.Ac.Uk/rolarr
76. Baik SH, Kim NK, Lim DR, Hur H, Min BS, Lee KY (2013) Oncologic outcomes and perioperative clinicopathologic results after robot-assisted tumor-specific mesorectal excision for rectal cancer. Ann Surg Oncol 20:2625–2632
77. Choi DJ, Kim SH, Lee PJ, Kim J, Woo SU (2009) Single-stage totally robotic dissection for rectal cancer surgery: technique and short-term outcome in 50 consecutive patients. Dis Colon Rectum 52:1824–1830
78. Pigazzi A, Luca F, Patriti A, Valvo M, Ceccarelli G, Casciola L et al (2010) Multicentric study on robotic tumor-specific mesorectal excision for the treatment of rectal cancer. Ann Surg Oncol 17:1614–1620

60. Delaney CP, Lynch AC, Senagore AJ, Fazio VW (2003) Comparison of robotically performed and traditional laparoscopic colorectal surgery. Dis Colon Rectum 46:1633–1639
61. deSouza AL, Prasad LM, Park JJ, Marecik SJ, Blumetti J, Abcarian H (2010) Robotic assistance in right hemicolectomy: is there a role? Dis Colon Rectum 53:1000–1006
62. deSouza AL, Prasad LM, Ricci J, Park JJ, Marecik SJ, Zimmern A et al (2011) A comparison of open and robotic total mesorectal excision for rectal adenocarcinoma. Dis Colon Rectum 54:275–282
63. Kang SK, [illegible] Robotic colorectal surgery [illegible] Colon Rectum [illegible]

Research Gaps in Pancreatic Cancer Research and Comparative Effectiveness Research Methodologies

Haejin In and Mitchell C. Posner

Abstract

Despite advances in cancer care, pancreatic adenocarcinoma remains one of the most lethal tumors. Most patients with pancreatic cancer are diagnosed with late stage disease, and approximately 6 % of patients are alive 5 years after diagnosis. Of the 10–20 % of patients who are candidates for resection and multi-modality therapy, most will succumb to the disease with 5-year survival rates only reaching approximately 25 % (Lim et al. in Annals of surgery 237(1):74–85, 2003 [1]; Trede et al. in Annals of surgery 211(4):447–458, 1990 [2]; Crist et al. in Annals of surgery 206(3):358–365, 1987 [3]). Clearly, there is a need to improve the management of this disease. To identify gaps in research and formulate strategies to address these issues, we designed a framework to encompass the scope of research for pancreatic cancer. In this chapter, we will examine each topic heading within this framework for gaps in knowledge and present research strategies focusing on diverse comparative effectiveness research (CER) methodologies to address the identified gaps.

Keywords

Pancreatic cancer research · Pancreatic cancer treatment · Comparative effectiveness research · Databases · Tumor registries · Big data · Adaptive clinical trials · Expertise-based clinical trials

H. In (✉)
Departments of Surgery and Epidemiology, Albert Einstein College of Medicine, Bronx, NY, USA
e-mail: Haejin.In@einstein.yu.edu

M.C. Posner
Division of Surgical Oncology, Department of Surgery, University of Chicago, Chicago, IL, USA

K.Y. Bilimoria et al. (eds.), *Comparative Effectiveness in Surgical Oncology*, Cancer Treatment and Research 164, DOI 10.1007/978-3-319-12553-4_10

Contents

1 Pancreas Cancer Research Framework

The management of a patient with pancreatic cancer involves two interrelated, yet separate components of care. The first component is care directly related to cancer such as surgery, chemotherapy and radiation. The second component is care of a patient whose tumor specifically resides in the pancreas, such as the surgical technique for pancreas resection and patient selection for pancreatic surgery. Research of pancreatic cancer parallels these aspects of care, and utilizes various research methodologies that allow these research topics to be explored (Fig. 1). Pancreas research methodologies will be discussed in the context of addressing research gaps.

1.1 Cancer Directed Care

Cancer directed care concerns issues of cancer detection, tumor factors, tumor targeted treatments, and subsequent cancer care.

Cancer detection involves topics such as screening, accurate diagnosis of pancreatic disease, and confirmation of malignancy. Research in this area includes identification of appropriate groups for screening, improvement of screening modalities, and development of innovative methods to detect malignancy in certain pancreatic lesions, such as small pancreatic lesions (<1 cm) or pancreatic cystic disease.

Tumor factors relate to the topics of tumor behavior and the interaction between the tumor and treatments. Research in this field includes defining tumor characteristics that have prognostic and predictive value. Identification of novel diagnostic biomarkers might improve our ability to predict outcomes and improve our ability to

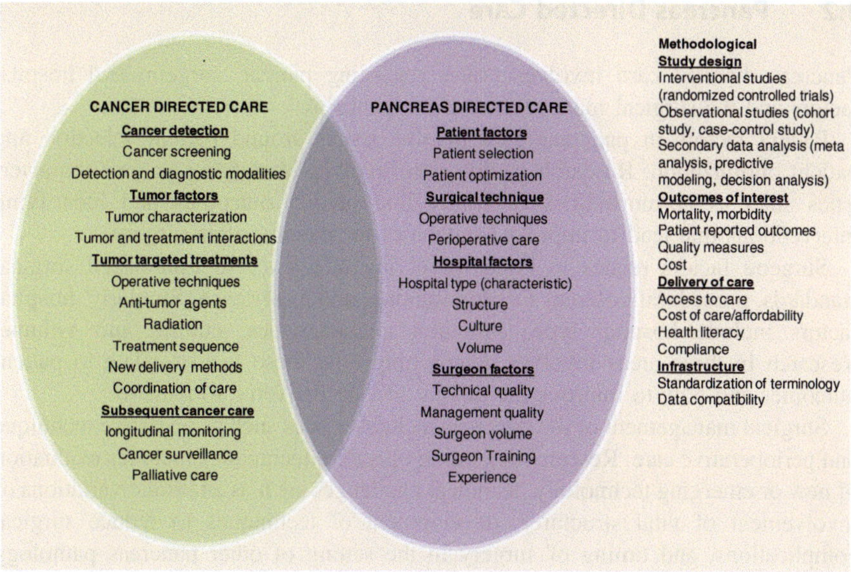

Fig. 1 Pancreas cancer research framework

balance the harms and benefit of treatments. Discovery of markers that predict outcome response to certain agents will increase the efficiency of treatment delivery.

Research pertaining to tumor-directed therapy involves identification of targeted agents, their application such as the sequence of administration (neoadjuvant vs. adjuvant therapy), the optimal combination of treatments and the role and extent of surgery.

Subsequent cancer care relates to issues involving cancer surveillance and palliative care. Research within these topics involves developing methods to improve longitudinal tracking of patients, defining the optimal method and timing of cancer surveillance, developing treatments for late stage cancer symptoms, and improving measurement of relevant outcomes in the palliative setting [survival vs. quality of life (QOL)].

Of these topics in cancer directed care, six high priority research gaps have been identified and will be discussed in this chapter. The topics are as follows;

1. Optimal chemotherapy regimens
2. Value of radiotherapy
3. Role of pre- versus peri- versus post-operative therapy
4. Value of vascular and multi-visceral resection
5. Resectable versus borderline resectable versus locally advanced unresectable tumors
6. Management of intraductal papillary mucinous neoplasm (IPMN)

1.2 Pancreas Directed Care

Pancreas directed care involves issues regarding patient, surgeon and hospital factors and the surgical management of the pancreas.

Patient factors in pancreas care involve issues around patient selection and patient optimization. Research in this area involves identifying patient characteristics such as co-morbidities or frailty that predict outcomes and identifying interventions that lead to improved outcomes for patients after surgery.

Surgeon factors relates to issues involving adherence to established surgical standards, procedural volume, surgeon training, and experience. Similarly, hospital factors include hospital type, structural characteristics, culture and volume. Research in these areas involves determining how these factors relate to patient outcomes and how to improve the quality of care delivered to patients.

Surgical management of the pancreas includes issues such as operative technique and perioperative care. Research regarding operative techniques includes evaluation of new or emerging technology, technical challenges such as anatomic variations or involvement of vital structures, development of techniques to reduce surgical complications, and timing of surgery in the setting of other pancreas pathology (such as acute pancreatitis). Research pertaining to perioperative care includes issues such as pre-operative patient management, coordination of the surgical team, immediate post-operative care plan, and rapid surgical recovery strategies.

Of these topics in pancreas directed care, Three high priority research gaps have been identified and will be discussed in this chapter. The topics are as follows;

1. Anastomotic technique and prevention of pancreatic fistula
2. Use of peritoneal drains, octreotide, and prokinetic agents following pancreaticoduodenectomy
3. Minimally invasive surgery versus open surgery

2 Research Gaps in Cancer Directed Care

2.1 Optimal Chemotherapy Regimens

Trials have demonstrated modest improvements in survival with the administration of adjuvant therapy, mostly consisting of 5-fluorouracil (5-FU) or gemcitabine, with or without radiation (Table 1). While the benefit of adjuvant therapy compared to surgery alone has been clearly demonstrated, the optimal regimen remains in question. Additionally, while new therapeutic agents such as FOLFIRINOX (leucovorin, 5-FU, irinotecan and oxaliplatin) and gemcitabine with nab-paclitaxel have proved effective in the metastatic setting [4, 5], their effectiveness in the adjuvant setting has, as of yet, not been determined.

Randomized controlled trials (RCT) compare outcomes of participants randomly assigned to a new treatment group to those of participants assigned to a placebo or

Table 1 Summary of trials examining the benefit of adding adjuvant therapy

	Year	N	Randomization arms	Overall survival (months)	p-value
ESPAC-1 [11]	2004	289	Chemotherapy	20.6	0.009
			No chemotherapy	15.5	
Kosuge et al. [12]	2006	88	5-FU + cisplatin	15.8	0.904
			Surgery alone	12.5	
CONKO-001 [13]	2007	368	Gemcitabine	22.1	0.06
			Surgery alone	20.2	
EORTC 40891 [14]	2007	218	5-FU + XRT (40 Gy)	15.6	0.165
			Surgery alone	12.0	
RTOG 9704 [15]	2011	451	Gemcitabine + 5FU/XRT (50.4 Gy)	20.5	0.08
			5-FU + 5FU/XRT (50.4 Gy)	17.1	

control group. They are regarded as the gold standard for evaluating new treatments and gaining regulatory approval due to their characteristic ability to address selection bias. However, modern oncology drug development faces increasing challenges. The average cost of bringing a drug to market is estimated to be $800 million [6]. Because adjuvant trials require the enrollment of a large number of patients and long-term follow-up, the actual therapies they assess may take 10–20 years to gain marketing approval [6]. Yet despite these astronomical time and monetary expenses, a report of the 2003–2010 phase III oncology drug trials found that more than 66 % of oncology drug trials fail to reach statistical significance in their primary end point [7]. This leads to an ever increasing backlog of potential anti-cancer drugs with promising results from early phase trials that have been untested.

In traditional clinical trials, initial parameters of study design such as sample size are pre-specified. This often leads to underpowered or overpowered studies due to inaccurate estimates of parameters. Re-thinking trial designs to include the CER-focused concepts may provide a method to enhance the operational efficiency, analytic efficiency and generalizability of RCTs. One such trial design is an adaptive clinical trial.

An adaptive clinical trial [8] accumulates evidence during an ongoing trial and actively reviews design elements and parameters to increase operational efficiency as well as the probability that trial participants actually benefit from participation. Examples of such "adaptions" include changing interventions or intervention doses, altering the rate of patient recruitment, or adjusting the probability of being randomly assigned to the different arms based on patient covariate information. Adaptive clinical trials allow new interventions to be added and less effective ones to be dropped without restarting the entire trial. In turn, this facilitates the comparison of therapeutic alternatives most relevant to current clinical practice and improves the timeliness and clinical relevance of clinical trials.

Adaptive clinical trials can be used for the rapid testing and development of new treatments for pancreatic cancer. Trials in pancreatic cancer often suffer from insufficient participation due to the limited number of patients with the disease. Aside from the tremendous costs required to conduct these trials, the scarcity of patients available for enrollment make it extremely difficult to employ a traditional clinical trial to compare all new anti-cancer drugs being developed at any given time as well as different dosing regimens, drug combinations, sequences of treatment and differential drug effects based on tumor profiles. An adaptive clinical trial design in pancreatic cancer could be protocoled to rapidly test new drugs combinations, doses and sequences. To expedite the fast turn-around for drug comparisons, an intermediary outcome that is predictive of clinical outcomes should be chosen as the end-point of the trial. In breast cancer, for example, since measuring overall survival after neoadjuvant takes a very long time, a more short-term marker such as clinical response (CR) was used in the I-SPY II trial [9, 10]. Similarly, in a highly aggressive tumor like pancreatic cancer, outcomes such as cancer recurrence or disease free survival (DFS) could be used due to the short amount of time needed to achieve these end-points. New drugs could be graduated if there were a high Bayesian predictive probability of achieving improved outcomes over the comparison group and dropped if a low probability of achieving improved outcomes was demonstrated. The graduated regimens would need to be re-tested and compared with other graduated drugs until the best drug is identified.

2.2 The Value of Radiotherapy

Patterns of recurrence in pancreatic cancer include both locoregional failure and systemic metastasis, with locoregional failure occurring in 50–60 % of cases [16, 17]. Even in cases where patients received adjuvant chemotherapy after surgery, locoregional recurrence rates remain as high as 30–60 % [11, 18]. The addition of adjuvant chemoradiation has been reported to decrease local recurrence rates to 20–40 % [19, 20]. However, there have been limited number of randomized clinical trials (Table 2) and the added benefit of combining radiation with chemotherapy in the adjuvant setting has yet to be determined. Of the trials that included radiation therapy, only ESPAC-1 [11] directly compared the addition of radiation to

Table 2 Summary of adjuvant trials examining the benefit of adding radiation

	Year	*N*	Randomization arms	Overall survival (months)	*p*-value
GITSG [20, 26]	1985	43	5-FU + XRT (40 Gy)	20.0	0.03
			Surgery alone	10.9	
ESPAC-1 [11]	2004	541	Chemoradiation	15.9	0.05
			No chemoradiation	17.9	
EORTC 40891 [14]	2007	218	5-FU + XRT (40 Gy)	15.6	0.165
			Surgery alone	12.0	

chemotherapy. ESPAC-1 used a 2 × 2 factorial designed to examine the benefit of chemotherapy over no chemotherapy and chemoradiotherapy over no chemoradiotherapy. The trial found that the clinical outcomes of patients who received chemoradiation were worse than those who did not. However, this trial has been criticized for the large number of patients who did not receive the intended therapy, its lack of standardized pathology review, and its high local recurrence rate [21, 22]. The debate about whether radiation should be included in the adjuvant setting is thus ongoing. A recently completed phase II trial, the EORTC 40013, investigated the role of chemoradiation over gemcitabine alone in the adjuvant setting [14]. While not designed to show difference, this study suggested that chemoradiation might improve outcomes over chemotherapy alone. To address this question, the ROTC 0848 was opened to accrural in November of 2009. This phase III trial aims to examine the role of both Erlotinib and chemoraditation as adjuvant treatment for patients with resected head of pancreas adenocarcinoma [23]. To meet its target accrual of 950 patients, this study involves 350 study locations, and is anticipated to close in year 2020.

While the final results of these trials will shed some light on this question, RCTs are extremely costly and time consuming, and results often needs be confirmed through multiple sources before being accepted into practice. Adaptive clinical trials, as explained above, could also be used to provide evidence to address this question in an efficient and effective manner. Another method would be to perform an analysis of data collected either for this purpose in mind, or for other purposes, such as cancer registry data. Cancer registries collect information on patient demographics, cancer stage, tumor characteristics and outcomes [24, 25]. Some cancer registries such as Surveillance, Epidemiology and End Results Program (SEER) and National Cancer Data Base (NCDB) also collect information on first course of treatment that could potentially be used to compare treatment effects. This data can be used to compare patients who did and did not have radiation as a part of their first course of treatment. While these cancer registries collect information about whether patients did not or did not received specific categories of treatment, such as chemotherapy, radiation therapy or hormonal therapy, they typically lack details about the precise chemotherapeutic regimens that were used. To supplement these shortcomings, the NCDB has a mechanism to request further information from hospitals at an ad hoc basis (http://www.facs.org/cancer/publicncdb.html). All Commission on Cancer (CoC)-approved cancer programs are mandated to participate in these special studies. This ad hoc data could be used to collect detailed information on factors that could influence outcomes, such as type of chemotherapy used, surgical details (drains, pylorus saving, duct to mucosa, ductal stenting, post-operative octerotide use), and perioperative outcomes (surgical complications). Such data could be used in conjunction with existing data regarding patient and tumor characteristics and radiation treatment details. Data analysis, such as cohort studies, case-control studies and regression analysis, could be applied to this data to determine differences in outcomes while controlling for all known biases.

2.3 Pre- Versus Peri- Versus Post-operative Therapy

The ideal timing of additional therapy in relation to surgery continues to be debated. For borderline resectable pancreatic disease, there has been recent convergence of expert opinions towards a recommendation for neoadjuvant therapy. The Americas Hepato-Pancreato-Biliary Association (AHPBA)/Society of Surgical Oncology (SSO)/Society for Surgery of the Alimentary Tract (SSAT) Consensus Statement for combined modality treatment of pancreatic cancer [27] states "patients with borderline resectable pancreas cancer should be treated with neoadjuvant therapy, ideally in the context of a clinical trial." For resectable pancreatic cancer no scientific evidence exists to determine the optimal sequencing of surgery in relation to the administration of systemic and/or radiation therapy.

The advantages of neoadjuvant therapy include early treatment of micrometastatic disease, and providing added time in which to identify patients with aggressive disease biology that will not benefit from surgery. Additionally, neoadjuvant therapy is a logical strategy to mitigate high rates of positive margins, while assuring that the patient will receive chemotherapy without the potential for post-operative delay or non-administration. Surgery following neoadjuvant therapy also provides tissue that can be compared with pre-treatment biopsy specimens, providing a valuable opportunity to study the direct tissue and molecular effects of therapy.

Unfortunately, it is difficult to examine the effects of neoadjuvant therapy using large databases. Except for some clinical trial databases or institutional databases, information regarding specific chemotherapeutic regimens is rarely collected even within cancer registry databases such as NCDB and SEER. Many patients receive chemotherapy in a facility that is different from the original treating hospital, making it difficult to obtain treatment data. Furthermore, there are often changes to treatment regimens during the course of treatment and inconsistent documentation by physicians administering chemotherapy.

On the other hand, information about radiation is often contained in large databases such as the NCDB and SEER. In the NCDB, start and end date of radiation, radiation treatment target (anatomic location, e.g. breast), radiation treatment modality (e.g. external beam, photons, etc.), regional dose (e.g. 50 Gy), boost treatment modality, and dosing information are collected and available to researchers for analysis.

While retrospective data analysis can provide supportive data, the benefit of neoadjuvant therapy for resectable pancreatic cancer will likely be best answered by well-conducted clinical trials. Fortunately, interest in the role of neoadjuvant therapies for pancreatic cancer has recently been growing. A query of ClinicalTrials.gov produced 43 trials examining the role of surgery plus some form of additional therapy for resectable and borderline resectable pancreatic cancers. Of these, 30 trials specifically examined the role of neoadjuvant therapy for resectable pancreatic cancer (Table 3). We anticipate that the maturation of these trials will provide further guidance in approaching these patients.

Table 3 Neoadjuvant therapy trials for resectable pancreatic cancer (queried May 2014)

Trial registration date	Patient eligibility criteria	ID	Status	Phase	Experimental treatment	Primary outcome
Oct 2005	Resectable	NCT00243854	Completed	1	Neoadjuvant hypofractioned radiotherapy concurrently with weekly gemcitabine and an EGFR tyrosine-kinase inhibitor (OSI-774, Tarceva)	Side effects that will prevent surgery following this therapy
Jan 2007	Resectable and borderline resectable	NCT00426738	Ongoing, but not recruiting	2	Neoadjuvant gemcitabine and oxaliplatin with radiation therapy	Two year disease free survival rate
Feb 2007	Resectable	NCT00438256	Ongoing, but not recruiting	1/2	Neoadjuvant proton beam XRT +capecitabine (4 dosing arms)	Feasibility and tolerability
Apr 2007	Resectable or borderline resectable	NCT00456599	Ongoing, but not recruiting	2	Neoadjuvant gemcitabine and oxaliplatin with radiation therapy	Two-year disease free survival
Jun 2007	Resectable	NCT00490360	Completed	2	Neoadjuvant chemotherapy with gemcitabine /cisplatin	Resectability rate > 70 % after restaging
Sep 2007	"Radiographically resectable pancreatic cancer, as determined by a surgical oncology"	NCT00536874	Ongoing, but not recruiting	2	Neoadjuvant gemcitabine and oxaliplatin	Overall survival at 18 months
Nov 2007	Resectable	NCT00557492	Ongoing, but not recruiting	2	Neoadjuvant bevacizumab and gemcitabine in combination with sequential rapid fractionation radiotherapy	R0 resection rate and rate of complete pathologic response

(continued)

Table 3 (continued)

Trial registration date	Patient eligibility criteria	ID	Status	Phase	Experimental treatment	Primary outcome
Feb 2008	Resectable and borderline resectable	NCT00609336	Ongoing, but not recruiting	2	Induction chemotherapy, neoadjuvant chemoradiotherapy, surgical resection and adjuvant chemotherapy.	Median overall survival of patients with adenocarcinoma of the pancreas
May 2009	Resectable	NCT00892242	Ongoing, but not recruiting	2	Zoledronic acid	Safety and feasibility
Dec 2009	Resectable	NCT01027221	Recruiting	1/2	Neoadjuvant photonradiation	Determination of an active local external beam radiotherapy dose leading to a maximal number of tumor infiltrating T-cells
May 2010	Resectable	NCT01130701	Withdrawn prior to enrollment	2	Neoadjuvant capecitabine, panitumumab and radiation	3 year progression-free survival
Sep 2010	Resectable	NCT01314027	Currently recruiting	3	Neoadjuvant (gemcitabine/oxaliplatin) + adjuvant chemotherapy (gemcitabine)	Progression-free survival
Feb 2011	Resectable	NCT01298011	Ongoing, but not recruiting	2	Gemcitabine and Nab-paclitaxel (Abraxane)	Grade III/IV histological response in tumor specimen rate after induction therapy
Mar 2011	Resectable or borderline resectable	NCT01333332	Recruiting	2	Capecitabine, radiation	Safety/Efficacy study

(continued)

Table 3 (continued)

Trial registration date	Patient eligibility criteria	ID	Status	Phase	Experimental treatment	Primary outcome
Jun 2011	Resectable	NCT01372735	Not yet open	1/2	Neoadjuvant short course IMRT	Local recurrence rate
Jul 2011	Resectable	NCT01389440	Ongoing, but not recruiting	2	Neoadjuvant treatment with gemcitabine and erlotinib followed by Gemcitabine, Erlotinib and radiotherapy in patients with resectable pancreatic adenocarcinoma	Percentage of ancients undergoing with neoadjuvant chemoradiotherapy and R0 resection
Jul 2011	Resectable	NCT01494155	Recruiting	2	Accelerated short course radiation therapy with proton beam capecitabine and hydroxychloroquine	Progression-free survival
Aug 2011	Resectable	NCT01419002	Terminated due to low recruitment rate	3	Neoadjuvant RTx	Local recurrence free survival
Sep 2011	Resectable or borderline resectable	NCT01446458	Recruiting	1	Modified FOLFIRINOX, SBRT	Maximum tolerated total dose of stereotactic body radiation
Nov 2011	Resectable and borderline resectable	NCT01470417	Ongoing, but not recruiting	2	Neoadj nab-paclitaxel/ gemcitabine + RT (in resectable patients)	Biochemical response rate, Radiographic response rate, pathologic downstaging and margin status
Dec 2011	Resectable	NCT01521702	Currently recruiting	3	Neoadjuvant gemcitabine/ oxaliplatin plus adjuvant gemcitabine	Progression-free survival

(continued)

Table 3 (continued)

Trial registration date	Patient eligibility criteria	ID	Status	Phase	Experimental treatment	Primary outcome
Dec 2011	Resectable or borderline resectable	NCT01726582	Recruiting	2	"personalized" therapy	Resectability Rate
May 2012	Allpts	NCT01760252	Recruiting	2	Capecitabine, oxaliplatin and irinotecan (CAPOXIRI)	Treatment adherence rate (TAR)
Aug 2012	Resectable	NCT01660711	Recruiting	2	FOLFIRINOX chemotherapy	Percentage of patients able to complete the full course of preoperative chemotherapy and undergo a resection
Sep 2012	Resectable	NCT01783054	Recruiting	2	Gemcitabine and abraxane.	Tumor Response
Jun 2013	Resectable	NCT01900327	Not yet open	3	Neoadjuvant chemoradiotherapy (CRT) (Gemcitabine, external beam) followed by curative surgery + adj Gem	3-Year survival rate
Aug 2013	Resectable	NCT01918644	Recruiting	1	(SBRT, capecitabine, and surgery)	Incidence of dose-limiting toxicity
Jan 2014	Resectable	NCT02030860	Recruiting	2/3	gemcitabine/abraxane with or without paricalcitol prior to surgery	Number of adverse events
Jan 2014	Resectable	NCT02047513	Not yet open	2	Neoadj nab-paclitaxel/gemcitabine + surgery + adj nab-paclitaxel/gemcitabine	DFS
Apr 2009	Resectable	NCT00889187	Terminated for excess toxicity	1/2	Capecitabine + accelerated short course radiation	Feasibility and tolerability

2.4 Value of Vascular and Multi-Visceral Resection

The pancreas resides in close anatomic quarters with many vital structures. As a result, pancreatic tumors often involve structures other than the pancreas, such as major vessels and adjacent organs, which are traditionally regarded to signal aggressive tumor biology compromising the benefit of resection. However, some surgeons have challenged this paradigm, suggesting instead that involvement of these vital structures reflects the tumor's precarious location rather than its aggressiveness.

Superior mesenteric vein (SMV) and portal vein (PV) resection and reconstruction during pancreaticoduodenectomy (PD) are generally considered to be reasonable surgical options for pancreatic cancers abutting or invading the SMV or PV. However, outcomes of these complex procedures remain controversial. Ramacciato et al. [28] and Chua and Saxena [29] found low operative mortality rates, ranging from 0 to 7 %, and 5-year survival rates around 12 %, suggesting that SMV-PV resection was a safe and feasible option that provided survival benefits similar to that of PD without venous involvement. Conversely, Worni et al. [30] using the National Inpatient Sample database found higher rates of intraoperative (OR 1.94, $p = 0.001$) and postoperative (OR 1.36, $p = 0.008$) complications than patients who underwent pancreatic resection alone. Likewise, Castleberry et al. [31] using the National Surgical Quality Improvement Program (NSQIP) database found that vascular reconstruction was associated with a doubling of post-operative mortality (5.7 % vs. 2.9 %, OR 2.1, $p = 0.008$) and increased morbidity (39.9 % vs. 33.3 %, OR 1.36, $p = 0.02$).

Arterial resections and multi-visceral resections for pancreatic cancers are similarly contentious surgical issues. Current guidelines define arterial involvement of the superior mesenteric artery, common hepatic artery and celiac artery as criteria of unresectability [32]. Yet as surgical resection remains the most effective therapeutic intervention for pancreatic cancer, the value of more radical resections continues to be debated. A systemic review and meta-analysis by Mollberg et al. [33] found simultaneous arterial resections to have higher perioperative mortality and lower 1-year survival than non-arterial resections, but more favorable survival compared to patients who did not undergo resection at all. Two recent studies of multi-visceral resection (MVR) revealed that patients undergoing MVR had a higher incidence of surgical morbidity but similar mortality and long-term survival compared to patients undergoing standard PD, and improved long-term outcomes compared to patients receiving palliative bypass (16 months vs. 6 months, $p < 0.0001$).

While the questions about the roles of PV and SMV, arterial and multi-visceral resections for pancreatic cancer may form three separate debates, all share a fundamental underlying question: Is involvement of these structures a sign of the tumor's biological aggressiveness or is it simply a bystander result of the tumor's close proximity to these structures?

Attempting to answer to this question is difficult because two different related issues need to be examined concurrently. First, we must address whether a tumor's

Table 4 2 × 2 matrix breakdown of the issues involved in determining if vessel or visceral involvement leads to worst outcomes

	Vessel or visceral involvement	No vessel or visceral involvement
Surgery of the vessel or visceral	(A)	(B)
No surgery of the vessel or visceral	(C)	(D)

involvement of vascular or visceral structures has an effect on long-term prognosis. Second, we must understand whether the addition of vascular or visceral resection leads to worse outcomes (Table 4). Because retrospective analyses have typically compared patients with vascular involvement who have undergone radical surgery (A) to patients without vascular involvement who did not undergo radical surgery (D), the validity of the comparison is questionable. Ideally, we would be able to examine the outcomes between patients with or without vessel or visceral involvement among patients who underwent extensive surgery (A vs. B), or among those who did not undergo extensive surgery (C vs. D). However, performing extended surgery on a patient without vascular involvement (B) or not doing surgery on a patient who has vascular involvement (C) would not be deemed ethical in a clinical trial setting and therefore cannot be compared in this way.

One strategy to realistically and effectively determine the benefit of extended resection would be to create a registry that would allow the collection of robust clinical data to control for all variables potentially confounding the outcomes. Specific tumor characteristics such as the tumor's location within the pancreas, its relationship to surrounding anatomy, and details about the extent to which particular vessels are involved would be collected. Additional variables including tumor size and number, location of positive lymph nodes, patient factors such as comorbidities, frailty, socioeconomic status and age, surgical factors such as operative technique, use of drains, and extent of lymph node dissection, operative factors such as time and estimated blood loss (EBL), and operative outcomes such as complications and length of stay would need to be collected according to predetermined definitions. Data should not only be collected on patients with vessel or visceral involvement, but also on those without vessel or visceral involvement who did or did not undergo surgery, so that resulting models can accurately estimate the effect of vessel or visceral involvement while controlling for confounding variables.

However, precise classification of vessel involvement can be challenging. It typically includes an assessment of the location of the tumor, the length of the involved segment of the vessel, and the circumference of the involved segment vessel. To perform large-scale comparative effectiveness research for pancreatic cancer involving major vessels, we need a standardized method that can be universally used to objectively describe and categorize the tumor and its relation to vital structures.

One approach could be to utilize computerized analysis of medical images [34]. Computerized analysis has the potential to define and categorize imaging studies for pancreatic cancer and develop computer-based algorithms to classify the subtypes of pancreatic cancers. Currently, there is ongoing research investigating the use of automated quantitative analysis of digitalized radiologic images. In oncology, computer-aided diagnosis (CAD) [35] has been investigated for breast, lung and colon cancers. For breast cancer, the use of CAD has been found to increased detection rates and is now used as a part of routine screening in many hospitals. Enabling the technology to accurately distinguish between the pancreatic cancer and normal tissue, developing algorithms to categorize each subtype, and incorporating this technology into main stream imaging systems would make it possible to establish an objective method of classifying subtypes of pancreatic cancer. The development of an objective method to categorize tumors would in turn allow for pooling of data from multiple sources and accurate investigation of this rare disease.

2.5 Resectable Versus Borderline Resectable Versus Locally Advanced Unresectable Tumors

Resection is the only chance for long-term survival for patients with pancreatic cancer, and therefore classifying a patient inoperable has substantial survival and emotional implications. As such, there has been increasing emphasis on identifying which tumors are amenable to negative margin resection and increasing the pool of potentially resectable patients.

The term 'borderline resectable" was introduced to identify patients that were not clearly resectable but had a probability of resection with negative margins. In 2008, the AHPBA, SSO, SSAT, MD Anderson Cancer Center (MDACC) and the Gastrointestinal Symposium Steering Committee [36], convened a consensus conference to define borderline resectable pancreatic cancer [27]. The criteria for labeling a tumor "borderline resectable" were, (1) no distant metastasis, (2) venous involvement of SMA or portal vein which allows safe resection and reconstruction, (3) gastroduodenal artery (GDA) encasement up to the hepatic artery without extension into the celiac axis, and (4) tumor abutment of the SMA not to exceed 180° of the vessel wall circumference (Table 4). This definition was then used to set NCCN guidelines (Table 5).

Even with these detailed consensus guidelines attempting to adequately classify tumor involvement, ambiguity still exists due to lack of clarity in distinguishing between resectable tumors from borderline resectable tumors, and borderline resectable tumors from locally advanced, unresectable tumors. For example, tumor abutment of the celiac axis lies somewhere between borderline resectable and unresectable as it represents neither circumferential tumor involvement nor tumor extension. Similarly, abutment of the hepatic artery without encasement lies somewhere between the resectable and borderline resectable definitions. Depending on subjective interpretations of the provider or the situation in which the terminology is being used, one can choose a narrow definition of borderline resectable

Table 5 AHPBA/SSO/SSAT Consensus statement regarding the definition of resectable, borderline resectable and unresectable pancreatic adenocarcinoma (adopted from Callery et al. Ann Surg Oncol 2009)

	Resectable	Borderline resectable	Unresectable
Distant met	No	No	Yes
PV-SMV	No	Tumor abutment, with or without venous deformity. Limited encasement (short segment occlusion with suitable vessel for anastomosis above and below)	Major venous thrombosis, extending for several centimeters
SMA	No	Tumor abutment <180°	Circumferential encasement
Celiac axis	No	No tumor extension	Circumferential encasement
Hepatic artery	No	Encasement of short segment	Circumferential encasement

tumors that only includes patients that definitively meet the established criteria or a broad definition that includes all patients that are not clearly resectable or clearly unresectable. Additionally, since pre-operative determination of resectablity relies on CT imaging, differences in CT imaging techniques based on the timing of contrast injection, speed and resolution of the CT scanner, and data processing capabilities can affect diagnostic accuracy.

Our inability to reliably group these patients into these subsets greatly hinders our ability to compare treatment effects among these groups. To address this concern, when the Alliance for Clinical Trials in Oncology recently opened a phase II trial examining the worth of preoperative chemotherapy and radiation therapy before surgery for borderline pancreatic cancer patients (ClinicalTrials.gov identifier: NCT01821612), the study design incorporated a central review of CT/MRI scans to confirm that the tumor fits their criteria of borderline resectablility. Similarly, computerized analysis of digital images can be used to objectively classify and group patients into comparable cohorts. For clinical trials, this method could be used to take the place of central review and to classify patients according to a particular trial protocol.

As we enter the era of "big data" where every piece of technology, including EMRs and digitally driven technologies for imaging and physiological monitoring, produces data that can be captured and stored for future use, we must rethink our paradigm of using hand-collected structured data for research purposes. As Big Data methodologies mature, the paradigm for how we classify borderline resectability and its treatments will likely need to evolve. The classification of borderline resectability will no longer be limited to pre-determined standards, but instead can use granular unstructured imaging data to create new definitions of resectability and develop sub-groups that are better able to inform treatment decisions and prognosis. These new groupings could be applied to large aggregate datasets from multiple institutions and research facilities to perform comparative effectiveness research. The results of this research could then be used to build an algorithm that could be directly utilized via clinical EMRs to provide point-of-care recommendations for treatment decisions such as which patients should get upfront surgery and which should receive neoadjuvant therapy.

2.6 Management of IPMN

The appropriate management of incidentally discovered asymptomatic pancreatic cysts is an increasingly encountered dilemma for pancreatic surgeons. Pancreatic cysts are being identified at an upwards rate of 2.6 % of CT scans [37] and 13.5 % of MRIs [38] performed for non-pancreas related symptoms. There has also been a marked shift in pathologic diagnosis of these cysts over time, and in a large series of 851 resected pancreatic cysts from a single institution, mucinous cystic neoplasm (MCN) and serous cystadenoma (SCA) represented the dominant neoplasm before 1990, whereas IPMN now accounts for 50 % of resected cases [39]. IPMNs have become a routine challenge for surgeons due to difficulties in accurately distinguishing IPMN from other types of pancreatic cystic tumors and in preoperatively determining if an IPMN is harboring or destined to become a malignancy.

Imaging alone is inadequate to accurately diagnose IPMN. CT alone was found to accurately identify the type of pancreatic cyst in only 24–61 % of cases [40–42]. In a study by Correa-Gallego et al. [43], 20 % of patients who underwent surgery for presumed branch duct IPMN (BD-IPMN) actually had main pancreatic duct involvement or an alternative diagnosis on final pathology. The current radiographic definition of BD-IPMN as a cyst that communicates with the pancreatic duct may also be flawed, as 9 % of serous cystadenomas and 18 % of mucinous cyst adenomas were also found to communicate with the main pancreatic duct [44, 45]. The addition of cyst fluid analysis for carcinoembryonic antigen (CEA), amylase and cytology has markedly improved our ability to distinguish between different types of cysts. Measurement of cystic fluid CEA levels is able to distinguish mucinous tumors from serous tumors with a 79 % sensitivity and 84 % specificity [46]. Cyst amylase levels allow IPMNs to be distinguished from pseudocysts. However, neither CEA nor amylase is helpful in differentiating between the mucinous tumors, IPMNs and MCNs, and have no predictive value for determining malignancy [47].

Accuracy of diagnosis is considered imperative for pancreatic cystic lesions because of the risk of cancer linked with certain cysts. However, diagnosis alone is not enough to predict malignancy risk accurately. Currently, we have a limited understanding of the degree to which factors such as presence of mural nodules, cyst size, communication with the main pancreatic duct, main pancreatic duct dilation, and cyst wall thickening actually influence malignant potential. We similarly lack a comprehensive understanding of the natural history of the disease, making it unclear which tumors already are or will ultimately become malignant and therefore have an impact on survival.

Consensus guidelines from Sendai, Japan were published to direct the management of patients with IPMN [48]. Key factors were identified that were associated with a high risk of malignancy in order to select which patients should or should not undergo surgical resection. However, studies looking at the accuracy of the guidelines have found that while they were able to reliably predict which tumors contained no malignancy (high negative predictive value), they were poor at predicting which tumors did harbor a malignancy [very low positive predictive value (approximately 20 %)], meaning that many patients who undergo surgery for a presumed malignancy in accordance with the guidelines would often not actually have one [49, 50]. The strict use of these guidelines to determine who should undergo resection may lead to unnecessary surgery with its associated risks of morbidity and mortality.

Currently existing databases that collect enough information to study this rare disease, such as administrative data or clinical registries, are not appropriate for this purpose. IPMN without malignancy has not clearly been established as a pre-malignant condition, and is currently not collected in cancer registries. IPMN also does not have a unique diagnosis code and cannot be queried for analysis in an administrative database. These databases additionally lack details about imaging findings or pancreas specific information such as tumor location. Single institution databases specifically designed to answer these questions are unlikely to be able to amass enough patient information to find significant differences among these already rare events. Additionally, home-grown datasets generally use definitions that are neither universally accepted nor standardized, making it difficult for the information to be applicable in other settings.

A multi-institutional, national pancreas specific registry should be created to collect clinically rich information that can be used to further our understanding of IPMN. The registry should collect detailed information on pre-operative imaging findings, cystic fluid analysis results, tumor specific biomarkers, serologic markers, intra-operative findings, pathologic results, treatment and follow-up data (recurrence and survival). The registry should have the flexibility to allow the collection of additional variables as new information becomes available, and should also have a tissue bank that can collect cystic fluid, serum and surgical specimens for future analysis. Patient specific factors such as comorbidities, socioeconomic status and frailty should also be recorded to allow for adequate adjustments when doing calculations of survival. QOL information can be collected to conduct studies on patient-centered outcomes. Surgical outcomes, such as short-term morbidities, readmission and death, can be collected to assess new technologies.

This information would allow us to improve our understanding of the natural history of the pancreatic cystic lesions, identify factors associated with malignancy, and use regression models to improve our understanding of the impact of these factors. Moreover, this data will allow for the creation of risk models for a variety of outcomes of interest. Risk models could then be used to predict the risk of malignancy, recurrence and long-term survival. These risk models can be incorporated into decision aids that account for a person's willingness to take health risks or patient co-morbidities to conclude whether surgery or surveillance should be recommended. Newer technology, such as ablative technologies for IPMN, could be evaluated for safety and efficacy and cost effectiveness analysis can be used to determine if the incremental benefit of such technologies is worth the cost. Finally a robust serum/fluid/tissue bank would be a rich resource for high throughput molecular analysis that would likely fine tune our ability to accurately tailor therapy to those patents either harboring or destined to develop a malignancy and avoid surgery in patients without premalignant or malignant pathology.

3 Research Gaps in Pancreas Directed Care

3.1 Anastomotic Technique and Prevention of Fistula

The most significant morbidity associated with pancreatic surgery is pancreatic duct leak, either from the pancreaticoenteric anastomosis after a pancreatic head resection or from the pancreatic stump after a distal pancreatectomy. Soft pancreatic texture and small pancreatic duct diameter are the most significant risk factors for pancreatic leak, otherwise known as "pancreatic fistula". Other risk factors include blood loss, increased operative time and presence of cardiovascular disease [51].

There have been numerous clinical trials focused on comparing surgical techniques in order to minimize pancreatic leaks after the removal of the pancreatic head. While total pancreatectomy [52] and duct occlusion [53] have been abandoned because of their high rate of complications, the superiority of any anastomotic technique, such as end-to-side, end-to-end [54], duct-to-mucosa and invagination [55], pancreaticojejunostomy, pancreaticogastrotomy and pylorus-preserving pancreaticojejunostomies [56–62] has not been conclusively demonstrated. Intraoperative or external stenting of the pancreatic duct and the use of a topical fibrin glue sealant on the anastomosis have also been investigated with similarly inconclusive results. Results from a Cochrane review of five randomized control trials with a total of 656 patients undergoing pancreaticduodenectomy showed that the use of stents overall did not improve outcomes, but external stents may be beneficial [63].

Investigations into methods of preventing pancreatic fistulas after distal pancreatectomies, including hand-sewn closure with or without selective duct ligation [64], transection and closure with stapling device [65], transection with various energy devices [66–68], reinforcement of the pancreatic stump with fibrin glue seal [62, 69], seromuscular patches [70, 71], or pancreaticoenteric anastomosis [72, 73] with prophylactic transpapillary pancreatic stent insertion [74] have been conducted with similarly inconclusive results.

While there have been numerous clinical trials comparing various surgical techniques to prevent pancreatic fistulas, these trials have suffered from the flaws common to many surgical trials. Surgical trials tend to enroll inadequate patient numbers, utilize unrealistic power calculations, use study endpoints derived from poor or non-standardized definitions, or inadequately blind subjects and observers to the randomization arm [75–77].

A unique aspect of surgical trials is the fact that individual surgeons have learning curves for any newly adopted technical procedure. It is impossible, then, to eliminate performance bias using conventional randomized control techniques [77]. An alternative to the conventional RCT that can overcome this issue is the expertise-based randomized control trial.

This concept was first conceptually described in 1980 by Van der Linden, who suggested randomizing participants to clinicians committed to performing different intentions. More recently, Devereaux promoted the use of the expertise-based randomized controlled trial as a superior alternative to conventional RCTs [78] by eliminating differential expertise bias. Differential expertise bias occurs when a disproportionate number of cases are performed by surgeons with expertise in one procedure over another. The trial results will be biased towards the procedure with the greater number of experts because "experts" tend to have improved outcomes over non-experts.

Expertise-based randomized control trial randomizes patients to surgeons with expertise in one technique or the other technique instead of to the intervention itself. For example, a patient would be randomized to either a surgeon with expertise in the duct-to-mucosa technique or a surgeon who is an expert at the invagination technique. This is in contrast to a conventional RCT, where the patient would be assigned to one intervention or another, and the surgeon would be expected to perform the intervention regardless of their operative expertise. Expertise-based RCT can address many problems that arise from conventional trial design for surgical interventions.

First, differential expertise bias can be directly addressed. Surgeons will perform only the procedure in which they have expertise, thus avoiding the problem of differential expertise. Second, such a design mitigates the unintentional but often encountered surgeons' opinions about one procedure over another that may lead to differential recording of data, repeated measurements, and interpretation of outcomes [78]. Third, surgeon initiated crossover is reduced due to limited surgeon expertise of the assigned procedure [79]. Finally, surgeon recruitment into clinical trials may improve as more surgeons may be willing to participate because they would only be required to perform techniques already mastered and that they are comfortable with, thereby also alleviating potential ethical distress associated with the expectation of performing a less familiar technique [80].

For pancreatic surgery techniques, expertise-based randomized control trial has the potential to provide an ideal method to compare surgical techniques without having to face the very steep learning curve that comes with any pancreatic surgery. Traditional methods to balance the groups such as stratification can be applied to the study design to address the patients' desires to be treated in a certain geographic locations or in certain settings (e.g., university hospital). For example, regions of

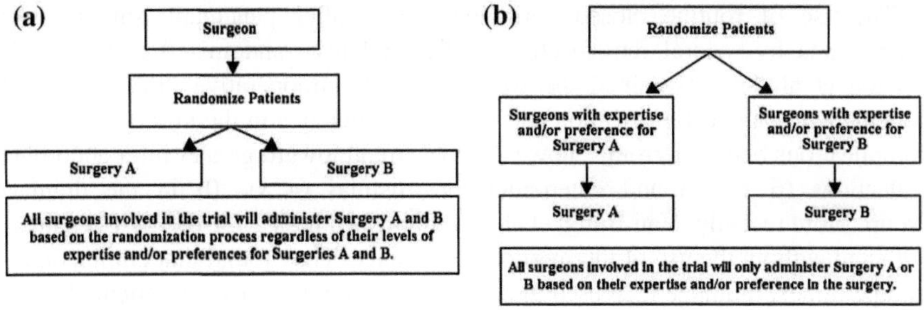

Fig. 2 Expertise-based randomized control trials [78, 81]. Comparisons of (**A**) conventional randomized clinical trial (RCT) and (**B**) expertise-based RCT designs are shown. In the conventional randomized clinical trial (**A**), patients are randomized to one of two surgeries (Surgery A or Surgery B), and surgeons administer Surgery A to some participants and Surgery B to others regardless of the surgeon's level of expertise and/or preference. In an alternative RCT design (B), patients are randomized to surgeons with expertise in Surgery A who are committed to performing only Surgery A or to surgeons with expertise in Surgery B who are committed to performing only Surgery B. This alternative design is referred to as an expertise-based RCT [81].

care can be stratified so patients can stay in the same geographic area regardless of randomization. There is clearly a tremendous need for more well-designed surgical trials (Fig. 2).

3.2 Drains, Octreotide and Prokinetic Agents Following Pancreaticoduodenectomy

Perioperative management practices associated with pancreatic resection that can also influence outcome include the use of intra-abdominal drains and prophylactic octreotide. The use of octerotide had been advocated to provide prophylaxis against the formation of pancreatic leaks while the use of drains is promoted as a method to decrease the complications associated with pancreatic leaks. Perioperative octreotide has been shown to be effective in preventing pancreatic fistula in some trials [82–85], while in others [86, 87] no difference has been demonstrated. In a Cochrane review of the role of octreotide for pancreatic surgery [88], Koti et al. identified 17 trials involving 2,143 patients, and found a lower incidence of postoperative complications (RR 0.7, 95 % CI 0.62–0.82) including pancreatic fistula (RR 0,64, 95 % CI 0.53–0.78), but no difference in perioperative mortality (RR 1.04, 95 % CI −2.54–0.46), reoperation rate (RR 1.14, 95 % CI 0.56–2.36) or hospital stay (MD −1.04 days, 95 % CI −2.54–0.46). However, when RCTs that examined clinically meaningful fistulas (grade B & C) were assessed, there was no difference in outcomes between the patients who did get octreotide and those who did not.

The use of routine closed peritoneal drains after pancreatic surgery been investigated by several retrospective studies and two randomized clinical trials. Conlon et al. [89] examined the routine use of intraoperative drainage in 179 patients with pancreatic resection and found no difference in the number or type of complications between groups, however saw a trend toward greater intra-abdominal collections (6 vs. 2) and enterocutaneous fistulas (4 vs. 0) in the drainage group. More recently, Van Buren et al. [90] published their RCT of 137 PD patients with and without the use of intraperitoneal drainage. They found that elimination of intraperitoneal drainage increased the number of complications per patient [1 (0−2) vs. 2 (1−4), $p = 0.029$], increased the number of patients who had at least 1 ≥ grade 2 complication [52 % vs. 68 %, $p = 0.047$] and had a higher average complication severity [2 (0−2) vs. 2 (1−3), $p = 0.027$]. Notably, this trial was stopped early due to the increased mortality from 3 to 12 % observed in the patients undergoing PD without intraperitoneal drainage.

For both these topics, the lack of robust data results in variability in practice patterns. A deficiency of studies with large sample sizes or population-based studies provide fertile ground for the use of CER methodology. Administrative databases capture billable events and provide a wealth of information including the ability to longitudinally track patient activities and costs associated with each event. They also facilitate the examination of indirect influences, such as location of care, availability of services, time between services, and cost of treatments, as well as of outcomes such as delivery of treatments, resource utilization, discharge location, length of stay and readmission. The use of an administrative database such as Medicare may be ideal to conduct comparative effectiveness research addressing whether octreotide can prevent pancreatic fistulas. The Medicare database, which provides billing information for all inpatient procedures for patients eligible for Medicare coverage, would be able to identify patients who were billed for octreotide and patients who were not. Billing information would also be able to provide information on outcomes such as length of stay and a variety of clinically meaningful events, such as reoperation, percutaneous drainage, and administration of antibiotics. Databases such as these can be used alone or in conjunction with databases that provide direct clinical data, such as institutional clinical data or tumor registries. For cancer patients, the SEER-linked Medicare data would provide detailed tumor information such as histology and staging, an operative summary, and information on adjuvant treatment, all of which could then be used to risk-stratify patients.

3.3 Minimally Invasive Surgery Versus Open Surgery

The safety of pancreatic resections has continued to improve in recent years with mortality rates of less than 5 % now reported in most series [91] and reflect modern advancements in surgical technique, better perioperative support, improved patient selection, and concentration of cases within high-volume centers.

The utility of minimally invasive approaches such as laparoscopy and robotic-assisted surgery, continue to be assessed for distal pancreatectomy and pancreaticoduodenectomy. At present, there are no RCT comparing minimally invasive approaches to open approaches, and data is only available from case reports, smaller case series, and a limited number of retrospective multicenter studies. While no clear conclusions can be drawn from these small observational studies the attractiveness of minimally invasive pancreatic resections is inescapable. In theory, patients undergoing minimally invasive pancreatic resection would be expected to have less scarring, less post-operative pain, fewer wound complications, an earlier return to normal activity with the potential to better tolerate and complete adjuvant chemotherapy regimens. Kooby et al. [92] examined records from 212 patients who underwent DP for pancreatic adenocarcinoma of which 11 % were approached laparoscopically. In the matched analysis, they found no difference in positive margin rates, number of nodes examined, number of patients with at least 1 positive node or overall survival, but did find that the hospital stay was 2 days shorter in the laparoscopically resected group. Similarly, Venkat et al. [93] found lower blood loss and reduced length of stay in laparoscopic distal pancreatectomy compared to open.

Unlike resections for distal pancreas lesions, studies examining the benefit of minimally invasive techniques for head of pancreas disease have more limited. Kuroki et al. [94] found no difference in terms of operative time or complications, but did find that the laparoscopic pancreaticduodenectomy group had less blood loss than the open surgical group. A meta-analysis by Nigri et al. [95] looked at 8 studies comparing open vs a minimally invasive approach to pancreaticoduodenectomies and found that minimally invasive approaches resulted in lower post-operative complications rates, less intraoperative blood loss, and shorter hospital stays, but notably longer operative times. Studies reporting robotic techniques have recently emerged and systematic literature reviews by Ciroocchi et al. of robotic distal pancreatectomy [96] and robotic pancreaticoduodenectomy [97] concluded that there was insufficient evidence to draw firm conclusions.

One method to examine this issue would be to utilize the expertise-based randomized control trial as described above. A trial comparing open versus minimally invasive approaches would be ideal for this type of design. Patients would be randomly assigned to have their surgery performed by a surgeon who was an expert in one technique or the other. This study design would eliminate expertise-bias created from the steep learning curve that exists for minimally invasive techniques as well as surgeon and patient biases for one technique over the other. Recruiting patients to a trial comparing open techniques to minimally invasive techniques remain extremely challenge for any RCT design due to strong pre-existing surgeon and patient preferences. Surgeons may have well-established opinions about one technique over another, making it difficult to maintain equipoise and recruit their patients for trials. Patients often consider "newer" surgeries to be "better" surgeries and often opt out of trials, especially if they have sought out a particular physician specifically for the ability to undergo the newer type of surgery. However, while newer techniques may provide short term benefits, long-term oncologic outcomes often remain unproven. Whatever it be an adaptive, expertise-based or traditional clinical trial, randomized clinical trials provide the only way to ensure no systematic differences, both known and unknown, are present between comparator groups and RCTs remain the gold standard for comparing interventions [98].

However, there are many situations where RCTs are not feasible, either due to time or monetary reasons. In these situations, a prospectively collected database utilizing similar principals as the expertise-based randomized control trial design described above may be an alternative way to compare open to minimally invasive techniques. The database would collect information from physicians that are an expert in one or the other technique. Only information from patients that were felt to be eligible for either surgery would be entered into this database, and patient enrollment would be designated prior to surgery to minimize selection bias. Detailed data regarding patient demographics, comorbidities and tumor status would be collected to verify that both groups were similar. Patients would proceed to get the surgery that was already being offered to them and would get treated according to the surgeon's protocol. Long term outcomes of interest would be collected. This "expertise-based prospective database design" would eliminate many of the difficulties of conducting a RCT examining open technique to a minimally invasive technique. Importantly, there would be no issues with lack of statistical power due to poor accrual and no issues with differences in level of expertise due to the steep learning curves involved with learning the minimally invasive technique. Surgeon participation would be greatly enhanced since there would be no burden of learning new techniques and surgeons would not be asked to abandon their operative preferences. Prospectively assigning patients to be entered into the database before the surgery would minimize most biases and make "expertise-based prospective database design" a compelling comparative effectiveness study.

4 Conclusion

There are many gaps in our understanding of the most effective way to manage pancreatic cancer patients. Comparative effectiveness research methodologies offer a way to address these research gaps by expanding our sources of information and engaging in innovative research designs. While only one research methodology has been presented for each of the research gaps in this chapter, these methodologies are not limited to these indications alone. Most of these methods can also be applied to other research gaps and readers are encouraged to apply the CER methodologies presented in this chapter to other meaningful clinical questions to ultimately improve the quality of patient care.

References

1. Lim JE, Chien MW, Earle CC (2003) Prognostic factors following curative resection for pancreatic adenocarcinoma: a population-based, linked database analysis of 396 patients. Ann Surg 237(1):74–85
2. Trede M, Schwall G, Saeger HD (1990) Survival after pancreatoduodenectomy. 118 consecutive resections without an operative mortality. Ann Surg 211(4):447–458
3. Crist DW, Sitzmann JV, Cameron JL (1987) Improved hospital morbidity, mortality, and survival after the Whipple procedure. Ann Surg 206(3):358–365
4. Conroy T, Desseigne F, Ychou M, Bouche O, Guimbaud R, Becouarn Y, Adenis A, Raoul JL, Gourgou-Bourgade S, de la Fouchardiere C et al (2011) FOLFIRINOX versus gemcitabine for metastatic pancreatic cancer. N Engl J Med 364(19):1817–1825
5. Von Hoff DD, Ervin T, Arena FP, Chiorean EG, Infante J, Moore M, Seay T, Tjulandin SA, Ma WW, Saleh MN et al (2013) Increased survival in pancreatic cancer with nab-paclitaxel plus gemcitabine. N Engl J Med 369(18):1691–1703
6. DiMasi JA, Hansen RW, Grabowski HG (2003) The price of innovation: new estimates of drug development costs. J Health Econ 22(2):151–185
7. DiMasi JA, Grabowski HG (2007) Economics of new oncology drug development. J Clin Oncol (official journal of the American Society of Clinical Oncology) 25(2):209–216
8. Berry DA (2012) Adaptive clinical trials in oncology. Nat Rev Clin Oncol 9(4):199–207
9. Barker AD, Sigman CC, Kelloff GJ, Hylton NM, Berry DA, Esserman LJ (2009) I-SPY 2: an adaptive breast cancer trial design in the setting of neoadjuvant chemotherapy. Clin Pharmacol Ther 86(1):97–100
10. Printz C (2013) I-SPY 2 may change how clinical trials are conducted: researchers aim to accelerate approvals of cancer drugs. Cancer 119(11):1925–1927
11. Neoptolemos JP, Stocken DD, Friess H, Bassi C, Dunn JA, Hickey H, Beger H, Fernandez-Cruz L, Dervenis C, Lacaine F et al (2004) A randomized trial of chemoradiotherapy and chemotherapy after resection of pancreatic cancer. N Engl J Med 350(12):1200–1210
12. Kosuge T, Kiuchi T, Mukai K, Kakizoe T (2006) A multicenter randomized controlled trial to evaluate the effect of adjuvant cisplatin and 5-fluorouracil therapy after curative resection in cases of pancreatic cancer. Jpn J Clin Oncol 36(3):159–165
13. Oettle H, Neuhaus P, Hochhaus A, Hartmann JT, Gellert K, Ridwelski K, Niedergethmann M, Zulke C, Fahlke J, Arning MB et al (2013) Adjuvant chemotherapy with gemcitabine and long-term outcomes among patients with resected pancreatic cancer: the CONKO-001 randomized trial. JAMA J Am Med Assoc 310(14):1473–1481
14. Van Laethem JL, Hammel P, Mornex F, Azria D, Van Tienhoven G, Vergauwe P, Peeters M, Polus M, Praet M, Mauer M et al (2010) Adjuvant gemcitabine alone versus gemcitabine-based chemoradiotherapy after curative resection for pancreatic cancer: a randomized EORTC-40013-22012/FFCD-9203/GERCOR phase II study. J Clin Oncol (official journal of the American Society of Clinical Oncology) 28(29):4450–4456
15. Bowsher RR, Wolny JD, Frank BH (1992) A rapid and sensitive radioimmunoassay for the measurement of proinsulin in human serum. Diabetes 41(9):1084–1090
16. Griffin JF, Smalley SR, Jewell W, Paradelo JC, Reymond RD, Hassanein RE, Evans RG (1990) Patterns of failure after curative resection of pancreatic carcinoma. Cancer 66(1):56–61
17. Tepper J, Nardi G, Sutt H (1976) Carcinoma of the pancreas: review of MGH experience from 1963 to 1973. Analysis of surgical failure and implications for radiation therapy. Cancer 37 (3):1519–1524
18. Oettle H, Post S, Neuhaus P, Gellert K, Langrehr J, Ridwelski K, Schramm H, Fahlke J, Zuelke C, Burkart C et al (2007) Adjuvant chemotherapy with gemcitabine vs observation in patients undergoing curative-intent resection of pancreatic cancer: a randomized controlled trial. JAMA J Am Med Assoc 297(3):267–277
19. Whittington R, Bryer MP, Haller DG, Solin LJ, Rosato EF (1991) Adjuvant therapy of resected adenocarcinoma of the pancreas. Int J Radiat Oncol Biol Phys 21(5):1137–1143

20. (1987) Further evidence of effective adjuvant combined radiation and chemotherapy following curative resection of pancreatic cancer. Gastrointestinal tumor study group. Cancer 59(12):2006–2010
21. Abrams RA, Lillemoe KD, Piantadosi S (2001) Continuing controversy over adjuvant therapy of pancreatic cancer. Lancet 358(9293):1565–1566
22. Choti MA (2004) Adjuvant therapy for pancreatic cancer–the debate continues. N Engl J Med 350(12):1249–1251
23. Clinical trials.gov—ROTC 0848. http://www.rtog.org/ClinicalTrials/ProtocolTable/StudyDetails.aspx?study=0848
24. National cancer data base (NCDB). http://www.facs.org/cancer/ncdb/
25. Surveillance epidemiology and end results (SEER). http://seer.cancer.gov/
26. Kalser MH, Ellenberg SS (1985) Pancreatic cancer. Adjuvant combined radiation and chemotherapy following curative resection. Arch Surg 120(8):899–903 (Chicago, Ill : 1960)
27. Callery MP, Chang KJ, Fishman EK, Talamonti MS, Traverso WL, Linehan DC (2009) Pretreatment assessment of resectable and borderline resectable pancreatic cancer: expert consensus statement. Ann Surg Oncol 16(7):1727–1733
28. Ramacciato G, Mercantini P, Petrucciani N, Romano C, Nigri G, Aurello P, D'Angelo F, Ravaioli M, Del Gaudio M, Cucchetti A et al (2010) Pancreatic carcinoma presenting with invasion of the vena porta or the superior mesenteric vein: our experience and review of the literature. Minerva Chir 65(6):587–599
29. Chua TC, Saxena A (2010) Extended pancreaticoduodenectomy with vascular resection for pancreatic cancer: a systematic review. J Gastrointest Surg (official journal of the Society for Surgery of the Alimentary Tract) 14(9):1442–1452
30. Worni M, Castleberry AW, Clary BM, Gloor B, Carvalho E, Jacobs DO, Pietrobon R, Scarborough JE, White RR (2013) Concomitant vascular reconstruction during pancreatectomy for malignant disease: a propensity score-adjusted, population-based trend analysis involving 10,206 patients. JAMA Surg 148(4):331–338
31. Castleberry AW, White RR, De La Fuente SG, Clary BM, Blazer DG III, McCann RL, Pappas TN, Tyler DS, Scarborough JE (2012) The impact of vascular resection on early postoperative outcomes after pancreaticoduodenectomy: an analysis of the american college of surgeons national surgical quality improvement program database. Ann Surg Oncol 19(13):4068–4077
32. National comprehensive cancer network (NCCN) Oncology Outcomes Database. http://www.nccn.org/network/business_insights/outcomes_database/outcomes.aspx
33. Mollberg N, Rahbari NN, Koch M, Hartwig W, Hoeger Y, Buchler MW, Weitz J (2011) Arterial resection during pancreatectomy for pancreatic cancer: a systematic review and meta-analysis. Ann Surg 254(6):882–893
34. Doi K (2007) Computer-aided diagnosis in medical imaging: historical review, current status and future potential. Comput Med Imaging Graph (the official journal of the Computerized Medical Imaging Society) 31(4–5):198–211
35. Shiraishi J, Li Q, Appelbaum D, Doi K (2011) Computer-aided diagnosis and artificial intelligence in clinical imaging. Semin Nucl Med 41(6):449–462
36. Vauthey JN, Dixon E (2009) AHPBA/SSO/SSAT consensus conference on resectable and borderline resectable pancreatic cancer: rationale and overview of the conference. Ann Surg Oncol 16(7):1725–1726
37. Laffan TA, Horton KM, Klein AP, Berlanstein B, Siegelman SS, Kawamoto S, Johnson PT, Fishman EK, Hruban RH (2008) Prevalence of unsuspected pancreatic cysts on MDCT. AJR Am J Roentgenol 191(3):802–807
38. Lee KS, Sekhar A, Rofsky NM, Pedrosa I (2010) Prevalence of incidental pancreatic cysts in the adult population on MR imaging. Am J Gastroenterol 105(9):2079–2084
39. Valsangkar NP, Morales-Oyarvide V, Thayer SP, Ferrone CR, Wargo JA, Warshaw AL, Fernandez-del Castillo C (2012) 851 resected cystic tumors of the pancreas: a 33-year experience at the Massachusetts general hospital. Surgery 152(3):S4–S12

40. Khashab MA, Shin EJ, Amateau S, Canto MI, Hruban RH, Fishman EK, Cameron JL, Edil BH, Wolfgang CL, Schulick RD et al (2011) Tumor size and location correlate with behavior of pancreatic serous cystic neoplasms. Am J Gastroenterol 106(8):1521–1526
41. Bassi C, Salvia R, Molinari E, Biasutti C, Falconi M, Pederzoli P (2003) Management of 100 consecutive cases of pancreatic serous cystadenoma: wait for symptoms and see at imaging or vice versa? World J Surg 27(3):319–323
42. Feller E, Schiffman FJ (1990) Extrahepatic biliary obstruction by lymphoma. Arch Surg (Chicago, Ill : 1960) 125(11):1507–1509
43. Correa-Gallego C, Ferrone CR, Thayer SP, Wargo JA, Warshaw AL, Fernandez-Del Castillo C (2010) Incidental pancreatic cysts: do we really know what we are watching? Pancreatology (official journal of the International Association of Pancreatology (IAP) [et al]) 10(2–3):144–150
44. Kimura W, Moriya T, Hirai I, Hanada K, Abe H, Yanagisawa A, Fukushima N, Ohike N, Shimizu M, Hatori T et al (2012) Multicenter study of serous cystic neoplasm of the Japan pancreas society. Pancreas 41(3):380–387
45. Yamao K, Yanagisawa A, Takahashi K, Kimura W, Doi R, Fukushima N, Ohike N, Shimizu M, Hatori T, Nobukawa B et al (2011) Clinicopathological features and prognosis of mucinous cystic neoplasm with ovarian-type stroma: a multi-institutional study of the Japan pancreas society. Pancreas 40(1):67–71
46. Brugge WR, Lewandrowski K, Lee-Lewandrowski E, Centeno BA, Szydlo T, Regan S, del Castillo CF, Warshaw AL (2004) Diagnosis of pancreatic cystic neoplasms: a report of the cooperative pancreatic cyst study. Gastroenterology 126(5):1330–1336
47. Al-Rashdan A, Schmidt CM, Al-Haddad M, McHenry L, Leblanc JK, Sherman S, Dewitt J (2011) Fluid analysis prior to surgical resection of suspected mucinous pancreatic cysts. A single centre experience. J Gastrointest Oncol 2(4):208–214
48. Tanaka M, Fernandez-del Castillo C, Adsay V, Chari S, Falconi M, Jang JY, Kimura W, Levy P, Pitman MB, Schmidt CM et al (2012) International consensus guidelines 2012 for the management of IPMN and MCN of the pancreas. Pancreatology (official journal of the International Association of Pancreatology (IAP) [et al]) 12(3):183–197
49. Pelaez-Luna M, Chari ST, Smyrk TC, Takahashi N, Clain JE, Levy MJ, Pearson RK, Petersen BT, Topazian MD, Vege SS et al (2007) Do consensus indications for resection in branch duct intraductal papillary mucinous neoplasm predict malignancy? A study of 147 patients. Am J Gastroenterol 102(8):1759–1764
50. Tang RS, Weinberg B, Dawson DW, Reber H, Hines OJ, Tomlinson JS, Chaudhari V, Raman S, Farrell JJ (2008) Evaluation of the guidelines for management of pancreatic branch-duct intraductal papillary mucinous neoplasm. Clin Gastroenterol Hep (the official clinical practice journal of the American Gastroenterological Association) 6(7):815–819; quiz 719
51. Mann CD, Palser T, Briggs CD, Cameron I, Rees M, Buckles J, Berry DP (2010) A review of factors predicting perioperative death and early outcome in hepatopancreaticobiliary cancer surgery. HPB (the official journal of the International Hepato Pancreato Biliary Association) 12(6):380–388
52. Bhayani NH, Miller JL, Ortenzi G, Kaifi JT, Kimchi ET, Staveley-O'Carroll KF, Gusani NJ (2014) Perioperative outcomes of pancreaticoduodenectomy compared to total pancreatectomy for neoplasia. J Gastrointest Surg (official journal of the Society for Surgery of the Alimentary Tract) 18(3):549–554
53. Tran K, Van Eijck C, Di Carlo V, Hop WC, Zerbi A, Balzano G, Jeekel H (2002) Occlusion of the pancreatic duct versus pancreaticojejunostomy: a prospective randomized trial. Ann Surg 236(4):422–428; discussion 428
54. Sikora SS, Posner MC (1995) Management of the pancreatic stump following pancreaticoduodenectomy. Br J Surg 82(12):1590–1597
55. Aston SJ, Longmire WP Jr (1974) Management of the pancreas after pancreaticoduodenectomy. Ann Surg 179(3):322–327

56. Bassi C, Falconi M, Molinari E, Salvia R, Butturini G, Sartori N, Mantovani W, Pederzoli P (2005) Reconstruction by pancreaticojejunostomy versus pancreaticogastrostomy following pancreatectomy: results of a comparative study. Ann Surg 242(6):767–771, discussion 771–763
57. Yeo CJ, Cameron JL, Maher MM, Sauter PK, Zahurak ML, Talamini MA, Lillemoe KD, Pitt HA (1995) A prospective randomized trial of pancreaticogastrostomy versus pancreaticojejunostomy after pancreaticoduodenectomy. Ann Surg 222(4):580–588; discussion 588–592
58. Duffas JP, Suc B, Msika S, Fourtanier G, Muscari F, Hay JM, Fingerhut A, Millat B, Radovanowic A, Fagniez PL (2005) A controlled randomized multicenter trial of pancreatogastrostomy or pancreatojejunostomy after pancreatoduodenectomy. Am J Surg 189(6):720–729
59. Tran KT, Smeenk HG, van Eijck CH, Kazemier G, Hop WC, Greve JW, Terpstra OT, Zijlstra JA, Klinkert P, Jeekel H (2004) Pylorus preserving pancreaticoduodenectomy versus standard Whipple procedure: a prospective, randomized, multicenter analysis of 170 patients with pancreatic and periampullary tumors. Ann Surg 240(5):738–745
60. Seiler CA, Wagner M, Bachmann T, Redaelli CA, Schmied B, Uhl W, Friess H, Buchler MW (2005) Randomized clinical trial of pylorus-preserving duodenopancreatectomy versus classical Whipple resection-long term results. Br J Surg 92(5):547–556
61. Lin PW, Shan YS, Lin YJ, Hung CJ (2005) Pancreaticoduodenectomy for pancreatic head cancer: PPPD versus Whipple procedure. Hepatogastroenterology 52(65):1601–1604
62. Suc B, Msika S, Fingerhut A, Fourtanier G, Hay JM, Holmieres F, Sastre B, Fagniez PL (2003) Temporary fibrin glue occlusion of the main pancreatic duct in the prevention of intra-abdominal complications after pancreatic resection: prospective randomized trial. Ann Surg 237(1):57–65
63. Dong Z, Xu J, Wang Z, Petrov MS (2013) Stents for the prevention of pancreatic fistula following pancreaticoduodenectomy. Cochrane Database Syst Rev 6:CD008914
64. Bilimoria MM, Cormier JN, Mun Y, Lee JE, Evans DB, Pisters PW (2003) Pancreatic leak after left pancreatectomy is reduced following main pancreatic duct ligation. Br J Surg 90 (2):190–196
65. Diener MK, Seiler CM, Rossion I, Kleeff J, Glanemann M, Butturini G, Tomazic A, Bruns CJ, Busch OR, Farkas S et al (2011) Efficacy of stapler versus hand-sewn closure after distal pancreatectomy (DISPACT): a randomised, controlled multicentre trial. Lancet 377 (9776):1514–1522
66. Suzuki Y, Fujino Y, Tanioka Y, Hori Y, Ueda T, Takeyama Y, Tominaga M, Ku Y, Yamamoto YM, Kuroda Y (1999) Randomized clinical trial of ultrasonic dissector or conventional division in distal pancreatectomy for non-fibrotic pancreas. Br J Surg 86(5):608–611
67. Kawai M, Tani M, Yamaue H (2008) Transection using bipolar scissors reduces pancreatic fistula after distal pancreatectomy. J Hepato-biliary-pancreatic Surg 15(4):366–372
68. Hartwig W, Duckheim M, Strobel O, Dovzhanskiy D, Bergmann F, Hackert T, Buchler MW, Werner J (2010) LigaSure for pancreatic sealing during distal pancreatectomy. World J Surg 34(5):1066–1070
69. Suzuki Y, Kuroda Y, Morita A, Fujino Y, Tanioka Y, Kawamura T, Saitoh Y (1995) Fibrin glue sealing for the prevention of pancreatic fistulas following distal pancreatectomy. Arch Surg (Chicago, Ill: 1960) 130(9):952–955
70. Olah A, Issekutz A, Belagyi T, Hajdu N, Romics L Jr (2009) Randomized clinical trial of techniques for closure of the pancreatic remnant following distal pancreatectomy. Br J Surg 96 (6):602–607
71. Moriura S, Kimura A, Ikeda S, Iwatsuka Y, Ikezawa T, Naiki K (1995) Closure of the distal pancreatic stump with a seromuscular flap. Surg Today 25(11):992–994
72. Wagner M, Gloor B, Ambuhl M, Worni M, Lutz JA, Angst E, Candinas D (2007) Roux-en-Y drainage of the pancreatic stump decreases pancreatic fistula after distal pancreatic resection. J Gastrointest Surg (official journal of the Society for Surgery of the Alimentary Tract) 11 (3):303–308

73. Kleeff J, Diener MK, Z'Graggen K, Hinz U, Wagner M, Bachmann J, Zehetner J, Muller MW, Friess H, Buchler MW (2007) Distal pancreatectomy: risk factors for surgical failure in 302 consecutive cases. Ann Surg 245(4):573–582
74. Fischer CP, Bass B, Fahy B, Aloia T (2008) Transampullary pancreatic duct stenting decreases pancreatic fistula rate following left pancreatectomy. Hepatogastroenterology 55(81):244–248
75. Ridgway PF, Guller U (2009) Interpreting study designs in surgical research: a practical guide for surgeons and surgical residents. J Am Coll Surg 208(4):635–645
76. Strobel O, Buchler MW (2013) The problem of the poor control arm in surgical randomized controlled trials. Br J Surg 100(2):172–173
77. Doerr-Harim C, Bruckner T, Diener MK, Knebel P (2014) Insights into surgical trials: methodological challenges and solutions. Langenbeck's Arch Surg/Deut Ges Chir 399 (3):273–278
78. Devereaux PJ, Bhandari M, Clarke M, Montori VM, Cook DJ, Yusuf S, Sackett DL, Cina CS, Walter SD, Haynes B et al (2005) Need for expertise based randomised controlled trials. BMJ (Clinical research ed) 330(7482):88
79. DeTurris SV, Cacchione RN, Mungara A, Pecoraro A, Ferzli GS (2002) Laparoscopic herniorrhaphy: beyond the learning curve. J Am Coll Surg 194(1):65–73
80. Sibai T, Carlisle H, Tornetta P 3rd (2012) The darker side of randomized trials: recruitment challenges. J Bone Joint Surg Am 94(1):49–55
81. Bednarska E, Bryant D, Devereaux PJ (2008) Orthopaedic surgeons prefer to participate in expertise-based randomized trials. Clin Orthop Relat Res 466(7):1734–1744
82. Montorsi M, Zago M, Mosca F, Capussotti L, Zotti E, Ribotta G, Fegiz G, Fissi S, Roviaro G, Peracchia A et al (1995) Efficacy of octreotide in the prevention of pancreatic fistula after elective pancreatic resections: a prospective, controlled, randomized clinical trial. Surgery 117 (1):26–31
83. Friess H, Beger HG, Sulkowski U, Becker H, Hofbauer B, Dennler HJ, Buchler MW (1995) Randomized controlled multicentre study of the prevention of complications by octreotide in patients undergoing surgery for chronic pancreatitis. Br J Surg 82(9):1270–1273
84. Pederzoli P, Bassi C, Falconi M, Camboni MG (1994) Efficacy of octreotide in the prevention of complications of elective pancreatic surgery. Italian Study Group. Br J Surg 81(2):265–269
85. Buchler M, Friess H, Klempa I, Hermanek P, Sulkowski U, Becker H, Schafmayer A, Baca I, Lorenz D, Meister R et al (1992) Role of octreotide in the prevention of postoperative complications following pancreatic resection. Am J Surg 163(1):125–130; discussion 130–121
86. Yeo CJ, Cameron JL, Lillemoe KD, Sauter PK, Coleman J, Sohn TA, Campbell KA, Choti MA (2000) Does prophylactic octreotide decrease the rates of pancreatic fistula and other complications after pancreaticoduodenectomy? Results of a prospective randomized placebo-controlled trial. Ann Surg 232(3):419–429
87. Lowy AM, Lee JE, Pisters PW, Davidson BS, Fenoglio CJ, Stanford P, Jinnah R, Evans DB (1997) Prospective, randomized trial of octreotide to prevent pancreatic fistula after pancreaticoduodenectomy for malignant disease. Ann Surg 226(5):632–641
88. Koti RS, Gurusamy KS, Fusai G, Davidson BR (2010) Meta-analysis of randomized controlled trials on the effectiveness of somatostatin analogues for pancreatic surgery: a Cochrane review. HPB (the official journal of the International Hepato Pancreato Biliary Association) 12(3):155–165
89. Conlon KC, Labow D, Leung D, Smith A, Jarnagin W, Coit DG, Merchant N, Brennan MF (2001) Prospective randomized clinical trial of the value of intraperitoneal drainage after pancreatic resection. Ann Surg 234(4):487–493; discussion 493–484
90. Van Buren G, 2nd, Bloomston M, Hughes SJ, Winter J, Behrman SW, Zyromski NJ, Vollmer C, Velanovich V, Riall T, Muscarella P et al (2014) A randomized prospective multicenter trial of pancreaticoduodenectomy with and without routine intraperitoneal drainage. Ann Surg 259 (4):605–612
91. Hackert T, Buchler MW (2013) Pancreatic cancer: advances in treatment, results and limitations. Dig Dis (Basel, Switzerland) 31(1):51–56

92. Kooby DA, Hawkins WG, Schmidt CM, Weber SM, Bentrem DJ, Gillespie TW, Sellers JB, Merchant NB, Scoggins CR, Martin RC, 3rd et al (2010) A multicenter analysis of distal pancreatectomy for adenocarcinoma: is laparoscopic resection appropriate? J Am Coll Surg 210(5):779–785, 786–777
93. Venkat R, Edil BH, Schulick RD, Lidor AO, Makary MA, Wolfgang CL (2012) Laparoscopic distal pancreatectomy is associated with significantly less overall morbidity compared to the open technique: a systematic review and meta-analysis. Ann Surg 255(6):1048–1059
94. Kuroki T, Adachi T, Okamoto T, Kanematsu T (2012) A non-randomized comparative study of laparoscopy-assisted pancreaticoduodenectomy and open pancreaticoduodenectomy. Hepatogastroenterology 59(114):570–573
95. Nigri G, Petrucciani N, La Torre M, Magistri P, Valabrega S, Aurello P, Ramacciato G (2014) Duodenopancreatectomy: Open or minimally invasive approach? Surg (Journal of the Royal Colleges of Surgeons of Edinburgh and Ireland)
96. Cirocchi R, Partelli S, Coratti A, Desiderio J, Parisi A, Falconi M (2013) Current status of robotic distal pancreatectomy: a systematic review. Surg Oncol 22(3):201–207
97. Cirocchi R, Partelli S, Trastulli S, Coratti A, Parisi A, Falconi M (2013) A systematic review on robotic pancreaticoduodenectomy. Surg Oncol 22(4):238–246
98. Sibbald B, Roland M (1998) Understanding controlled trials. Why are randomised controlled trials important? BMJ (Clinical research ed) 316(7126):201

Comparative Effectiveness in Hepatic Malignancies

Andrew J. Page, David Cosgrove and Timothy M. Pawlik

Abstract

The benefits of applying comparative effectiveness research (CER) strategies to the management of cancer are important. As the incidence of cancer increases both in the United States and worldwide, accurate analysis of which tests and treatments should be applied in which situations is critical, both in terms of measurable and meaningful clinical outcomes and health care costs. In the last 20 years alone, multiple controversies have arisen in the diagnosis and treatment of primary and metastatic tumors of the liver, making the management of liver malignancies a prime example of CER. Contributing factors to the development of these controversies include improvements in molecular characterization of these diseases and technological advances in surgery and radiology. The relative speed of these advances has outpaced data from clinical trials, in turn making robust data to inform clinical practice lacking. Indeed, many of the current treatment recommendations for the management of liver malignancies are based primarily on retrospective data. We herein review select CER issues concerning select decision-making topics in the management of liver malignancies.

Keywords

Comparative effectiveness · Hepatocellular carcinoma · Colorectal metastasis · Hepatectomy · Neuroendocrine metastasis

A.J. Page · T.M. Pawlik (✉)
Division of Surgical Oncology, John L. Cameron Professor of Alimentary Tract Surgery, Department of Surgery, Johns Hopkins Hospital, 600 N. Wolfe Street, Baltimore, MD 21287, USA
e-mail: tpawlik1@jhmi.edu

D. Cosgrove
Department of Medical Oncology, Johns Hopkins Hospital, Baltimore, MD, USA

K.Y. Bilimoria et al. (eds.), *Comparative Effectiveness in Surgical Oncology*, Cancer Treatment and Research 164, DOI 10.1007/978-3-319-12553-4_11

Contents

1 Hepatocellular Carcinoma (HCC)

Hepatocellular carcinoma (HCC) is the seventh most common cancer in the world and its incidence is increasing [1, 2]. The presentation of patients with HCC is broad, both in terms of tumor burden and extent of liver dysfunction. Tumor burden may range from small and solitary HCC, to multinodular and metastatic disease; the degree of liver dysfunction can also be extensive with cirrhosis, or be absent without any evidence of liver function compromise. The management of HCC must be directed to patients anywhere along this spectrum, and includes systemic chemotherapy, non-resection local therapies (NRLT), liverl resection (LR), and liver transplant (LT). Given the broad spectrum of presentation, combined with multiple emerging treatment modalities, expectedly, there are CER dilemmas.

1.1 Unresectable HCC: The Role of Local Therapies

Unfortunately, many patients with HCC present with disease that is unresectable secondary either to advanced stage, or with evidence of liver dysfunction that cannot tolerate resection. For those patients with advanced HCC that is unresectable, less invasive therapies like NRLT have been incorporated into the management of HCC. The common examples of NRLTs include percutaneous ethanol injection (PEI), radiofrequency ablation (RFA), transarterial chemoembolization (TACE), drug-eluting bead transarterial chemoembilzation (DEB-TACE), and transarterial radio-embolization (TARE) with yttrium-90 (Y90). Over the past 20 years, each type of these therapies has been studied and applied to patients with varying levels of disease burden and liver dysfunction. Recently, the comparative data supporting the use of these less-invasive therapies in unresectable HCC has grown rapidly.

Prior to the 1990s, there was no evidence-based algorithm for applying local therapies in HCC and most guidelines were based on small retrospective reviews [3, 4]. This was especially true for unresectable patients with a low burden of disease, but who had evidence of significant cirrhosis. In 2003, Lencioni et al. [5] were one of the first groups to examine the role of NRLT in a prospective randomized study involving patients with HCC deemed to be not appropriate for LT or LR. In a sample of 102 patients, all patients with cirrhosis and single HCC <5 cm or three HCCs each <3 cm were randomized to PEI or RFA. At 2 years, the authors noted that patients treated with RFA had a trend toward improved overall survival and significantly better recurrence-free survival compared with patients treated with PEI (98 % vs. 88 %, p = 0.138, and 96 % vs. 62 %, RR = 0.17, p = 0.002, respectively). On multivariate analysis, RFA remained an independent prognostic factor associated with an improvement in local recurrence-free survival (RR 0.20, p = 0.015). Lin et al. [6] reported similar trends in a larger prospective trial with longer follow-up in which the authors noted improvements in both overall survival and recurrence-free survival with RFA. At 3 years, overall survival was 74 % versus 51 % (p = 0.31), with recurrence-free survival (43 % vs. 21 %; p = 0.038) also favoring the RFA versus PEI group. While overall survival was equivocal, the aggregate data seemed to support RFA over PEI for small HCC in terms of recurrence-free survival.

Some patients will present with HCC that has progressed to a more advanced stage where ablation cannot be utilized. In this scenario, the HCC typically has reached a larger size and transitioned to receive the majority of its blood flow from the hepatic artery [7]. With the HCC being larger in size, treatments like RFA and PEI do not have the same efficacy as when the lesion is smaller [8, 9]. As such, alternative NRLTs that utilize the vascular supply of the HCC to deliver therapy have been incorporated into the management of more advanced HCC. These intra-arterial therapies include bland embolization, embolization with chemotherapy (TACE), or embolization with drug-eluting beads with chemotherapy (DEB-TACE).

There are a number of CER issues relating to intra-arterial therapy of HCC, including but not limited to: (1) what type of chemotherapy (if any) should be given with TAE, (2) is there a role for DEB, (3) what agent should be used for embolization, (4) how many treatments or sessions should be offered, and (5) which patients will benefit from this type of therapy. Despite the many questions around the evolving treatment modalities for advanced HCC, some data do exist to guide our current understanding for the role of intra-arterial therapies for more advanced HCC. One early study, performed by the D'Etude [10] evaluated the effect of TACE on unresectable, larger HCC compared with conservative treatment/best supportive care. The authors noted that TACE reduced tumor growth (decreased >50, 16 % vs. 5 %, p = 0.001) and decreased serum AFP (decreased >50, 23 % vs. 8 %, p = 0.001). The effect of TACE on overall survival was not pronounced, with 4-year overall survival of 12 % versus 15 % (p = 0.13). Other studies have explored the role of TACE in unresectable HCC and similarly failed to demonstrate a dramatic improvement in survival with intra-arterial therapy [11–14]. In a separate study, however, Llovet et al. [15] demonstrated that TACE did indeed lead to a survival benefit. In this prospective study, patients with advanced HCC (i.e. lesions not amenable to resection or transplantation) were randomized to TACE, bland embolization, or conservative therapy/best supportive care. The investigators noted an overall survival benefit for TACE over bland embolization and conservative therapy (2-year overall survival: 63 % vs. 50 % vs. 27 %, respectively; $p = 0.009$). On multivariate analysis, TACE was the only variable independently associated with survival (OR 0.45, $p = 0.02$). The authors attributed this improvement to strict patient selection, gelfoam as their embolization agent, and doxorubicin as the chemotherapeutic agent. The trial was stopped early so that patients in this setting could receive TACE. Based on these data, TACE is now part of the standard therapeutic armamentarium for patients with advanced HCC [16–18].

1.2 Imaging and Tumor Response After Local Therapies

An area that has evolved dramatically both in terms of technological advancement and CER has been the adoption of standardized and objective radiological response criteria after NRLT. Radiologic response to local therapies is critical to the management of HCC as it may be a surrogate marker for survival [19]. The two earliest suggested recommendations for standardization of objective response to NRLT were the World Health Organization (WHO) criteria and the Response Evaluation Criteria in Solid Tumors (RECIST) guidelines [20, 21]. Both of these guidelines were based on tumor response being correlated with changes in tumor size. However, treatment with these types of NRLT of HCC often results in change in tumor vascularity and viability, but not necessarily changes in tumor size. As such, the WHO and RECIST criteria have been criticized as being limited and unreliable. Subsequently, the European Association for the Study of the Liver (EASL) and the American Association for the Study of Liver Diseases (AASLD) proposed additional guidelines to assess tumor response following NRLT [22, 23]. These criteria specifically took into account tumor necrosis by examining the reduction in viable tumor area using contrast-enhanced radiologic imaging. Viable tumor was defined as the part of the tumor that took up contrast in the arterial phase, while the role of overall tumor size was made a secondary consideration in the assessment of the tumor response [23]. Another proposed set of criteria to assess response include the modified RECIST (mRECIST) criteria, which bases assessment of overall response on target lesions characteristics noted on contrast enhanced imaging, non-target lesions response, and the presence or absence of new lesions. The field of imaging assessment for tumor response after NRLT will continue to evolve as treatment and radiological modalities improve and will need to be a topic of future CER.

1.3 Resectable HCC: Non-resection Local Therapies Versus Resection

Patients with HCC may present with early stage disease/resectable lesion and optimal liver function with minimal to no comorbidities. For these patients, LR represents a potential therapeutic option. The long-term outcome with certain

NRLT, such as ablation that can spare higher risk surgical patients from potential perioperative complications, is not well-defined and represents a subject of CER interest [24, 25]. Chen et al. [24] compared LR versus RFA for patients with a solitary small HCC. In this prospective series, 180 patients were randomized to RFA or LR. Inclusion criteria for the study were solitary HCC <5 cm in diameter, no vascular involvement, no evidence of liver dysfunction, and patients had to be suitable for either LR or RFA. At 4 years, overall survival was equivalent among patients undergoing RFA or LR at 65.9 % versus 64.0 %, respectively. In terms of disease-free survival, results were also similar with 4-year recurrence-free survival being 48.2 % versus 51.6 %, respectively. The authors concluded that RFA and LR were equally effective in the treatment of solitary and small HCC, with RFA being associated with decreased morbidity. Huang et al. [25] also prospectively examined the issue of LR versus RFA, but with expanded guidelines and came to different conclusions. In this study, patients with 3 lesions <3 cm or one lesion <5 cm were included. LR had improved survival and decreased recurrence over RFA. The 5-year overall survival was 54.8 % versus 75.7 % for RFA and LR, respectively (p = 0.001). In terms of disease-free survival, the same trend of better outcomes with LR over RFA was observed (5-year disease-free survival: 51.3 % vs. 28.7 %, respectively; p = 0.024). Direct comparisons of the different outcomes in the Chang and Huang studies is difficult as the studies varied in their inclusion criteria. Of note, in the Huang study, patients were not blinded to their treatment plan and 7 patients chose LR over RFA. In addition, the tumor size of the HCC was different between groups and the rate of loss of follow-up between groups was higher in the LR group (15.6 % vs. 6.1 %, $p < 0.05$). The comparison of these studies represents a key component to CER—understanding differences in study design, inclusion/exclusion criteria, as well as recognizing limitations in analysis. Furthermore, applying this CER perspective is necessary as more treatment modalities become available, e.g. the role of microwave versus RFA [26].

1.4 Resection Versus Transplant

Another source of treatment of CER interest is the debate over when to offer LR versus LT for early HCC. Theoretically, for most patients with HCC, LT represents the best treatment for survival because it removes both the tumor and underlying liver disease. There are, however, obstacles preventing LT from being offered to all patients with HCC including a limited availability of donor organs [27]. Historically in the 1980s and 1990s, the broad criteria utilized in organ allocation for patients with HCC led to a variety of outcomes for patients transplanted with HCC. In fact, the 90-day mortality, tumor recurrence, and long-term survival were not equivalent among all patients who were transplanted and some results were actually quite poor [28]. As such, attempts were made to identify the specific subset of patients who would benefit the most from LT [29]. In the seminal report by Mazzaferro et al. [30] the authors reported on a subset of patients with specific HCC characteristics who were proposed as a select patient population who would benefit from LT. This so-called “Milan criteria” included patients with one lesion smaller than 5 cm, up to 3 lesions smaller than 3 cm, no extra-hepatic manifestations, and no vascular invasion [30]. Since the adoption of the Milan criteria, additional guidelines have been suggested to broaden the inclusion of patients eligible for LT [31, 32]. These proposed guidelines include increasing the acceptable tumor size for transplantation. The ideal patient population to benefit from LT is still evolving and only with persistent CER re-assessment will refinements in the allocation system be possible.

Despite the identification of patient populations who benefit from LT, there are still limitations of donor organ availability, making application of LT to all patients with HCC not feasible. In turn, LR is a feasible alternative for some patients. Improvements in patient selection and perioperative management have made LR safe and relatively effective. While patients with end-stage liver disease and early stage tumors are most appropriate for LT, patients with compensated liver disease and early stage tumors can be appropriate for LT or LR. Choosing LT or LR for patients with compensated cirrhosis and early stage HCC remains challenging and often debated. In a retrospective review, Margarit et al. [33] examined the issue of when to offer LT versus LR for patients with early stage HCC and compensated cirrhosis. In this study, the authors reviewed patients with a single tumor <5 cm and Child’s class A liver disease and noted 10-year disease-free survival was worse after LR versus LT (18 % vs. 56 %, $p = 0.001$), with mean disease-free survival of 52 months versus 86 months, respectively ($p = 0.04$). Only 2.7 % in the LT group had local, hepatic recurrence versus 48.6 % in the LR cohort ($p = 0.001$). In terms of overall survival, there were no differences between the two groups (46 % vs. 36 %, LR vs. LT, $p = 0.3$) (Fig. 1a). Other studies have examined the same topic, with larger cohorts and intention-to-treat analyses [34–37] (Table 1). For example, Bellavance et al. [38] reported on 245 patients who underwent hepatic resection and 134 patients who underwent liver transplantation for early stage HCC. All patients had well-compensated cirrhosis. Compared with transplantation, patients undergoing resection had larger tumors and a higher incidence of microscopic vascular invasion. Transplantation was associated with better 5-year disease-free and overall survival compared with resection (Fig. 1b). Hepatitis status, presence of microscopic vascular invasion, and tumor size were predictors for recurrence, while the presence of microscopic vascular invasion and tumor size conferred an increased risk of death. The disease-free survival advantage with transplantation was more pronounced in hepatitis C patients compared with non-hepatitis and hepatitis B patients. The overall survival advantage with transplantation persisted in cases of solitary lesions ≤3 cm, but was attenuated in patients with a MELD score ≤8.

Final consensus on the comparative debate between LR and LT for early stage HCC with compensated liver disease remains lacking. While disease-free survival is clearly better among patients undergoing LT, the relative overall survival benefit of LT over LR remains ill defined. While LT has benefits over LR, it remains unclear whether patients who recur following LR can be salvaged with LT and experience the same long-term survival [39–41]. Prospective, randomized studies taking into

Fig. 1 **a**, **b** Actuarial patient survival after liver resection and liver transplant. Used with permission [33, 38]

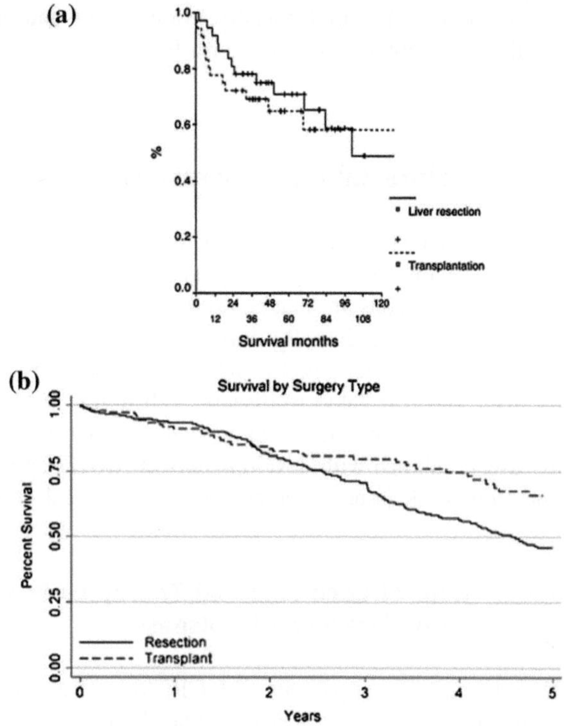

Table 1 Summary of studies examining liver resection versus liver transplant for early hepatocellular cancer

First author (year)	Treatment groups	Total patients	Childs A/B/C or average MELD	Mean maximal tumor size (cm)	5-year disease free survival (%)	5-year overall survival (%)
Figueras (2000) [35]	Resection	35	31/4/0	4.8	31	51
	Transplant	85	43/35/7	2.8	60	60
Margarit (2005) [33]	Resection	37	37/0/0	3.2	39	70
	Transplant	36	36/0/0	3.0	64	65
Poon (2007) [34]	Resection	204	195/9/0	<5	42	68
	Transplant	43	8/15/20	<5	84	81
Del Gaudio (2008) [36]	Resection	80	55/14/0	3.1	41	66
	Transplant	293	23/139/131	1.3	71	73
Bellavance (2008) [38]	Resection	245	9.1	NR	40	48[a]
	Transplant	134	11.0		82	79[a]
Lee (2010) [111]	Resection	130	113/17/0	4.5	50	52
	Transplant	78	35/43/0	3.8	75	68
Koniaris (2011) [37]	Resection	106	7.3	6.1	45	53
	Transplant	257	12.9	3.0	60	62

Adapted from and used with permission [110]
NR not reported
[a] For solitary lesions, ≤3 cm

account tumor size, multifocality, waitlist time and organ availability, and comorbidities, with appropriate long-term follow-up are needed to better address the LR versus LT debate.

2 Colorectal Liver Metastases

In the United States, colorectal metastases to the liver (CRLM) are probably the most common secondary malignancy involving the liver [42]. Approximately 140,000 Americans are diagnosed with colon cancer annually, with more than half of these patients eventually developing metastases [43]. Most of these metastases are found in the liver, and the presentation may vary from disease that is isolated to the liver and resectable to disease with tumor burden that is extensive and unresectable [44]. Given the heterogeneity of this patient population with metastatic disease, combined with developments in NRLTs and a paucity of prospective data, numerous CER issues have arisen in the surgical oncology literature.

2.1 Role of Loco-regional Therapies in Patients with Unresectable Disease

Unfortunately, most patients with CRLM have unresectable disease [45]. There are numerous reasons why a patient may be unresectable and not be an appropriate candidate for LR, including multiple small tumors, vascular involvement of the tumor, a small future liver remnant (FLR), medical comorbidities, or extra-hepatic disease. Typically patients with unresectable disease are treated with systemic therapy, with an associated median survival of 2 years and 5-year survival around 10–15 % [46, 47]. For those patients with liver predominant or liver only disease that is unresectable, local therapies may have a possible therapeutic role over systemic therapy. These options include RFA, TARE with Yttrium-90 microspheres, TACE with irinotecan eluting beads (DEBIRI), and hepatic artery infusion (HAI) pumps [48, 49].

The role for RFA has been examined frequently as one of the more common alterative or adjunct therapeutic options for patients with unresectable advanced disease [50–55]. Siperstein et al. [56] examined a retrospective cohort of patients with unresectable CRLMs that were treated with RFA. A unique strength to this study was its extensive 10-year follow-up. In the cohort of 234 patients—all of whom were treated with RFA—the 5-year survival was 18.4 %, which the authors noted was better than the 5-year survival or 10 % for historical controls treated with systemic therapy alone [57]. In a separate study, as part of the Intergroup 40,004 trial contrast, Ruers et al. [58] reported their findings for patients with unresectable CRLM. In this prospective study, the investigators compared systemic FOLFOX-based chemotherapy combined with RFA versus systemic therapy alone for patients with advanced CRLM. The authors noted that 30-month overall survival was similar: 61.7 % in the combined arm versus 57.6 % in the systemic therapy alone arm (p = NS). Median overall survival was also similar: 40.5 months in the systemic arm versus 45.3 months in the combined treatment arm (p = NS). While overall survival was the same in both groups, 3-year progression free survival was worse in the systemic alone arm (10.6 % vs. 27.6 %, HR = 0.63, p = 0.025). Therefore, the authors concluded that overall survival for patients with unresectable disease treated with systemic therapy alone versus ablation plus systemic therapy was similar, while progression free survival was improved with the use of ablation.

Other local therapies have also shown promise, however the data supporting their use is not as robust and therefore is a focus on CER. One such therapy is the HAI pump. First proposed in 1984, the role for HAI has been controversial, and its efficacy has been compared to systemic therapies in multiple prospective studies [59–62]. Many of these studies, however, have been criticized due to low sample size, patient cross-over, and the single-center nature of the trials [63]. In an effort to address these issues, Kemeny et al. [63] prospectively compared HAI pump therapy with systemic therapy in a large multi-institutional trial that did not allow cross-over. The authors reported that overall survival was improved for patients who received HAI versus systemic chemotherapy (median, 24.4 months vs. 20 months, p = 0.0034). Additionally, response rates were higher (47 % vs. 24 %, p = 0.012) and time to hepatic progression was longer (9.8 months vs. 7.3 months, p = 0.034) with HAI therapy. While these data were promising, other studies have challenged the survival benefit of HAI. In a meta-analysis of 10 randomized controlled trials performed comparing HAI with systemic chemotherapy, Mocellin et al. recently suggested that there is no evidence supporting the use of HAI. In the pooled analysis, while tumor response rate was expectedly better in the HAI group (42.9 % vs. 18.4 %, RR 2.3, <0.001), overall survival was not different comparing HAI versus systemic therapy (15.9 months vs. 12.4 months, HR 0.9, p = 0.24, respectively). While HAI therapy may provide some benefit in the treatment of advanced colorectal liver metastasis, more CER is needed to determine the role for HAI.

Other newer local therapies such as TACE with irinotecan beads (DEBIRI) and TARE with Yttrium-90 (Y-90) have posed CER issues in the context of unresectable CRLM. There are emerging data for the use of transarterial DEBIRI in the treatment of unresectable liver metastasis [64–66]. Many studies, however, incorporate TACE or TARE only for patients who are refractory to systemic therapies. Martin et al. [66] reported 55 patients who had received prior systemic chemotherapy and who underwent DEBIRI treatment. In this series, response rates were 66 % at 6 months and 75 % at 12 months. TARE with Y-90 has also been investigated for patients refractory to chemotherapy [67, 68]. Cosimelli et al. [68] in a prospective multicenter phase II trial, evaluated the effect of TARE on patients who had failed previous oxaliplatin and ironotecan based chemotherapies. Based on RECIST criteria, 2 % had a complete response, 22 % a partial response, 24 % had stable disease, 44 % had progressive disease, and 8 % were non-evaluable. Because of these promising results, a phase III multicenter clinical trial, Efficacy Evaluation of TheraSphere following Failed First-Line Chemotherapy in Metastatic Colorectal Cancer (EPOCH) trial will soon open to elucidate the effect of TARE on not just response rates, but also overall survival. Final consensus on the optimal management of patients with unresectable CRLM is still developing, but progress is being made with emerging meta-analyses and prospective studies.

2.2 Ablation Versus Liver Resection

For the 10–25 % of patients with resectable CRLM, LR is the standard treatment approach with 5-year survival following surgery now approaching 60 % [42, 69, 70]. The role of ablation versus surgery among patients with CRLM potentially amenable to either therapy has been debated. The median overall survival associated with LR of CRLM reported in the literature ranges from 24 to 59 months whereas the data on survival following ablation are more limited [52, 71]. Several studies have sought to compare outcomes for patients who underwent ablation versus patients who underwent resection for CRLM [72–76]. Abdalla et al. [52] reported on 358 consecutive patients who underwent hepatic resection with or without RFA for CRLM. In this cohort, LR provided a significantly better overall 4-year survival over RFA alone, (65 % vs. 22 %, $p < 0.001$). Similarly, Hur et al. [77] noted a 5-year survival advantage for patients who underwent LR versus RFA (25.1 % for RFA vs. 50.0 % for LR). Based on the available data, it appears that patients managed with ablation have a worse outcome compared with patients who underwent hepatic resection (Table 2) [72, 74–76, 78].

The difference in the outcomes may, however, not be solely attributable to the type of therapy delivered (i.e. LR versus ablation), but also an issue of disparate underlying tumor biology among each patient population. Specifically, patients who undergo ablation as treatment for their CRLM often represent a distinct subgroup of patients with otherwise advanced disease who are not amenable to surgical extirpation [79]. In fact, many of the clinicopathologic features such as tumor size and number are often different in the group of patients receiving LR versus ablation. To achieve more comparable groups, subgroup analyses of patients undergoing either LR or ablation for CRLM have been performed, which have commonly been stratified by tumor number [78]. For example, Aloia et al. [78] examined a cohort of patients all of whom had only a solitary lesion. In this study, 150 patients treated with resection were compared with 30 patients treated with RFA. The authors reported that patients who underwent resection had a significantly better 5-year survival (resection: 71 % vs. RFA: 27 %; $p < 0.001$). However, patients managed with RFA likely had worse tumor biology as indicated by a higher proportion of patients with concomitant extrahepatic disease. In a separate study, Gleisner et al. [80] sought to examine how discordant clinicopathologic factors might play a crucial role in comparing patients who underwent resection versus ablation. Specifically, Gleisner et al. compared overall survival between patients who underwent resection with survival of patients who underwent RFA using three distinct statistical methods. The authors reported that patients managed with resection alone had an improved long-term overall survival compared with patients treated with

Table 2 Summary of studies comparing RFA with resection for colorectal liver metastases

First author (Year)	Treatment groups	Total patients	Mean maximal tumor size (cm)	Median time to local recurrence (months)	Median survival (months)	5-year local recurrence free survival	5-year overall survival
Oshowo (2003) [72]	RFA	25	3	NR	37	NR	52.6[a]
	Resection	20	4	NR	41		55.4[a]
Aloia (2006) [78]	RFA	30	3.0	18	NR	60	27
	Resection	150	3.5	31	NR	92	71
White (2007) [74]	RFA	22	2.4	NR	31	NR	0
	Resection	30	2.7	NR	80	NR	58
Berber (2008) [75]	RFA	68	3.7	NR	34	NR	30.0
	Resection	90	3.8	NR	57	NR	40.0
Lee (2008) [76]	RFA	37	2.25	NR	NR	42.6	48.5
	Resection	116	3.29	NR	NR	84.6	65.7
Hur (2009) [77]	RFA	25	2.5	NR	NR	69.7	25.5
	Resection	42	2.8	NR	NR	89.7	50.1
Reuter (2009) [113]	RFA	66	3.2	12.2	27.0	NR	NR
	Resection	126	5.3	31.1	36.4	NR	NR

Adapted and used with permission [112]
NR not reported
[a] At 3 years

resection plus ablation. The authors noted, however, that there were many differences in the clinicopathologic profile of each group. To examine the comparability of the baseline characteristics of the two treatment groups, Gleisner and colleagues utilized propensity score methodology. The authors noted that the aggregate distribution of the clinical and pathologic characteristics of patients undergoing resection alone versus RFA ± resection were markedly different and therefore direct comparisons of these groups may not be appropriate. The work of Gleisner and colleagues serves therefore to highlight the significant shortcomings of using retrospective data to compare outcomes following resection versus ablation in cohorts of patients who are very different and whose choice of treatment was undoubtedly based in part based of very different baseline characteristics.

In 2009, as part of an American Society of Clinical Oncology (ASCO) evidence-based review, Wong et al. [81] attempted to examine all data available at that time on ablation and LR for CRLM. The authors concluded that the available data were insufficient to form the basis of an evidence-based recommendation. Specifically, the authors noted that there was wide variability in 5-year survival (14–55 %) and local tumor recurrence (3.6–60 %) with ablation compared with LR. In turn, the investigators commented that the question of ablation versus LR could only be answered by a prospective, randomized trial. Such a trial, while ideal, would be challenging for a variety of reasons, most significantly, accrual would be required to be multi-institutional, and the ablation procedure itself would need to be standardized [45]. In an attempt to simulate such a trial, Khajanchee et al. [45] used a Markov and Monte Carlo analysis comparing RFA and LR. The authors reported that the model estimated 5-year survival among those patients who underwent LR over RFA alone to be 38.2 % versus 27.2 %, respectively. Five-year disease-free survival was also superior in the LR group (LR: 29.8 % vs. RFA: 15.5 %). While there are no prospective data comparing ablation with LR in the resectable population, from the limited data available, LR should remain the preferred approach with ablation being used as an adjunct second line therapy.

2.3 Systemic Therapy, Neoadjuvant Chemotherapy and the Disappearing Liver Metastasis

While local therapies such as ablation and resection are important treatment options for patients with CRLM, systemic chemotherapy plays a critical role in the multimodal therapy of these patients. Systemic therapy has the potential of treating micrometastatic disease, evaluating tumor response, and downstaging unresectable tumors to resectability. The benefits of chemotherapy come with some possible consequences, including hepatotoxicity such as sinusoidal dilation, steatosis, or steatohepatitis [47, 57, 82, 83].

In an attempt identify which patients may benefit the most from systemic chemotherapy, several predictive models have been designed to identify patients at high risk for recurrence after hepatectomy. Fong et al. [42] were one of the first groups to propose a clinical risk score for predicting recurrence and survival. This study identified several prognostic factors for recurrence including: extra-hepatic disease, node-positive primary tumor, disease free interval from primary to metastases <12 months, CEA level >200, largest hepatic tumor >5 cm, and number of hepatic tumors >1. Similarly, Adam et al. [84] also created a prognostic model, examining initially unresectable CRLM that received chemotherapy and that were downstaged to resectability. In this study, the investigators identified a rectal primary, ≥3 CRLMs, maximum CRLM size of ≥10 cm, and CA19-9 >100 as independent factors of poor prognosis. Capussotti et al. [85] in 2007 suggested their own prognostic model. These authors identified patients with T4 primary colon cancers, metastases with infiltration of neighboring structures, and patients with more than three metastases as being potential indicators of poor prognosis and, in turn, may indicate a potential benefit from systemic chemotherapy. Despite these large retrospective series, there are still no specific consensus guidelines to indicate which patients with resectable CLRM should receive systemic chemotherapy either in the adjuvant or neoadjuvant setting [86].

Among the cohort of patients treated with neoadjuvant or preoperative systemic chemotherapy, there are several CER issues that remain debatable. Most data would suggest that those patients who have progressive disease on preoperative chemotherapy have a very poor prognosis [84]. Whether these patients should categorically be refused potential surgery even if the disease is technically still resectable remains controversial. Among patients who have a response to neoadjuvant/preoperative chemotherapy, surgery is typically performed with the goal of resecting all sites of disease. Up to 10–25 % of patients with CRLM who are treated with preoperative chemotherapy, however, will have a complete response with radiographic "disappearance" of some or all CRLM lesions in the liver [87, 88]. The so called "disappearing liver metastasis" (DLM) raises a number of CER issues.

From a radiologic perspective, there is no consensus regarding which imaging modality (CT, MRI, FDG-PET, or FDG-PET-CT) is most appropriate to determine whether the DLM is simply "missing" due to low sensitivity of the chosen imaging modality versus whether it has truly "disappeared." Most medical oncologists and surgeons currently use CT in the treatment of patients with CRLM. The widespread use of dual phase helical CT is based on clinician familiarity and a high degree of reproducibility with excellent sensitivity and specificity up to 90 % when diagnosing CRLM [89, 90]. In the setting of a DLM, when the liver has been exposed to systemic chemotherapy—often many cycles—the background liver can appear darker with less contrast between the liver and any hypovascular metastases [91]. PET-CT has been considered as adjunct to CT alone, however PET-CT has limited sensitivity in its ability to detect lesions <1 cm and chemotherapy decreases hexokinase activity, thereby inhibiting glucose uptake for CRLM [92, 93]. Recently, there has been increasing data to suggest that MRI should be the imaging modality of choice in the setting of DLM. MRI, has increased sensitivity compared with CT, particularly in the setting of chemotherapy induced hepatic parenchymal changes (Fig. 2) [88]. In a recent meta-analysis, van Kessel et al. [94] compared various imaging modalities in the detection of CRLM after preoperative chemotherapy and found that the sensitivity of MRI was 85.7 % versus 69.9 % for CT, 54.5 % for PET, and 51.7 % for PET-CT. As such, MRI seems to be the imaging modality of choice for patients treated with preoperative chemotherapy—especially those with DLM. Future CER to understand better the role of different imaging modalities in treating patients with CRLM will be needed.

In addition to radiological issues in management of DLM, there is also is also a lack of consensus about the surgical management of DLM. As with other CER dilemmas, this primarily stems from the lack of reliable data. van Vledder et al. [87] attempted to examine the question of how to manage DLM using retrospective data; the authors noted that patients with untreated DLM had an increased local recurrence rate compared with patients who underwent LR of the DLM (p = 0.04). Despite these findings, the 1-, 3-, and 5-year overall survival was not different for patients undergoing LR versus those patients who had DLM left in situ (92.3 % vs. 93.8 %, 70.8 % vs. 63.5 %, 46.2 % vs. 63.5 % respectively) (Fig. 3a, b). The CER issues raised by the management of DLM were recently addressed by Bischof et al. [88]. In their review of DLM, the authors concluded that among patients who had a complete radiographic response, only 20–50 % had a durable long-term remission.

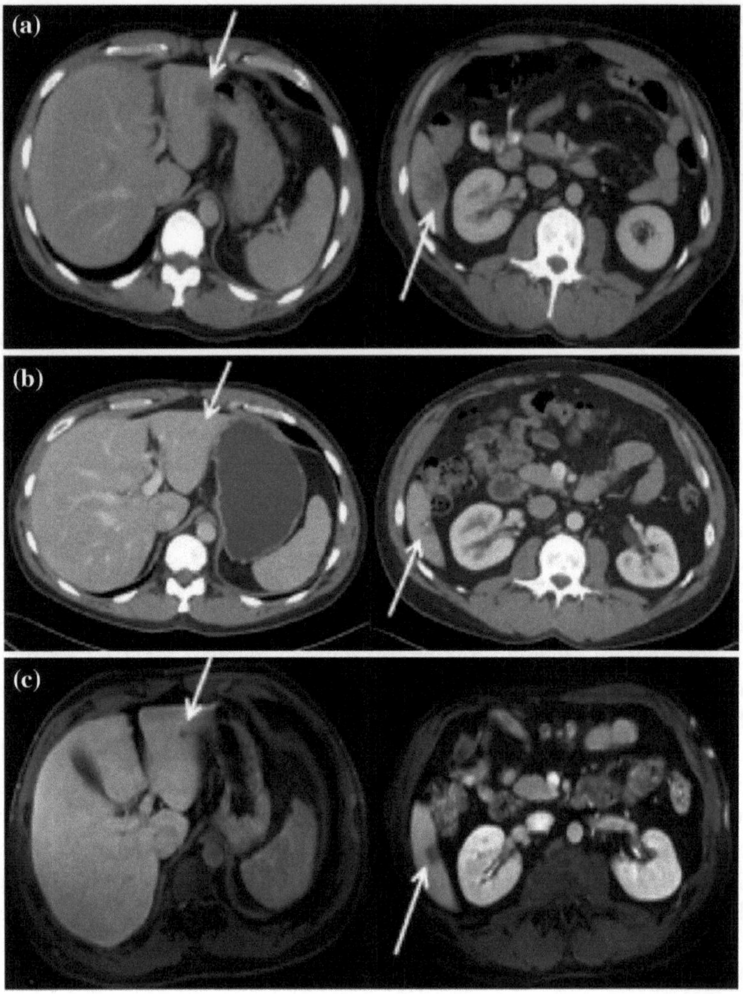

Fig. 2 **a** Computed tomography (CT) image demonstrating colorectal liver metastases in segments II and VI (*arrows*) before systemic chemotherapy. **b** After 6 cycles of FOLFOX (folinic acid, 5-fluorouracil, oxaliplatin) therapy, CT showed that the lesion in segment II had 'disappeared', whereas the lesion in segment VI was significantly smaller and calcified. **c** Magnetic resonance imaging similarly identified the lesion in segment VI, but also demonstrated a residual 7-mm lesion in segment II. Used with permission [88]

In addition, among patients who had the DLM resected, residual tumor was present in 25–45 % of patients. Therefore, more CER is need to understand which patients need surgery for a DLM after receipt of preoperative chemotherapy.

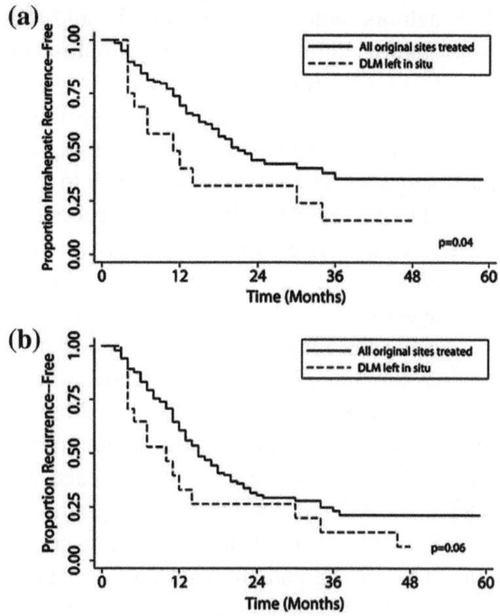

Fig. 3 **a** Kaplan–Meier curve of overall survival in patients with untreated DLM when compared to patients in whom all original disease sites were resected. **b** Kaplan–Meier curve showing overall survival in 99 patients with a complete or partial radiological response (RECIST) to preoperative chemotherapy stratified by the presence of untreated DLM. Used with permission [87]

3 Neuroendocrine Liver Metastases

Neuroendocrine tumors (NETs) represent another important topic in the context of liver surgery and CER. NETs are of particular interest as these tumors are increasing in incidence and 40–95 % of cases are metastatic at diagnosis [95]. Treatment strategies for NETs once they have metastasized to the liver (NELM) are similar to those employed for the aforementioned liver tumors, and options include systemic chemotherapy, various NRLT, and LR. Also similar to other hepatic tumors, there is an absence of data from rigorous trials [96]. To further exacerbate the issue of reliable long-term data is the often indolent biologic behavior of these tumors compared to other liver tumors [97].

3.1 Cytoreductive Therapy—Liver Resection and Non-surgical Local Therapies

While the standard of care for NELM is LR, the data guiding this recommendation are surprisingly limited. In 2000, Chamberlain et al. [98] argued in presenting the results of their surgical series that LR improved survival. In this study, the authors demonstrated on multivariate analysis that LR prolonged 5-year survival versus NRLT (bland embolization) and best supportive care (76 % vs. 50 % vs. <25 %, respectively; $p < 0.05$). In a separate study, Sarmiento et al. [99] from the Mayo Clinic reported on an experience with 170 patients who underwent LR for NELM.

The authors noted that overall 5- and 10-year survival were 61 and 35 %, respectively. Similarly, in a large multi-center study, Mayo et al. [100] reported excellent long-term results following surgery with 5- and 10-year survival of 74 and 51 %, respectively. As such, based on these data, surgical resection of NELM is widely utilized as it is believed to offer patients improved long-term survival. While most surgeons agree with an approach to resect patients with a low-disease burden, the role of surgical debulking of patients with larger disease-burdens is more controversial. For example, some groups have even suggested that patients with a high tumor burden may have a survival benefit after palliative debulking, as long as the majority (>75–80 %) of the liver disease can be removed [99, 101].

Despite the long-term survival associated with LR for NELM, recurrence following surgical management of NELM is almost universal. Specifically, in the largest retrospective review to date by Mayo et al. [100] the authors reported a 94 % recurrence at 5 years and 99 % recurrence rate at 10 years. Because of this remarkably high incidence of recurrence, there has been an increased interest in NRLT for NELM, including such intra-arterial therapies (IAT) as TACE and TARE. In a large, multi-institutional respective review, Mayo et al. [102] compared outcomes among patients with NELM based on treatment by LR versus IAT. Not surprisingly, the authors noted significant differences in the baseline characteristics of patients who underwent LR versus IAT, with the IAT group having more hormonally active tumors (48 % vs. 28 %, $p < 0.001$) and a larger hepatic tumor burden (>25 %: 76 % vs. 52 %, $p < 0.001$). The selection bias obviously calls into question any conclusions that can be drawn from retrospective comparisons of these two treatment modalities and highlights the CER challenges in answering this question. The authors did attempt to address the issue of selection bias by using propensity score matching. Propensity scoring provides a means to design and analyze a nonrandomized, retrospective dataset in an attempt to mimic some of the characteristics of a randomized controlled trial [103]. In the study, quintiles were created from their entire cohort with similar clinicopathologic characteristics and used in a matched analysis. With propensity matching, the authors noted that the analytic cohort comparing LR versus IAT groups now had much similar baseline characteristics. While LR was still associated with an improved survival over IAT, the difference was less pronounced (Fig. 4a, b). Furthermore, on stratified analyses, it was noted that symptomatic patients with a small burden of liver disease benefited the most from surgery. While symptomatic patients with a large burden of liver disease (>25 % hepatic tumor involvement) had improved median survival with LR over IAT (87 months vs. 51 months, $p < 0.001$, respectively), patients who were asymptomatic did not seemingly benefit from surgery resection (LR, 16.7 months vs. IAT, 18.5 months, $p = 0.78$). While propensity matching can assist with the comparison of groups with disparate baseline characteristics, more effective methodology and prospective trials will be necessary to answer better the CER question around which patients benefit from LR versus IAT.

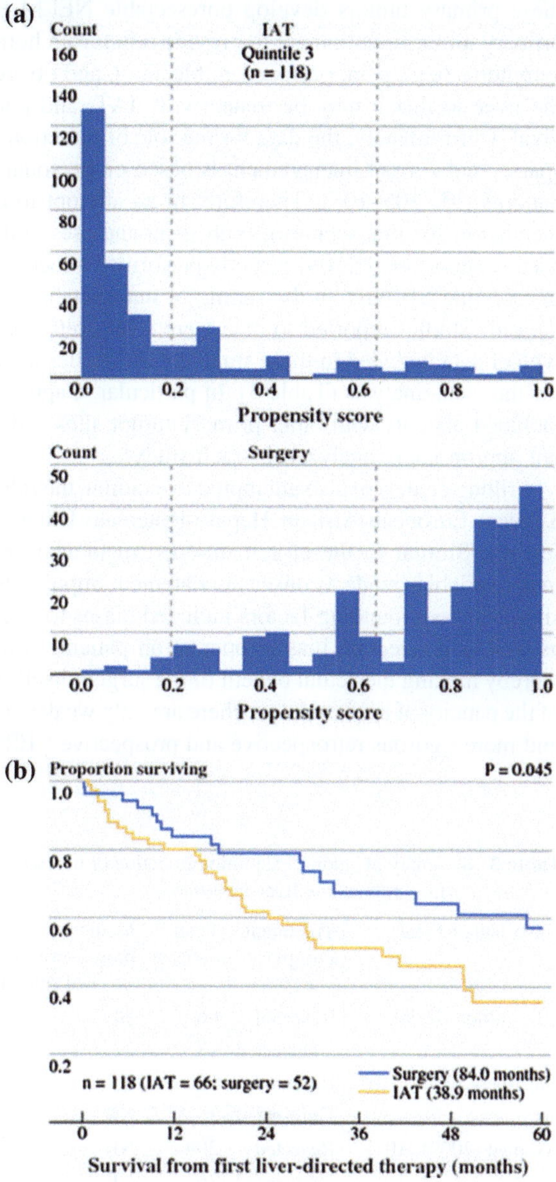

Fig. 4 **a** Histograms demonstrating the distribution of the propensity scores in the surgical and intra-arterial therapy (*IAT*) patient cohorts. The area of greatest overlap (quintile 3) corresponds to group of patients most likely have undergone either treatment based on baseline characteristics. **b** Overall survival of propensity-matched patients in quintile 3 stratified by receipt of surgery versus IAT. Used with permission [102]

3.2 Role of Resecting the Small Bowel Primary in the Unresectable NELM Setting

An additional area of CER contention is the question whether to leave an asymptomatic small bowel (SB) primary NET in place in the setting of unresectable NELMs. For patients with SB-NET, this scenario is not uncommon, as 15–80 % of these primary tumors develop unresectable NELM [104]. The proposed goals of primary tumor resection are to provide relief from hormonal and local tumor-related symptoms (e.g., pain, perforation, bleeding, and obstruction), limit disease solely to the liver so that it may be treated with IAT, and potentially improve overall survival. Unfortunately, the data for the role of resection in this scenario is particularly sparse, and current management is based on personal experience and local practice patterns [95, 105–108]. Therefore, in an attempt to create evidence-based recommendation for this scenario, both meta-analyses and consensus panels have been used. Capurso et al. [109] recently performed a meta-analysis and examined the role of resecting SB-NET in the setting of unresectable NELM. The authors found that the only studies reported to date were solely retrospective and that the quality and type of data included in these small cohort studies did not meet the inclusion criteria for the meta-analysis (Table 3). In particular, Capuso et al. noted that some studies included patients with other primary tumor sites and the role of resection was also not appropriately analyzed in each study.

Frilling et al. [96] also attempted to examine the role of primary tumor resection in a recent European-African Hepato-Pancreato-Biliary (E-AHPBA) consensus conference. Similar to the aforementioned meta-analysis, the authors concluded that many variables made a consensus statement impossible. The investigators noted that significant confounding factors included biases to operate on less advanced tumors, as well as a selection bias to operate on patients with better performance status—thereby making the actual benefit of the surgery itself impossible to discern. Because of the paucity of unbiased data, there are only weak evidence to recommend resection and more rigorous retrospective and prospective CER studies are needed.

Table 3 Summary of studies examining resection or unresected primary midgut carcinoid tumors in patients with unresectable liver metastases

First author (year)	Treatment groups	Total patients	Median progression-free survival (months)	Median overall survival (months)	5-year survival
Givi (2006) [106]	Resected	66	54	108	81
	Unresected	18	27	50	21
Strosberg (2009) [105]	Resected	100	NR	110	NR
	Unresected	35	NR	88	NR
Ahmed (2009) [107]	Resected	209	NR	119	74
	Unresected	76	NR	57	46
Norlen (2012) [108]	Resected	493	NR	NR	75
	Unresected	86	NR	NR	28

Adapted and used with permission [109]

4 Conclusion

Examining current treatment recommendations through the prism of CER is challenging and humbling, as it sheds light on areas that lack robust data and rigorous analysis. The management of liver malignancies is an ideal example of how CER has led to reliable treatments, but also where progress is urgently needed. When prospective, randomized controlled trials can be completed, these data will remain the gold standard for practice. However, in those scenarios where such trials are not feasible, clinicians must be cautious when adopting conclusions drawn from retrospective analyses.

References

1. El-Serag HB, Mason AC (1999) Rising incidence of hepatocellular carcinoma in the United States. N Engl J Med 340(10):745–750
2. Yang JD, Roberts LR (2010) Hepatocellular carcinoma: a global view. Nat Rev Gastroenterol Hepatol 7(8):448–458
3. Bruix J, Sherman M, Llovet JM et al (2001) Clinical management of hepatocellular carcinoma. Conclusions of the Barcelona-2000 EASL conference. J Hepatol 35(3):421–430
4. Livraghi T, Goldberg SN, Lazzaroni S, Meloni F, Solbiati L, Gazelle GS (1999) Small hepatocellular carcinoma: treatment with radio-frequency ablation versus ethanol injection. Radiology 210(3):655–661
5. Lencioni RA, Allgaier H-P, Cioni D et al (2003) Small hepatocellular carcinoma in cirrhosis: randomized comparison of radio-frequency thermal ablation versus percutaneous ethanol injection1. Radiology 228(1):235–240
6. Lin S, Lin C, Lin C, Hsu C, Chen Y (2005) Randomised controlled trial comparing percutaneous radiofrequency thermal ablation, percutaneous ethanol injection, and percutaneous acetic acid injection to treat hepatocellular carcinoma of 3 cm or less. Gut 54(8):1151–1156
7. Caturelli E, Siena DA, Fusilli S et al (2000) Transcatheter arterial chemoembolization for hepatocellular carcinoma in patients with cirrhosis: evaluation of damage to nontumorous liver tissue—long-term prospective study 1. Radiology 215(1):123–128
8. Veltri A, Moretto P, Doriguzzi A, Pagano E, Carrara G, Gandini G (2006) Radiofrequency thermal ablation (RFA) after transarterial chemoembolization (TACE) as a combined therapy for unresectable non-early hepatocellular carcinoma (HCC). Eur Radiol 16(3):661–669
9. Livraghi T (2003) Radiofrequency ablation, PEIT, and TACE for hepatocellular carcinoma. J Hepato-Biliary-Pancreatic Surg 10(1):67–76
10. d'Etude G, Hépatocellulaire TDC (1995) A comparison of lipiodol chemoembolization and conservative treatment for unresectable hepatocellular carcinoma. N Engl J Med 332:1256–1261
11. Lin D, Liaw Y, Lee T, Lai C (1988) Hepatic arterial embolization in patients with unresectable hepatocellular carcinoma—a randomized controlled trial. Gastroenterology 94 (2):453–456
12. Pelletier G, Roche A, Ink O et al (1990) A randomized trial of hepatic arterial chemoembolization in patients with unresectable hepatocellular carcinoma. J Hepatol 11 (2):181–184
13. Madden M, Krige J, Bailey S et al (1993) Randomised trial of targeted chemotherapy with lipiodol and 5-epidoxorubicin compared with symptomatic treatment for hepatoma. Gut 34 (11):1598–1600

14. Llovet JM, Fuster J, Bruix J (1999) Intention-to-treat analysis of surgical treatment for early hepatocellular carcinoma: resection versus transplantation. Hepatology 30(6):1434–1440
15. Llovet JM, Real MI, Montaña X et al (2002) Arterial embolisation or chemoembolisation versus symptomatic treatment in patients with unresectable hepatocellular carcinoma: a randomised controlled trial. Lancet 359(9319):1734–1739
16. Sergio A, Cristofori C, Cardin R et al (2008) Transcatheter arterial chemoembolization (TACE) in hepatocellular carcinoma (HCC): the role of angiogenesis and invasiveness. Am J Gastroenterol 103(4):914–921
17. Pinter M, Hucke F, Graziadei I et al (2012) Advanced-stage hepatocellular carcinoma: transarterial chemoembolization versus sorafenib. Radiology 263(2):590–599
18. Becker G, Soezgen T, Olschewski M, Laubenberger J, Blum HE, Allgaier H-P (2005) Combined TACE and PEI for palliative treatment of unresectable hepatocellular carcinoma. World J Gastroenterol 11(39):6104
19. Bhagat N, Reyes DK, Lin M, et al. (2013) Phase II study of chemoembolization with drug-eluting beads in patients with hepatic neuroendocrine metastases: high incidence of biliary injury. Cardiovasc Intervent Radiol: 1–11
20. Miller A, Hoogstraten B, Staquet M, Winkler A (1981) Reporting results of cancer treatment. Cancer 47(1):207–214
21. Therasse P, Arbuck SG, Eisenhauer EA et al (2000) New guidelines to evaluate the response to treatment in solid tumors. J Natl Cancer Inst 92(3):205–216
22. Llovet JM, Bruix J (2008) Novel advancements in the management of hepatocellular carcinoma in 2008. J Hepatol 48:S20–S37
23. Bruix J, Sherman M (2011) Management of hepatocellular carcinoma: an update. Hepatology 53(3):1020–1022
24. Chen M-S, Li J-Q, Zheng Y et al (2006) A prospective randomized trial comparing percutaneous local ablative therapy and partial hepatectomy for small hepatocellular carcinoma. Ann Surg 243(3):321
25. Huang J, Yan L, Cheng Z et al (2010) A randomized trial comparing radiofrequency ablation and surgical resection for HCC conforming to the Milan criteria. Ann Surg 252(6):903–912
26. Qian G-J, Wang N, Shen Q et al (2012) Efficacy of microwave versus radiofrequency ablation for treatment of small hepatocellular carcinoma: experimental and clinical studies. Eur Radiol 22(9):1983–1990
27. Merion RM, Pelletier SJ, Goodrich N, Englesbe MJ, Delmonico FL (2006) Donation after cardiac death as a strategy to increase deceased donor liver availability. Ann Surg 244(4):555
28. Earl TM, Chapman WC (2013) Hepatocellular carcinoma: resection versus transplantation. In: Seminars in liver disease. Thieme Medical Publishers, Stuttgart, pp 282–292
29. Yao F, Xiao L, Bass N, Kerlan R, Ascher N, Roberts J (2007) Liver transplantation for hepatocellular carcinoma: validation of the UCSF-expanded criteria based on preoperative imaging. Am J Transplant 7(11):2587–2596
30. Mazzaferro V, Regalia E, Doci R et al (1996) Liver transplantation for the treatment of small hepatocellular carcinomas in patients with cirrhosis. N Engl J Med 334(11):693–700
31. Yao F (2008) Liver transplantation for hepatocellular carcinoma: beyond the Milan criteria. Am J Transplant 8(10):1982–1989
32. Belghiti J, Durand F (2011) Criteria for liver transplantation for hepatocellular carcinoma: what is an acceptable outcome? Liver Int 31(s1):161–163
33. Margarit C, Escartín A, Castells L, Vargas V, Allende E, Bilbao I (2005) Resection for hepatocellular carcinoma is a good option in Child-Turcotte-Pugh class A patients with cirrhosis who are eligible for liver transplantation. Liver Transpl 11(10):1242–1251
34. Poon RT, Fan ST, Lo CM, Liu CL, Wong J (2007) Difference in tumor invasiveness in cirrhotic patients with hepatocellular carcinoma fulfilling the Milan criteria treated by resection and transplantation: impact on long-term survival. Ann Surg 245(1):51

35. Figueras J, Jaurrieta E, Valls C et al (2000) Resection or transplantation for hepatocellular carcinoma in cirrhotic patients: outcomes based on indicated treatment strategy. J Am Coll Surg 190(5):580–587
36. Del Gaudio M, Ercolani G, Ravaioli M et al (2008) Liver transplantation for recurrent hepatocellular carcinoma on cirrhosis after liver resection: University of Bologna experience. Am J Transplant 8(6):1177–1185
37. Koniaris LG, Levi DM, Pedroso FE et al (2011) Is surgical resection superior to transplantation in the treatment of hepatocellular carcinoma? Ann Surg 254(3):527–538
38. Bellavance EC, Lumpkins KM, Mentha G et al (2008) Surgical management of early-stage hepatocellular carcinoma: resection or transplantation? J Gastrointest Surg 12(10):1699–1708
39. Belghiti J, Cortes A, Abdalla EK et al (2003) Resection prior to liver transplantation for hepatocellular carcinoma. Ann Surg 238(6):885
40. Poon RT-P, Fan ST, Lo CM, Liu CL, Wong J (2002) Long-term survival and pattern of recurrence after resection of small hepatocellular carcinoma in patients with preserved liver function: implications for a strategy of salvage transplantation. Ann Surg 235(3):373–382
41. Belghiti J, Carr B, Greig P, Lencioni R, Poon R (2008) Treatment before liver transplantation for HCC. Ann Surg Oncol 15(4):993–1000
42. Fong Y, Fortner J, Sun RL, Brennan MF, Blumgart LH (1999) Clinical score for predicting recurrence after hepatic resection for metastatic colorectal cancer: analysis of 1001 consecutive cases. Ann Surg 230(3):309
43. Tzeng C-WD, Aloia TA (2013) Colorectal liver metastases. J Gastrointest Surg 17(1):195–202
44. Mansour J, Fong Y (2007) Timing of the liver resection for patients with synchronous metastases: practical and outcome considerations. Ann Surg Oncol 14(9):2435–2436
45. Khajanchee YS, Hammill CW, Cassera MA, Wolf RF, Hansen PD (2011) Hepatic resection vs minimally invasive radiofrequency ablation for the treatment of colorectal liver metastases: a Markov analysis. Arch Surg 146(12):1416
46. Kopetz S, Chang GJ, Overman MJ et al (2009) Improved survival in metastatic colorectal cancer is associated with adoption of hepatic resection and improved chemotherapy. J Clin Oncol 27(22):3677–3683
47. Saltz LB, Clarke S, Díaz-Rubio E et al (2008) Bevacizumab in combination with oxaliplatin-based chemotherapy as first-line therapy in metastatic colorectal cancer: a randomized phase III study. J Clin Oncol 26(12):2013–2019
48. Narayanan G, Barbery K, Suthar R, Guerrero G, Arora G (2013) Transarterial chemoembolization using DEBIRI for treatment of hepatic metastases from colorectal cancer. Anticancer Res 33(5):2077–2083
49. Martin RC, Joshi J, Robbins K, Tomalty D, O'Hara R, Tatum C (2009) Transarterial chemoembolization of metastatic colorectal carcinoma with drug-eluting beads, irinotecan (DEBIRI): multi-institutional registry. J Oncol 2009:539795
50. Mulier S, Miao Y, Mulier P et al (2005) Electrodes and multiple electrode systems for radiofrequency ablation: a proposal for updated terminology. Eur Radiol 15(4):798–808
51. Goldberg SN, Hahn PF, Tanabe KK et al (1998) Percutaneous radiofrequency tissue ablation: does perfusion-mediated tissue cooling limit coagulation necrosis? J Vasc Interv Radiol 9 (1):101–111
52. Abdalla EK, Vauthey J-N, Ellis LM et al (2004) Recurrence and outcomes following hepatic resection, radiofrequency ablation, and combined resection/ablation for colorectal liver metastases. Ann Surg 239(6):818
53. Mulier S, Ruers T, Jamart J, Michel L, Marchal G, Ni Y (2009) Radiofrequency ablation versus resection for resectable colorectal liver metastases: time for a randomized trial? Dig Surg 25(6):445–460
54. Mulier S, Ni Y, Jamart J, Ruers T, Marchal G, Michel L (2005) Local recurrence after hepatic radiofrequency coagulation: multivariate meta-analysis and review of contributing factors. Ann Surg 242(2):158–171

55. Gillams A, Lees W (2009) Five-year survival in 309 patients with colorectal liver metastases treated with radiofrequency ablation. Eur Radiol 19(5):1206–1213
56. Siperstein AE, Berber E, Ballem N, Parikh RT (2007) Survival after radiofrequency ablation of colorectal liver metastases: 10-year experience. Ann Surg 246(4):559–567
57. Wicherts DA, Miller R, de Haas RJ et al (2008) Long-term results of two-stage hepatectomy for irresectable colorectal cancer liver metastases. Ann Surg 248(6):994–1005
58. Ruers T, Punt C, Van Coevorden F et al (2012) Radiofrequency ablation combined with systemic treatment versus systemic treatment alone in patients with non-resectable colorectal liver metastases: a randomized EORTC Intergroup phase II study (EORTC 40004). Ann Oncol 23(10):2619–2626
59. Kemeny N, Daly J, Oderman P et al (1984) Hepatic artery pump infusion: toxicity and results in patients with metastatic colorectal carcinoma. J Clin Oncol 2(6):595–600
60. Hohn DC, Stagg RJ, Friedman MA et al (1989) A randomized trial of continuous intravenous versus hepatic intraarterial floxuridine in patients with colorectal cancer metastatic to the liver: the Northern California Oncology Group trial. J Clin Oncol 7(11):1646–1654
61. Chang AE, Schneider PD, Sugarbaker PH, Simpson C, Culnane M, Steinberg SM (1987) A prospective randomized trial of regional versus systemic continuous 5-fluorodeoxyuridine chemotherapy in the treatment of colorectal liver metastases. Ann Surg 206(6):685
62. Lorenz M, Müller H-H (2000) Randomized, multicenter trial of fluorouracil plus leucovorin administered either via hepatic arterial or intravenous infusion versus fluorodeoxyuridine administered via hepatic arterial infusion in patients with nonresectable liver metastases from colorectal carcinoma. J Clin Oncol 18(2):243
63. Kemeny NE, Niedzwiecki D, Hollis DR et al (2006) Hepatic arterial infusion versus systemic therapy for hepatic metastases from colorectal cancer: a randomized trial of efficacy, quality of life, and molecular markers (CALGB 9481). J Clin Oncol 24(9):1395–1403
64. Fiorentini G, Aliberti C, Tilli M et al (2012) Intra-arterial infusion of irinotecan-loaded drug-eluting beads (DEBIRI) versus intravenous therapy (FOLFIRI) for hepatic metastases from colorectal cancer: final results of a phase III study. Anticancer Res 32(4):1387–1395
65. Martin RC II, Scoggins CR, Tomalty D et al (2012) Irinotecan drug-eluting beads in the treatment of chemo-naive unresectable colorectal liver metastasis with concomitant systemic fluorouracil and oxaliplatin: results of pharmacokinetics and phase I trial. J Gastrointest Surg 16(8):1531–1538
66. Martin RC, Joshi J, Robbins K et al (2011) Hepatic intra-arterial injection of drug-eluting bead, irinotecan (DEBIRI) in unresectable colorectal liver metastases refractory to systemic chemotherapy: results of multi-institutional study. Ann Surg Oncol 18(1):192–198
67. Gray B, Van Hazel G, Hope M et al (2001) Randomised trial of SIR-Spheres® plus chemotherapy vs. chemotherapy alone for treating patients with liver metastases from primary large bowel cancer. Ann Oncol 12(12):1711–1720
68. Cosimelli M, Golfieri R, Cagol P et al (2010) Multi-centre phase II clinical trial of yttrium-90 resin microspheres alone in unresectable, chemotherapy refractory colorectal liver metastases. Br J Cancer 103(3):324–331
69. Nordlinger B, Guiguet M, Vaillant JC et al (1996) Surgical resection of colorectal carcinoma metastases to the liver: a prognostic scoring system to improve case selection, based on 1568 patients. Cancer 77(7):1254–1262
70. Fernandez FG, Drebin JA, Linehan DC, Dehdashti F, Siegel BA, Strasberg SM (2004) Five-year survival after resection of hepatic metastases from colorectal cancer in patients screened by positron emission tomography with F-18 fluorodeoxyglucose (FDG-PET). Ann Surg 240 (3):438
71. Berber E, Flesher N, Siperstein AE (2002) Laparoscopic radiofrequency ablation of neuroendocrine liver metastases. World J Surg 26(8):985–990
72. Oshowo A, Gillams A, Harrison E, Lees W, Taylor I (2003) Comparison of resection and radiofrequency ablation for treatment of solitary colorectal liver metastases. Br J Surg 90 (10):1240–1243

73. Aloia TA, Vauthey J-N, Loyer EM et al (2006) Solitary colorectal liver metastasis: resection determines outcome. Arch Surg 141(5):460–467
74. White R, Avital I, Sofocleous C et al (2007) Rates and patterns of recurrence for percutaneous radiofrequency ablation and open wedge resection for solitary colorectal liver metastasis. J Gastrointest Surg 11(3):256–263
75. Berber E, Tsinberg M, Tellioglu G, Simpfendorfer CH, Siperstein AE (2008) Resection versus laparoscopic radiofrequency thermal ablation of solitary colorectal liver metastasis. J Gastrointest Surg 12(11):1967–1972
76. Lee W-S, Yun SH, Chun H-K et al (2008) Clinical outcomes of hepatic resection and radiofrequency ablation in patients with solitary colorectal liver metastasis. J Clin Gastroenterol 42(8):945–949
77. Hur H, Ko YT, Min BS et al (2009) Comparative study of resection and radiofrequency ablation in the treatment of solitary colorectal liver metastases. Am J Surg 197(6):728–736
78. Aloia TA, Vauthey J-N, Loyer EM et al (2006) Solitary colorectal liver metastasis: resection determines outcome. Arch Surg 141(5):460
79. Tsai S, Pawlik TM (2009) Outcomes of ablation versus resection for colorectal liver metastases: are we comparing apples with oranges? Ann Surg Oncol 16(9):2422–2428
80. Gleisner AL, Choti MA, Assumpcao L, Nathan H, Schulick RD, Pawlik TM (2008) Colorectal liver metastases: recurrence and survival following hepatic resection, radiofrequency ablation, and combined resection-radiofrequency ablation. Arch Surg 143 (12):1204
81. Wong SL, Mangu PB, Choti MA et al (2010) American Society of Clinical Oncology 2009 clinical evidence review on radiofrequency ablation of hepatic metastases from colorectal cancer. J Clin Oncol 28(3):493–508
82. Goldberg RM, Sargent DJ, Morton RF et al (2004) A randomized controlled trial of fluorouracil plus leucovorin, irinotecan, and oxaliplatin combinations in patients with previously untreated metastatic colorectal cancer. J Clin Oncol 22(1):23–30
83. Vauthey J-N, Pawlik TM, Ribero D et al (2006) Chemotherapy regimen predicts steatohepatitis and an increase in 90-day mortality after surgery for hepatic colorectal metastases. J Clin Oncol 24(13):2065–2072
84. Adam R, Delvart V, Pascal G et al (2004) Rescue surgery for unresectable colorectal liver metastases downstaged by chemotherapy: a model to predict long-term survival. Ann Surg 240(4):644
85. Capussotti L, Luca VM, Ferrero A, Tesoriere RL, Ribero D, Polastri R (2007) Timing of resection of liver metastases synchronous to colorectal tumor: proposal of prognosis-based decisional model. Ann Surg Oncol 14(3):1143–1150
86. Pawlik TM, Cosgrove D (2011) The role of peri-operative chemotherapy for resectable colorectal liver metastasis: what does the evidence support? J Gastrointest Surg 15(3):410–415
87. van Vledder MG, de Jong MC, Pawlik TM, Schulick RD, Diaz LA, Choti MA (2010) Disappearing colorectal liver metastases after chemotherapy: should we be concerned? J Gastrointest Surg 14(11):1691–1700
88. Bischof D, Clary B, Maithel S, Pawlik T (2013) Surgical management of disappearing colorectal liver metastases. Br J Surg 100(11):1414–1420
89. Bhattacharjya S, Bhattacharjya T, Baber S, Tibballs J, Watkinson A, Davidson B (2004) Prospective study of contrast-enhanced computed tomography, computed tomography during arterioportography, and magnetic resonance imaging for staging colorectal liver metastases for liver resection. Br J Surg 91(10):1361–1369
90. Kamel IR, Choti MA, Horton KM et al (2003) Surgically staged focal liver lesions: accuracy and reproducibility of dual-phase helical CT for detection and characterization1. Radiology 227(3):752–757

91. Oliva MR, Mortele KJ, Segatto E et al (2006) Computed tomography features of nonalcoholic steatohepatitis with histopathologic correlation. J Comput Assist Tomogr 30 (1):37–43
92. Tan MC, Linehan DC, Hawkins WG, Siegel BA, Strasberg SM (2007) Chemotherapy-induced normalization of FDG uptake by colorectal liver metastases does not usually indicate complete pathologic response. J Gastrointest Surg 11(9):1112–1119
93. Fong Y, Saldinger PF, Akhurst T et al (1999) Utility of $_{18}$F-FDG positron emission tomography scanning on selection of patients for resection of hepatic colorectal metastases. Am J Surg 178(4):282–287
94. van Kessel CS, Buckens CF, van den Bosch MA, van Leeuwen MS, van Hillegersberg R, Verkooijen HM (2012) Preoperative imaging of colorectal liver metastases after neoadjuvant chemotherapy: a meta-analysis. Ann Surg Oncol 19(9):2805–2813
95. Modlin IM, Oberg K, Chung DC et al (2008) Gastroenteropancreatic neuroendocrine tumours. Lancet Oncol 9(1):61–72
96. Frilling A, Modlin IM, Kidd M et al (2014) Recommendations for management of patients with neuroendocrine liver metastases. Lancet Oncol 15(1):e8–e21
97. Hashim YM, Trinkaus KM, Linehan DC et al (2014) Regional lymphadenectomy is indicated in the surgical treatment of pancreatic neuroendocrine tumors (PNETs). Ann Surg 259(2):197–203
98. Chamberlain RS, Canes D, Brown KT et al (2000) Hepatic neuroendocrine metastases: does intervention alter outcomes? J Am Coll Surg 190(4):432–445
99. Sarmiento JM, Heywood G, Rubin J, Ilstrup DM, Nagorney DM, Que FG (2003) Surgical treatment of neuroendocrine metastases to the liver: a plea for resection to increase survival. J Am Coll Surg 197(1):29–37
100. Mayo SC, de Jong MC, Pulitano C et al (2010) Surgical management of hepatic neuroendocrine tumor metastasis: results from an international multi-institutional analysis. Ann Surg Oncol 17(12):3129–3136
101. McEntee G, Nagorney D, Kvols L, Moertel C, Grant C (1990) Cytoreductive hepatic surgery for neuroendocrine tumors. Surgery 108(6):1091–1096
102. Mayo SC, de Jong MC, Bloomston M et al (2011) Surgery versus intra-arterial therapy for neuroendocrine liver metastasis: a multicenter international analysis. Ann Surg Oncol 18 (13):3657–3665
103. Austin PC (2011) An introduction to propensity score methods for reducing the effects of confounding in observational studies. Multivar Behav Res 46(3):399–424
104. John BJ, Davidson BR (2012) Treatment options for unresectable neuroendocrine liver metastases. Expert Rev Gastroenterol Hepatol 6(3):357–369
105. Strosberg J, Gardner N, Kvols L (2009) Survival and prognostic factor analysis of 146 metastatic neuroendocrine tumors of the mid-gut. Neuroendocrinology 89(4):471–476
106. Givi B, Pommier SJ, Thompson AK, Diggs BS, Pommier RF (2006) Operative resection of primary carcinoid neoplasms in patients with liver metastases yields significantly better survival. Surgery 140(6):891–898
107. Ahmed A, Turner G, King B et al (2009) Midgut neuroendocrine tumours with liver metastases: results of the UKINETS study. Endocr Relat Cancer 16(3):885–894
108. Norlén O, Stålberg P, Öberg K et al (2012) Long-term results of surgery for small intestinal neuroendocrine tumors at a tertiary referral center. World J Surg 36(6):1419–1431
109. Capurso G, Rinzivillo M, Bettini R, Boninsegna L, Fave GD, Falconi M (2012) Systematic review of resection of primary midgut carcinoid tumour in patients with unresectable liver metastases. Br J Surg 99(11):1480–1486
110. Rahman A, Assifi MM, Pedroso FE et al (2012) Is resection equivalent to transplantation for early cirrhotic patients with hepatocellular carcinoma? A meta-analysis. J Gastrointest Surg 16(10):1897–1909
111. Lee KK, Kim DG, Moon IS, Lee MD, Park JH (2010) Liver transplantation versus liver resection for the treatment of hepatocellular carcinoma. J Surg Oncol 101(1):47–53

112. Wu Y-Z, Li B, Wang T, Wang S-J, Zhou Y-M (2011) Radiofrequency ablation vs hepatic resection for solitary colorectal liver metastasis: a meta-analysis. World J Gastroenterol: WJG 17(36):4143
113. Reuter NP, Woodall CE, Scoggins CR, McMasters KM, Martin RC (2009) Radiofrequency ablation vs. resection for hepatic colorectal metastasis: therapeutically equivalent? J Gastrointest Surg 13(3):486–491

Comparative Effectiveness Research in Urologic Cancers

Seth A. Strope

Abstract

Controversies abound in urologic cancers. While some work in comparative effectiveness research has been performed, most controversies remain unresolved. In this chapter, we examine the three most common urologic malignancies: Prostate cancer, kidney cancer, and bladder cancer. We will review progress made in comparative effectiveness research for each cancer and outline important topics where future research is needed.

Keywords

Prostate cancer · Kidney cancer · Bladder cancer · Screening · Surgical therapy · Medical therapy

Contents

S.A. Strope (✉)
Division of Urologic Surgery, Washington University School of Medicine,
St. Louis, MO, USA
e-mail: stropes@wudosis.wustl.edu

K.Y. Bilimoria et al. (eds.), *Comparative Effectiveness in Surgical Oncology*,
Cancer Treatment and Research 164, DOI 10.1007/978-3-319-12553-4_12

1 Prostate Cancer

As the most common urologic malignancy, prostate cancer is a substantial burden for patients and the health care system. From screening through treatment for metastatic disease, the best treatments for many aspects of prostate cancer are not known (Fig. 1). We will examine prostate cancer screening, treatment for localized prostate cancer, and treatment for metastatic disease.

1.1 Prostate Cancer Screening

Prostate cancer screening is highly controversial. The United States Preventative Services task force gave prostate cancer screening with PSA a D rating [1]. Conversely, the American Urological Society continues to endorse PSA based screening after informed decision making with patients [2]. Here, comparative effectiveness research has been performed to help inform the debate. Two large randomized studies, the Prostate Lung Colorectal and Ovarian (PLCO) trial and European Randomized Study of Screening for Prostate Cancer (ERSPC), came to conflicting conclusions about the efficacy of PSA based screening for preventing death from prostate cancer. The PLCO study showed no benefit to men in the screening arm versus the non-screening arm of the study at 7–10 years of follow up [3]. ERSPC showed that men in the PSA screening group had a 20 % reduction in prostate cancer mortality at a median of 9 years of follow up [4]. Controversy about PSA based

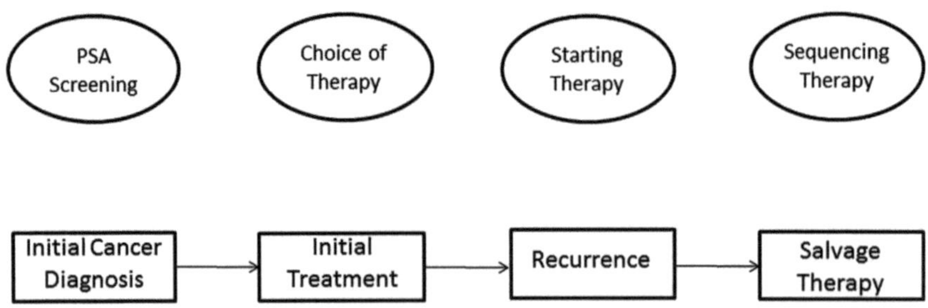

Fig. 1 Comparative effectiveness topics

screening continues due to the large number of men diagnosed with potentially non-lethal prostate cancer. Since most men diagnosed with prostate cancer in the United States receive treatment [5], a real risk of overtreatment exists. The risks of over-diagnosis and overtreatment are what led to the D rating from the USPSTF [1].

Screening could be improved through development of new tests to improve upon or replace PSA. New approaches, including PCA-3 [6], TMPRESS-erg fusion [7], and other genetic variations [8] have been explored as diagnostic tests for prostate cancer. The Early Disease Research Network is involved in efforts to improve these alternative tests and bring them to the point of clinical use. Should the results be promising for one or more of the markers, they will need robust CER efforts to determine which marker should be used in what screening situation. For instance, PCA-3 has FDA approval for use in the setting on an elevated PSA with a prior negative prostate biopsy to evaluate the need for a subsequent biopsy. As other markers become available, they could be directly tested against the existing approved marker in this setting. Additionally, studies are needed comparing new markers with PSA in unscreened populations. Currently, most new markers are tested as adjunct to PSA based screening. A challenge will be finding unscreened populations in which to perform this testing.

2 Treatment of Localized Disease

2.1 Observation, Active Surveillance, and Active Treatment of Prostate Cancer

With the high risk of over diagnosis of prostate cancer with SPA based screening, efforts have moved to changing the rates of overtreatment of disease that might not actively harm patients. Decreasing overtreatment requires comparative effectiveness research showing non-treatment of prostate cancer is as effective as active intervention. However, two studies of watchful waiting versus prostatectomy show some advantage to prostatectomy in higher risk men. The Scandinavian Prostate Cancer Study Group (SPCG-4) showed a mortality advantage to prostatectomy [9]. These men were typically diagnosed prior to the PSA era, and had more extensive disease than currently seen in practice. The Prostate Intervention Versus Observation Trial (PIVOT) study compared active intervention versus observation in patients treated in the Veterans Administration hospital system. Patients with low risk prostate cancer received no benefit from intervention, whereas men with intermediate or high risk disease appeared to receive some benefit [10]. Important criticisms against this study were the high background mortality rate in the study. Despite attempting to screen for healthy patients, the median survival for patients in the observation and intervention groups was only 10 years. The applicability of these results to other setting remains controversial.

Both SPCG-4 and PIVOT compared observation, not active surveillance, with treatment. Active surveillance differs from observation because men are followed regularly with PSA and biopsy and intervention instituted if higher risk disease develops during observation. No studies are available comparing active surveillance to intervention in a robust manner. Two trials, START and SPIRIT, were stopped due to poor enrollment. Only one in six patients consented for enrollment at a major center despite extensive patient education efforts [11]. An ongoing trial in the United Kingdom, ProtecT, will attempt to answer the role of active surveillance versus active treatment. This study enrolled over 3,000 participants and randomized them to prostatectomy, radiation therapy, or active surveillance [12]. Quality of life and survival results are expected in 2015, and may help guide decision making for men with prostate cancer.

2.2 Comparative Effectiveness of Prostate Cancer Therapies

Once men have chosen active intervention for prostate cancer, little comparative effectiveness evidence exists to guide them in selection of treatments. No trial has been published randomizing men to radiation or surgery, a deficit the ProtecT trial will correct. As such, all comparisons between the modalities have been observational studies. The PCOS trial provided early information about the side effects and quality of life after treatment by the different modalities, and now has shown a survival advantage for men treated with radical prostatectomy over those treated with radiation therapy [13]. Additional quality of life data has come from the PROSQA study showing distinct patterns to urinary and sexual function among men treated with prostatectomy, external-beam radiation therapy, and brachytherapy [14].

Despite these past efforts in prospective patient reported outcomes, major gaps remains in the understanding of efficacy of surgery versus radiation. Since the enrollment of men in the PCOS study in the 1990s, substantial changes have occurred in radiation therapy administration, including better image guidance, higher doses of radiation provided, and use of proton beam therapy. A new observational study, CEASAR attempts to rectify this knowledge gap [15]. The study enrolled over 3,000 men in a prospective cohort. Detailed information on demographics, treatment preferences, treatments received, and functional outcomes (urinary, sexual, and bladder) are being assessed. The study will provide updated information on the comparative effectiveness of the many different treatments for localized prostate cancer. Initially, these results will focus on differences in symptoms after treatment and the long term resolution or progression of these symptoms. Future plans include longer follow up to provide information on survival differences between different treatment modalities.

ProtecT and CEASAR will provide excellent data to help resolve controversies about active surveillance versus active treatment. However, even these well designed studies cannot answer all of the relevant questions regarding treatment versus active surveillance and surgery versus radiation. Further investigations based on the new findings from these studies will be needed. A concern will also be the applicability of the results of the ProtecT study to African–Americans. CEASAR has a broader enrollment, but the long term follow up for efficacy is planned, but not funded per their recent publication [15].

2.3 Comparative Effectiveness of Surgical Approaches for Prostate Cancer

Once patients make their decision regarding treatment modality, a new set of clinical questions emerges. Observational studies have addressed minimally invasive versus open approaches to radical prostatectomy. Early studies showed improved length of stay with minimally invasive approaches and lower use of blood transfusions. These improvements were balanced by higher rates of incontinence and erectile dysfunction [16]. Further investigations have failed to show significant differences in laparoscopic radical prostatectomy versus the use of robotic assistance [17]. Despite the paucity of data, most prostatectomies performed in the United States are done using a robotic assisted technique.

The spread of robotic prostatectomy reflects a common problem in surgical innovation. New technology disseminates before any comparative effectiveness studies show a benefit to the new technology. Once the technology has saturated the market, designing high quality comparative effectiveness studies becomes difficult. Here, the possibility of randomized controlled trials is unlikely due to patient preference and direct to consumer marketing. Unique prospective cohorts, with well defined data collection and study parameters, are needed to answer important comparative effectiveness questions.

2.4 Comparative Effectiveness of Radiation Therapy Modalities

Radiation therapy has an additional set of treatment choices, where the options lack solid comparative effectiveness data (Table 1). Current guidelines recommend 3-D conformal or intensity modulated radiation therapy with image guidance for

Table 1 Treatments and comparisons needed in radiation therapy for prostate cancer

Option	Comparison needed
Intensity modulated radiation therapy	Conformal beam radiation therapy
Brachytherapy	IMRT or CBT
Proton beam therapy	IMRT, CBT, or Brachytherapy

external beam radiation therapy with primary brachytherapy an alternative for patients with low risk cancers [18]. Aside from the previously mentioned studies comparing functional outcomes between brachytherapy and external beam radiation therapy, good studies exploring cancer control with the multiple different radiation modalities are lacking. For instance, no comparative effectiveness studies were done comparing conformal external beam radiation with IMRT [19], yet IMRT is the dominant form of external beam therapy used in the United States [20]. In a population based study using SEER-Medicare data, IMRT showed less gastrointestinal morbidity and fewer hip fractures than conformal radiation [21]. However, IMRT was associated with increased risk of erectile dysfunction. This study also compared IMRT to proton therapy and found less gastrointestinal complications with IMRT. The lack of data comparing different modalities is one place the CEASAR study may provide additional information [15]. However, one study alone cannot address all of the controversies in radiation options, and other well designed prospective or randomized studies will be needed.

2.5 Recurrent and Metastatic Prostate Cancer

For years the treatment of metastatic prostate cancer was simple and limited by available medications. Men with metastatic prostate cancer were treated by androgen deprivation, initially through orchiectomy and later through luteinizing hormone receptor agonists. After failure of these methods, men received best supportive care with no evidence that further androgen manipulation or chemotherapy helped improve outcomes. In the past ten years, treatment options for metastatic prostate cancer have grown enormously. The proper sequencing and use of these medications remains an area of active research. In this section, we discuss three important topics for comparative effectiveness research: how should men with a rising PSA after definitive therapy be treated, what medication should men with asymptomatic or mildly symptomatic metastatic disease be treated with, and what treatment should be provided to men with symptomatic metastatic disease.

A central unresolved question in prostate cancer therapy is when to initiate androgen deprivation therapy. This question exists both in patients who have PSA recurrence after prior radiation or surgical therapy, and in patients who are not candidates for definitive therapy, but have a rising PSA without evidence of metastatic disease. No studies currently address these issues. From prior case series, the time period from PSA detection to development of metastatic disease is estimated to be 5 years [22], and the PSA velocity during recurrence is an important predictor of metastatic disease and death [23]. NCCN guidelines acknowledge the lack of evidence about when to initiate ADT. Resolution of this issue will require unique data sets and examination, and are unlikely to be resolved with randomized trials.

Documentation of metastatic disease is another area of controversy. Since prostate cancer primarily recurs in bone, assessment for metastatic disease with

99mTc-medronate bone scans has been central for diagnosis. A newer modality, 18F-NaF PET has been developed. This technology has increased sensitivity for detection of bone metastases [24]. However, how this increased sensitivity impacts management of men with metastatic prostate cancer remains unresolved.

Once metastatic disease is documented, men with prostate cancer have multiple options for management. A continuing controversy involves the use of combined androgen blockage with a luteinizing hormone releasing hormone agonist combined with an anti-androgen versus LHRH agonist monotherapy. Furthermore, the role of LHRH antagonists versus agonists remains to be identified.

When the PSA rises during ADT therapy, patients are considered to have castration-recurrent prostate cancer. Treatment options vary based on the severity of patient symptoms. For patients with asymptomatic CRPC, level 1 evidence supports the use of Sipilucel-T and Abiraterone [25, 26]. A randomized trial of enzalutamide in this setting has also been completed and the results have been presented but publication of the results is still pending. For patients who are symptomatic, docetaxel and radium-223 have level one evidence supporting their use [27–29]. In addition, the trials with abiraterone and enzalutamide included men who were mildly symptomatic, while the trials with docetaxel included some asymptomatic men. With the substantial overlap between agents and the studies supporting the agents, no good evidence exists to support the sequencing of agents. Trials comparing the agents and alternative sequencing of agents are needed.

A final area of controversy exists in the treatment of men who progress after the use of docetaxel. Both enzalutimide and abiraterone have randomized trial evidence showing the improvement in patient survival in this setting [30, 31]. How one agent compares to the other remains undefined.

3 Bladder Cancer

For most patients with low grade and non-muscle invasive bladder cancer, treatments are routine and control the cancer with little risk of progression to metastatic disease and death. Most controversy for these patients exists in the proper sequence and amount of surveillance care patients receive. Among higher risk patients with high grade or muscle invasive disease, risk or recurrence and death is high. It is in these patients that current treatment options are limited and extensive controversies exist.

3.1 Non-muscle Invasive Bladder Cancer

Low grade, non-muscle invasive, bladder cancer is characterized by a high recurrence rate with a low rate of progression to muscle invasive disease or development of metastatic disease. These patients are managed by resection of the tumor through a transurethral approach followed by surveillance regimens. These surveillance regimens have proven controversial, with few patients receiving recommended care [32], and adherence with recommended care showing no benefits with overall or cancer specific survival [33]. Despite these controversies, no randomized trials exist to guide care. Practice continues based on best practices, and no trials are currently under way to address the issue.

One issue that has been well investigated in the non-muscle invasive bladder cancer population is the use of intravesical chemotherapy after resection. A single dose of intravesical chemotherapy increased recurrence free survival by 38 % in a recent meta analysis [34]. Medications used included mitomycin-c, epirubicin, peplomycin, THP-doxorubicin, and gemcitabine, with mitomycin-c and epirubicine showing the greatest efficacy compared to placebo or not active intervention. However, no CER study has been performed comparing one agent to another, making this an area where CER research could be employed.

3.2 Follow-up Care After Definitive Bladder Cancer Therapy

Bladder cancer patients who receive a radical cystectomy remain at high risk for recurrence and death from their disease. For these patients, the ideal follow up regimen is now known. Recommended follow up tests include CT or MRI scans [35], trans-rectal ultrasound [36], no imaging [37], voided cytology [35, 38] and urethral wash cytology [35, 38–40]. The performance of these follow up studies in patients treated with neoadjuvant or adjuvant chemotherapy is unknown [41, 42]. A recent analysis found urine testing after cystectomy and doctor visits positively impacted patient survival, but imaging tests had no impact [43]. While the observational data helps point towards beneficial modalities of therapy, further research comparing the effectiveness of different follow up patterns is needed to positively impact the outcomes for patients.

3.3 Comparative Effectiveness of Radiation and Surgery for Muscle Invasive Bladder Cancer

A final area of controversy is in bladder sparing protocols for muscle invasive bladder cancer versus radical cystectomy. Overall, curative therapy is used by only a fraction of patients with muscle invasive bladder cancer [44]. Trimodality therapy, combining transurethral resection of the tumor, radiation therapy and radio sensitizing chemotherapy provides an additional option to patients for cure of muscle invasive bladder cancer. Results of this therapy are comparable to those of radical cystectomy with five year survival rates of 48–65 % and bladder preservation rates of 70 % [45]. However, in the absence of comparative studies, the true effectiveness

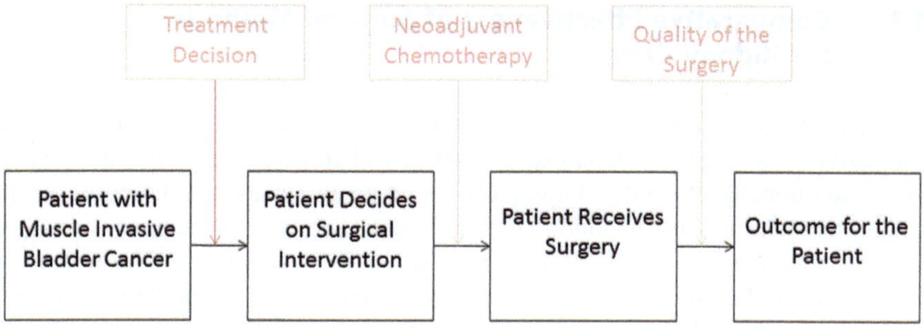

Fig. 2 Treatment decisions in muscle invasive bladder cancer

comparing trimodality therapy to radical cystectomy remains unknown. Issues of patient selection for each therapy and standardization of both surgical and radiation management need to be explored.

The comparative effectiveness of surgical versus radiation therapy for muscle invasive bladder cancer fits into a framework of decision making for patients with muscle invasive bladder cancer (Fig. 2). The initial treatment decision for surgery versus radiation or observation is followed by a decision regarding the use of neoadjuvant chemotherapy, and finally a set of variables related to the quality of the surgery. Each of these points requires robust research to answer questions about the effectiveness of the available interventions. For example, groups are trying to refine patient selection for neoadjuvant chemotherapy referral [46]. Other efforts are underway comparing the quality and effectiveness of robotic and open approaches to surgery. Finally a randomized clinical trial (S1011) assessing the extent of lymph node dissection is accruing patients in a cooperative group trial. Such efforts will help answer critical questions about the appropriateness of different surgical techniques and are needed for multiple aspects of the surgical management of bladder cancer.

4 Kidney Cancer

Recent expansions in the therapeutic options for patients with kidney cancer have raised important questions related to clinical effectiveness. Management of localized disease, metastatic disease with the primary kidney tumor in place, and metastatic disease that developed after prior nephrectomy are disease states where comparative effectiveness research is needed. In this next section, we discuss these controversies and the limitations in current understanding.

4.1 Comparative Effectiveness of Surgical Methods for Kidney Cancer

Localized kidney tumors are typically managed by surgical resection. Multiple alternatives, ranging from laparoscopic, open, and robotic approaches to surgery, exist. Additionally, the entire kidney can be removed versus just the portion containing the cancer. Further options for local control involve percutaneous or laparoscopic cryoablation of the tumor or radiofrequency ablation of the tumor. In addition to local control, many centers advocate observation of small renal masses, especially in the elderly or patients with extensive comorbidity. Some CER has been performed to inform patients and surgeons on the relative risks and benefits of each approach to management of localized kidney cancer.

Open radical versus partial nephrectomy were compared in a randomized trial started in 1992 and reported in 2011 [47]. The authors found that patients treated with radical nephrectomy had better overall survival at 10 years (81.1 %) than patients treated with partial nephrectomy (75.7 %) [47]. These results were controversial since prior observational data suggested worsened renal function among patients who received radical nephrectomy [48], and other evidence linked worsened renal function to increased mortality [49]. Adding to the controversy, a cohort study suggests improvement in mortality among patients who received partial instead of radical nephrectomy [50].

4.2 Intervention Versus Observation for Kidney Tumors

As seen in the example of radical versus partial nephrectomy, resolving the controversies in kidney cancer treatment will require new efforts at comparative effectiveness research. Central to these efforts is better defining who needs treatment versus observation. Some groups have been using biopsy of the kidney to help guide this therapy [51], but the concept has not been explored within a robust CER framework. Similar to prostate cancer, not all patients need active intervention, but determining the correct patient for intervention remains challenging. Additional efforts to better delineate the trade offs between ablative and extirpative therapy for patients receiving intervention are needed.

4.3 Cytoreductive Nephrectomy for Metastatic Kidney Cancer

In patients with kidney cancer who present with metastatic disease, the role of a cytoreductive nephrectomy was established by a pivotal study showing nephrectomy with interferon was associated with a 3 month median increase in survival compared to nephrectomy alone [52]. This initial finding has become controversial since INF is rarely used in current therapy and the use of cytoreductive nephrectomy has expanded beyond the limited population treated in the landmark study. In an observational cohort study spanning the INF and current treatment era, many patients were found to not have a survival benefit from cytoreductive nephrectomy [53]. Fortunately, two randomized clinical trials are accruing patients to help answer the effectiveness of cytoreductive nephrectomy combined with current medical therapy. The CARMENA trial randomizes patients to nephrectomy followed by sunitinib versus sunitinib alone. An alternative design is explored in the SURTIME trial. Patients are randomized to immediate nephrectomy versus initial treatment with sunitinib followed by nephrectomy. Both these trials enroll healthy patients with performance status of 0 or 1, leaving questions remaining about the efficacy of cytoreductive nephrectomy in patients with poor performance status and greater comorbidity.

4.4 Choice and Sequencing of Agents for Metastatic Kidney Cancer

With multiple agents approved for treatment of metastatic renal cell cancer, appropriate selection and sequencing remain active areas of concern. Currently tyrosine kinase inhibitors (sorafanib, sunitinib, pazopanib, axitinib), monoclonal antibody in combination with interferon (bevacizumab), and the inhibitors of the mammalian target of rapamycin (everolimus and temsirolimus) are available for the treatment of metastatic renal cell cancer [54]. Current guidelines recommend pazopanib, sunitinib, or bevacizumab with interferon as first line therapy for good or intermediate risk patients with clear cell renal cell cancer, and temsirolimus is the only agent recommended for high risk patients [55]. These studies were done either with placebo or interferon alpha as the comparator group. Only a few studies assess comparative effectiveness among the agents [56–58] (Table 2). Increasingly, new

Table 2 A few studies assessing comparative effectiveness among the agents

Agent	Study design	Comparison agent	Result
Axitinib	Open label randomized phase III study	Sorafenib	Progression free survival 10.2 months with axitinib versus 6.5 months with sorafenib. Not statistically significant and the side effect profile was different, but not improved [56]
Pazopanib	Phase III randomized non-inferiority study	Sunitinib	Pazopanib was non-inferior to sunitinib for progression and overall survival. Pazopanib had a superior side effect profile [58]
Sorafenib	Phase III randomized clinical trial	Tivozanib	Tivozanib had improved progression free survival [57]

Table 3 Comparative studies of second line therapy

Agent	Study design	Comparison agent	Result
Axitinib	Phase III randomized clinical trial	Sorafenib in a second line setting	Progression free survival was improved with axitinib, but no difference in overall survival was found [61]
Temsirolimus	Phase III randomized clinical trial	Sorafenib in a second line setting after prior sunitinib therapy	No differences were found in progression free survival and sorafenib had better overall survival [59]

agents used in the first line setting will need to prove superiority to existing therapy. The pazopanib versus sunitinib study provides a good example of a comparative effectiveness study can change clinical management. By comparing two of the recommended first line agents directly, the results of the study provide clear guidance on which agent should be used.

The ideal treatment of patients who progress on first line therapy is also unclear. The definition of progression is fluid, with recommendations provided in a recent review based on the time course of the disease [54]. Despite the challenges of defining progressive disease, multiple studies have been done directly comparing available agents in the second-line setting [59–61]. These studies suggest a role for axitinib over sorafenib in the second line therapy setting. However, studies directly comparing the most active agents have not been done (Table 3). With multiple agents available, further comparative studies are needed to accurately guide therapy.

References

1. Available from http://www.uspreventiveservicestaskforce.org/prostatecancerscreening.htm
2. Carter HB, Albertsen PC, Barry MJ et al (2013) Early detection of prostate cancer: AUA guideline. J Urol 190:419–426
3. Andriole GL, Crawford ED, Grubb RL 3rd et al (2009) Mortality results from a randomized prostate-cancer screening trial. N Engl J Med 360:1310–1319
4. Schroder FH, Hugosson J, Roobol MJ et al (2009) Screening and prostate-cancer mortality in a randomized European study. N Engl J Med 360:1320–1328
5. Cooperberg MR, Broering JM, Carroll PR (2010) Time trends and local variation in primary treatment of localized prostate cancer. J Clin Oncol 28:1117–1123
6. Crawford ED, Rove KO, Trabulsi EJ et al (2012) Diagnostic performance of PCA3 to detect prostate cancer in men with increased prostate specific antigen: a prospective study of 1,962 cases. J Urol 188:1726–1731
7. Park K, Dalton JT, Narayanan R et al (2014) TMPRSS2:ERG gene fusion predicts subsequent detection of prostate cancer in patients with high-grade prostatic intraepithelial neoplasia. J Clin Oncol 32:206–211
8. Zheng SL, Sun J, Wiklund F et al (2008) Cumulative association of five genetic variants with prostate cancer. N Engl J Med 358:910–919

9. Bill-Axelson A, Holmberg L, Filen F et al (2008) Radical prostatectomy versus watchful waiting in localized prostate cancer: the Scandinavian prostate cancer group-4 randomized trial. J Natl Cancer Inst 100:1144–1154
10. Wilt TJ, Brawer MK, Jones KM et al (2012) Radical prostatectomy versus observation for localized prostate cancer. N Engl J Med 367:203–213
11. Wallace K, Fleshner N, Jewett M, Basiuk J, Crook J (2006) Impact of a multi-disciplinary patient education session on accrual to a difficult clinical trial: the Toronto experience with the surgical prostatectomy versus interstitial radiation intervention trial. J Clin Oncol 24:4158–4162
12. Hoffman RM, Penson DF, Zietman AL, Barry MJ (2013) Comparative effectiveness research in localized prostate cancer treatment. J Comp Eff Res 2:583–593
13. Hoffman RM, Koyama T, Fan KH et al (2013) Mortality after radical prostatectomy or external beam radiotherapy for localized prostate cancer. J Natl Cancer Inst 105:711–718
14. Sanda MG, Dunn RL, Michalski J et al (2008) Quality of life and satisfaction with outcome among prostate-cancer survivors. N Engl J Med 358:1250–1261
15. Barocas DA, Chen V, Cooperberg M et al (2013) Using a population-based observational cohort study to address difficult comparative effectiveness research questions: the CEASAR study. J Comp Eff Res 2:445–460
16. Hu JC, Gu X, Lipsitz SR et al (2009) Comparative effectiveness of minimally invasive vs open radical prostatectomy. JAMA 302:1557–1564
17. Willis DL, Gonzalgo ML, Brotzman M, Feng Z, Trock B, Su LM (2012) Comparison of outcomes between pure laparoscopic vs robot-assisted laparoscopic radical prostatectomy: a study of comparative effectiveness based upon validated quality of life outcomes. BJU Int 109:898–905
18. Mohler JL, Kantoff PW, Armstrong AJ et al (2013) Prostate cancer, version 1.2014. J Natl Compr Canc Netw 11:1471–1479
19. Pugh TJ, Nguyen BN, Kanke JE, Johnson JL, Hoffman KE (2013) Radiation therapy modalities in prostate cancer. J Natl Compr Canc Netw 11:414–421
20. Jacobs BL, Zhang Y, Schroeck FR et al (2013) Use of advanced treatment technologies among men at low risk of dying from prostate cancer. JAMA 309:2587–2595
21. Sheets NC, Goldin GH, Meyer AM et al (2012) Intensity-modulated radiation therapy, proton therapy, or conformal radiation therapy and morbidity and disease control in localized prostate cancer. JAMA 307:1611–1620
22. Pound CR, Partin AW, Eisenberger MA, Chan DW, Pearson JD, Walsh PC (1999) Natural history of progression after PSA elevation following radical prostatectomy. JAMA 281:1591–1597
23. Freedland SJ, Humphreys EB, Mangold LA et al (2005) Risk of prostate cancer-specific mortality following biochemical recurrence after radical prostatectomy. JAMA 294:433–439
24. Poulsen MH, Petersen H, Hoilund-Carlsen PF, et al (2013) Spine metastases in prostate cancer: comparison of [Tc]MDP wholebody bone scintigraphy, [F]choline PET/CT, and [F] NaF PET/CT. BJU Int 114(6):818–823
25. Small EJ, Schellhammer PF, Higano CS et al (2006) Placebo-controlled phase III trial of immunologic therapy with sipuleucel-T (APC8015) in patients with metastatic, asymptomatic hormone refractory prostate cancer. J Clin Oncol 24:3089–3094
26. Ryan CJ, Smith MR, de Bono JS et al (2013) Abiraterone in metastatic prostate cancer without previous chemotherapy. N Engl J Med 368:138–148
27. Petrylak DP, Tangen CM, Hussain MH et al (2004) Docetaxel and estramustine compared with mitoxantrone and prednisone for advanced refractory prostate cancer. N Engl J Med 351:1513–1520
28. Tannock IF, de Wit R, Berry WR et al (2004) Docetaxel plus prednisone or mitoxantrone plus prednisone for advanced prostate cancer. N Engl J Med 351:1502–1512
29. Parker C, Nilsson S, Heinrich D et al (2013) Alpha emitter radium-223 and survival in metastatic prostate cancer. N Engl J Med 369:213–223

30. Scher HI, Fizazi K, Saad F et al (2012) Increased survival with enzalutamide in prostate cancer after chemotherapy. N Engl J Med 367:1187–1197
31. de Bono JS, Logothetis CJ, Molina A et al (2011) Abiraterone and increased survival in metastatic prostate cancer. N Engl J Med 364:1995–2005
32. Chamie K, Saigal CS, Lai J et al (2011) Compliance with guidelines for patients with bladder cancer: variation in the delivery of care. Cancer 117:5392–5401
33. Hollenbeck BK, Ye Z, Dunn RL, Montie JE, Birkmeyer JD (2009) Provider treatment intensity and outcomes for patients with early-stage bladder cancer. J Natl Cancer Inst 101:571–580
34. Perlis N, Zlotta AR, Beyene J, Finelli A, Fleshner NE, Kulkarni GS (2013) Immediate post-transurethral resection of bladder tumor intravesical chemotherapy prevents non-muscle-invasive bladder cancer recurrences: an updated meta-analysis on 2548 patients and quality-of-evidence review. Eur Urol 64:421–430
35. Sanderson KM, Cai J, Miranda G, Skinner DG, Stein JP (2007) Upper tract urothelial recurrence following radical cystectomy for transitional cell carcinoma of the bladder: an analysis of 1,069 patients with 10-year followup. J Urol 177:2088–2094
36. Volkmer BG, Kuefer R, Bartsch GC Jr, Gust K, Hautmann RE (2009) Oncological followup after radical cystectomy for bladder cancer-is there any benefit? J Urol 181:1587–1593 (discussion 1593)
37. Meissner C, Giannarini G, Schumacher MC, Thoeny H, Studer UE, Burkhard FC (2007) The efficiency of excretory urography to detect upper urinary tract tumors after cystectomy for urothelial cancer. J Urol 178:2287–2290
38. Raj GV, Bochner BH, Serio AM et al (2006) Natural history of positive urinary cytology after radical cystectomy. J Urol 176:2000–2005 (discussion 2005)
39. Solsona E, Iborra I, Rubio J, Casanova J, Dumont R, Monros JL (2003) Late oncological occurrences following radical cystectomy in patients with bladder cancer. Eur Urol 43:489–494
40. Kuroda M, Meguro N, Maeda O et al (2002) Stage specific follow-up strategy after cystectomy for carcinoma of the bladder. Int J Urol 9:129–133
41. Stein JP, Lieskovsky G, Cote R et al (2001) Radical cystectomy in the treatment of invasive bladder cancer: long-term results in 1,054 patients. J Clin Oncol 19:666–675
42. Madersbacher S, Hochreiter W, Burkhard F et al (2003) Radical cystectomy for bladder cancer today–a homogeneous series without neoadjuvant therapy. J Clin Oncol 21:690–696
43. Strope SA, Chang SH, Chen L, Sandhu G, Piccirillo JF, Schootman M (2013) Survival impact of followup care after radical cystectomy for bladder cancer. J Urol 190:1698–1703
44. Gore JL, Litwin MS, Lai J et al (2010) Use of radical cystectomy for patients with invasive bladder cancer. J Natl Cancer Inst 102(11):802–811
45. Chen RC, Shipley WU, Efstathiou JA, Zietman AL (2013) Trimodality bladder preservation therapy for muscle-invasive bladder cancer. J Natl Compr Canc Netw 11:952–960
46. Vemana G, Nepple KG, Vetter J, Sandhu G, Strope SA (2014) Defining the potential of neoadjuvant chemotherapy utilization as a quality indicator for bladder cancer care. J Urol 192:43–49
47. Van Poppel H, Da Pozzo L, Albrecht W et al (2011) A prospective, randomised EORTC intergroup phase 3 study comparing the oncologic outcome of elective nephron-sparing surgery and radical nephrectomy for low-stage renal cell carcinoma. Eur Urol 59:543–552
48. Huang WC, Levey AS, Serio AM et al (2006) Chronic kidney disease after nephrectomy in patients with renal cortical tumours: a retrospective cohort study. Lancet Oncol 7:735–740
49. Go AS, Chertow GM, Fan D, McCulloch CE, Hsu CY (2004) Chronic kidney disease and the risks of death, cardiovascular events, and hospitalization. N Engl J Med 351:1296–1305
50. Tan HJ, Norton EC, Ye Z, Hafez KS, Gore JL, Miller DC (2012) Long-term survival following partial vs radical nephrectomy among older patients with early-stage kidney cancer. JAMA 307:1629–1635

51. Halverson SJ, Kunju LP, Bhalla R et al (2013) Accuracy of determining small renal mass management with risk stratified biopsies: confirmation by final pathology. J Urol 189:441–446
52. Flanigan RC, Salmon SE, Blumenstein BA et al (2001) Nephrectomy followed by interferon alfa-2b compared with interferon alfa-2b alone for metastatic renal-cell cancer. N Engl J Med 345:1655–1659
53. Culp SH, Tannir NM, Abel EJ et al (2010) Can we better select patients with metastatic renal cell carcinoma for cytoreductive nephrectomy? Cancer 116:3378–3388
54. Escudier B, Gore M (2013) Sequencing therapy in metastatic renal cell cancer. Semin Oncol 40:465–471
55. Escudier B, Eisen T, Porta C, et al (2012) Renal cell carcinoma: ESMO clinical practice guidelines for diagnosis, treatment and follow-up. Ann Oncol 23(7):vii65–vii71
56. Hutson TE, Lesovoy V, Al-Shukri S et al (2013) Axitinib versus sorafenib as first-line therapy in patients with metastatic renal-cell carcinoma: a randomised open-label phase 3 trial. Lancet Oncol 14:1287–1294
57. Motzer RJ, Nosov D, Eisen T et al (2013) Tivozanib versus sorafenib as initial targeted therapy for patients with metastatic renal cell carcinoma: results from a phase III trial. J Clin Oncol 31:3791–3799
58. Motzer RJ, Hutson TE, Cella D et al (2013) Pazopanib versus sunitinib in metastatic renal-cell carcinoma. N Engl J Med 369:722–731
59. Hutson TE, Escudier B, Esteban E, et al (2013) Randomized phase III trial of temsirolimus versus sorafenib as second-line therapy after sunitinib in patients with metastatic renal cell carcinoma. J Clin Oncol 32(8):760–767
60. Rini BI, Escudier B, Tomczak P et al (2011) Comparative effectiveness of axitinib versus sorafenib in advanced renal cell carcinoma (AXIS): a randomised phase 3 trial. Lancet 378:1931–1939
61. Motzer RJ, Escudier B, Tomczak P et al (2013) Axitinib versus sorafenib as second-line treatment for advanced renal cell carcinoma: overall survival analysis and updated results from a randomised phase 3 trial. Lancet Oncol 14:552–562

Comparative Effectiveness Research in Gynecologic Oncology

Sonali Patankar, Ana I. Tergas and Jason D. Wright

Abstract

The field of gynecologic oncology is faced with a number of challenges including how to incorporate new drugs and procedures into practice, how to balance therapeutic efficacy and toxicity of treatment, how to individualize therapy to particular patients or groups of patients, and how to contain the rapidly rising costs associated with oncologic care. In this chapter we examine three common and highly debated clinical scenarios in gynecologic oncology: the initial management of ovarian cancer, the role of lymphadenectomy in the treatment of endometrial cancer, and the choice of adjuvant therapy for ovarian cancer.

S. Patankar · A.I. Tergas · J.D. Wright (✉)
Department of Obstetrics and Gynecology, Columbia University College of Physicians and Surgeons, New York, US
e-mail: jw2459@columbia.edu

S. Patankar
e-mail: ssp2157@cumc.columbia.edu

A.I. Tergas
e-mail: ait2111@columbia.edu

A.I. Tergas
Department of Epidemiology, Mailman School of Public Health, Columbia University, New York, US

J.D. Wright
Herbert Irving Comprehensive Cancer Center, Columbia University College of Physicians and Surgeons, New York, US

K.Y. Bilimoria et al. (eds.), *Comparative Effectiveness in Surgical Oncology*, Cancer Treatment and Research 164, DOI 10.1007/978-3-319-12553-4_13

Keywords
Gynecologic cancer · Endometrial cancer · Ovarian cancer · Chemotherapy · Lymphadenectomy

Contents

1 Introduction

Gynecologic oncology incorporates a diverse group of diseases of the female genital tract. Some tumor types, such as endometrial cancer, are commonly detected early and associated with a high cure rate. In contrast, other malignancies, such as ovarian cancer, are more commonly diagnosed after dissemination and are accompanied by a poorer overall prognosis. Treatment for nearly all of the gynecologic cancers incorporates a multimodal approach utilizing various combinations of surgery, chemotherapy, and radiation.

The field of gynecologic oncology is faced with a number of challenges including how to incorporate new drugs and procedures into practice, how to balance therapeutic efficacy and toxicity of treatment, how to individualize therapy to particular patients or groups of patients, and how to contain the rapidly rising costs associated with oncologic care. In this chapter we examine three common and highly debated clinical scenarios in gynecologic oncology: the initial management of ovarian cancer, the role of lymphadenectomy in the treatment of endometrial cancer, and the choice of adjuvant therapy for ovarian cancer.

2 Initial Management of Ovarian Cancer

2.1 Background

Epithelial ovarian cancer is a major cause of cancer-related mortality in women. The high mortality associated with ovarian cancer is due in large part to the lack of effective screening tests for the disease. While potential screening tests such as transvaginal ultrasonography and serum screening with CA125 have been evaluated in a number of prospective trials, these tests are associated with low specificity and often fail to detect ovarian tumors when they are confined to the ovary and potentially curable. The difficulty in diagnosis is further compounded by the fact that most women with early-stage tumors are asymptomatic and, as such, the majority of women already have dissemination of the tumor within the abdominal cavity and often beyond (stage III or IV), at the time of diagnosis.

Traditional management for advanced-stage ovarian is surgical. Surgery for ovarian tumors relies a procedure known as cytoreduction or debulking. The goal of cytoreductive surgery is removal of all gross tumor within the abdominal cavity. In addition to hysterectomy and bilateral salpingo-oophorectomy, the procedure often requires omentectomy, peritoneactomy and frequently resection of the abdominal viscera including small bowel resection, colectomy, rectosigmoid colectomy, splenectomy, partial hepatectomy, and diaphragm resection. Surgery is typically followed by chemotherapy, most commonly employing a platinum-based regimen. Survival is highly correlated with the amount of residual tumor at the completion of surgery [1, 2]. Patients are classified as having undergone optimal cytoreduction if the greatest dimension of the largest residual tumor nodule is <1 cm and as having undergone suboptimal cytoreduction if the largest residual tumor is >1 cm in diameter.

Despite the oncologic benefits of cytoreduction, the procedure can be associated with substantial perioperative morbidity [3]. One population-based report noted that major perioperative complications occured in nearly a quarter of women who undergo surgery for ovarian cancer [3]. Further, a systematic review reported that the perioperative mortality rate was nearly 4 % in women who underwent surgery [4]. Additional work has also shown that those women who experience major perioperative complications often have delayed receipt of chemotherapy, thereby potentially negating the beneficial effects of cytoreductive surgery [5, 6].

An alternative to primary cytoreductive surgery is neoadjuvant chemotherapy. Women who undergo neoadjuvant chemotherapy typically receive primary platinum and taxane based chemotherapy followed by interval cytoreduction and additional cytotoxic therapy postoperatively. Institutional series have noted that perioperative morbidity is often reduced in women who undergo neoadjuvant chemotherapy compared to those treated with a strategy of primary cytoreductive surgery [7, 8]. However, the reported survival rates in these observational studies are often inferior to survival outcomes from cooperative group trials and from some tertiary centers [9, 10].

2.2 Evidence

2.2.1 Evidence for Primary Cytoreduction

Despite the fact the surgical cytoreduction is the standard of care for advanced stage ovarian cancer, the procedure is not based on randomized controlled trial data. The concept of surgical cytoreduction originated in the 1970s with the goal of resecting all visible tumor within the abdominal cavity [11]. The rationale for tumor debulking was to not only improve symptoms for bulky abdominal disease, but also to reduce the potential of residual chemotherapy resistant tumor clones and improve response to chemotherapy [12].

The efficacy of surgical cytoreduction was based in large part on retrospective studies that suggested that survival was improved in women with lower residual tumor burden after surgery [1, 2]. The Gynecologic Oncology Group (GOG) performed a number of analyses that helped demonstrate this concept [2]. In one report of 294 patients with stage III ovarian cancer, the relative risk of death increased sequentially as the diameter of the largest residual tumor nodule increased. Compared to women with a residual disease <2 cm, the relative risk of death in those with a residual tumor diameter of 2–2.9 cm was 1.90 while the relative risk in those with the largest tumor nodule measuring 3–3.9 cm was 1.91 [2].

The importance of cytoreduction has been demonstrated in multiple institutional series as well as a meta-analysis of available data that suggested similar findings [1, 13–18]. Among 81 studies including women with advanced-stage ovarian cancer, each 10 % increase in maximal cytoreduction was associated with a 5.5 % increase in median survival [1]. One single institution study compared survival in their patients before and after a programmatic change in surgical approach that adopted aggressive primary surgery including upper abdominal surgery when necessary. Five-year survival improved from 35 to 47 % after the paradigm shift [15].

Cytoreductive surgery not only involves resection of the ovaries and uterus, but also often requires removal of other pelvic viscera. One concern with aggressive surgery is the risk of perioperative morbidity and mortality. A number of studies have attempted to model factors associated with perioperative complications including age, functional status and extent of cytoreduction [19, 20]. After completion of cytoreduction most women receive adjuvant chemotherapy.

2.2.2 Evidence for Neoadjuvant Chemotherapy

Much of the evidence describing the outcomes of neoadjuvant chemotherapy is based on retrospective institutional reports that have compared the outcomes of primary cytoreduction to a strategy of neoadjuvant chemotherapy [7, 8, 21–26]. Many of these studies have noted that neoadjuvant chemotherapy is associated with less perioperative morbidity and a higher rate of optimal cytoreduction than primary cytoreduction. A meta-analysis of 21 studies found that patients who received neoadjuvant chemotherapy were less likely to undergo a sub-optimal cytoreduction (pooled odds ratio 0.50; 95 % CI, 0.29–0.86) [22].

One report comparing 109 patients who underwent primary surgery to 63 women treated with neoadjuvant chemotherapy noted a higher rate of optimal cytoreduction in those treated with neoadjuvant chemotherapy (95 % vs. 71 %). Further, aggressive surgery was required in only 5 % of those women who received neoadjuvant chemotherapy compared to 25 % in the primary surgery group. The median overall survival in the neoadjuvant therapy group was 46 months, similar to the 47 months noted in the primary surgery patients [8].

A second institutional series identified 200 patients with advanced stage epithelial ovarian cancer and included 98 patients who had initial chemotherapy and 102 who underwent surgery. Surgical morbidity was similar between the two groups, however, optimal cytoreduction was more often achieved in patients who underwent neoadjuvant chemotherapy (86 % vs. 54 %, $P < 0.001$). In the survival analysis, optimal cytoreduction was the only independent predictor of improved of survival. Timing of cytoreduction, either as primary surgery or after neoadjuvant chemotherapy, was not associated with survival [7].

The only randomized controlled trial of primary surgery versus neoadjuvant chemotherapy was undertaken by the European Organization for Research and Treatment of Cancer (EORTC) and reported in 2010. The study randomized 670 patients with stage IIIC-IV epithelial ovarian cancer to primary cytoreduction followed by platinum-based chemotherapy or neoadjuvant platinum-based chemotherapy (Table 1). Optimal cytoreduction to a largest tumor diameter of <1 cm was achieved in 41.6 % of patients who underwent primary debulking compared to 80.6 % of those who received neoadjuvant therapy. Perioperative morbidity was lower in those who underwent neoadjuvant chemotherapy and the postoperative mortality rate was 0.7 % in patients who received neoadjvuant chemotherapy compared to 2.5 % in those randomized to primary surgery. Median overall survival was comparable between the two arms, 29 months in those who underwent primary surgery and 30 months in women who received neoadjuvant chemotherapy. The investigators concluded that neoadjuvant surgery was not inferior to primary cytoreduction [26].

Table 1 Randomized control trial of neoadjuvant chemotherapy versus primary cytoreduction for advanced stage ovarian cancer

Study	Arms	Subjects	Optimal cytoreduction (≤1 cm residual tumor) (%)	Perioperative mortality (%)	Median progression-free survival (months)	Median overall survival (months)
Vergote (2010)						
	Primary surgery	336	42	2.5	12	29
	Neoadjuvant chemotherapy	334	81	0.7	12	30

2.3 Areas of Uncertainty

Despite the data describing the potential benefits of neoadjuvant chemotherapy for advanced stage ovarian cancer, the topic remains controversial [27–29]. A survey of gynecologic oncologists in the US found that most used neoadjuvant chemotherapy infrequently with the majority of participants reporting use in <10 % of cases. Further, the majority of respondents to the survey reported that they felt that the evidence supporting neoadjuvant chemotherapy was insufficient [27].

An important argument against the use of neoadjuvant chemotherapy stems from comparison of outcomes of patients treated with primary surgery [9]. Survival estimates of many observational studies as well as the randomized controlled trial of neoadjuvant therapy have been inferior to survival data reported for primary surgery documented from institutional series and cooperative group trials [9, 10, 30]. For example, the GOG recently reported data from a phase III trial of women with stage III and IV ovarian cancer randomized to intravenous or intraperitoneal platinum and taxane based chemotherapy. Median overall survival in this trial was 50 months for intravenous chemotherapy and 66 months for intraperitoneal treatment [10]. Survival estimates from this and other trials is substantially longer than reported for either the neoadjuvant (30 months) or primary surgery arms of the EORTC trial [10, 30, 31].

The relatively poor survival as well as low overall rate of optimal cytoreduction in the EORTC trial have raised the concern that the results of this data are not applicable to patients in the US who have access to gynecologic oncologists skilled in performance of aggressive cytoreductive surgery [29]. A single institution report identified patients who met the eligibility criteria for the EORTC trial and who underwent primary cytoreductive surgery. In this report, the median overall survival was 50 months, superior to the overall survival of both the neoadjuvant and primary surgery arms of the EORTC study [9, 31].

A major limitation of the currently available data is that many observational studies comparing the outcomes of primary surgery and neoadjuvant chemotherapy are limited by strong selection bias [7, 8, 21–25, 32, 33]. Patients with poor prognostic factors including advanced age, higher grade, and stage and more medical comorbidities are often preferentially treated with neoadjuvant chemotherapy. In addition, more subtle differences in patient characteristics such as the volume and distribution of tumor often influence decision making. Measurement of these more subtle factors is problematic not only in studies using administrative data, but also in studies that directly abstract data from medical records. The strong selection bias in treatment choice and comparison to highly selected patients enrolled in cooperative group trials and treated at tertiary centers may result in biased conclusions [26].

2.4 Areas of Future Study

Clearly, additional randomized controlled trials comparing primary cytoreduction and neoadjuvant chemotherapy with interval surgery would be of great value. Trials that compare outcomes at tertiary referral centers where patients are treated by high-volume gynecologic oncologists as well as trials in community settings would both be of utility. Ideally these studies would include both "favorable" prognosis patients with advanced stage disease as well as women with larger volume disease.

While randomized controlled trials in this setting would be of great utility, undertaking these trials is challenging. First, among gynecologic oncologists there is often a strong bias towards one treatment approach over another, potentially limiting referral to trials. Second, enrollment into clinical trials in which patients are randomized to either a surgical intervention or to a non-surgical alternative is often problematic. Lastly, ovarian cancer is often a disease that is treated over the course of many years. Initial surgery and chemotherapy, regardless of the sequence, is typically followed by multiple lines of cytotoxic chemotherapy and often secondary surgery for recurrent disease. Imbalances in downstream treatment often make interpretation of trials focused on initial therapy difficult [34].

Given the difficulty in performing prospective, randomized trials, there has been great interest in using observational data to explore primary treatment for ovarian cancer. Studies using observational in this setting are limited by both selection bias and the influence of multiple measured and unmeasured confounders that influence both treatment selection and outcomes. Recent studies attempted to overcome some of these limitations using statistically methodology such as propensity score matching and instrumental variable analysis to limit the influence of selection bias and confounding. One report examined treatment outcomes in over 9,500 women with advanced-stage ovarian cancer. Using traditional regression analysis, survival was inferior in women who received neoadjuvant chemotherapy. However, after leveraging geographic variation in treatment as an instrumental variable to limit the effects of unmeasured confounding, there was no statistically significant difference in survival between those who received neoadjuvant chemotherapy and those women treated with primary cytoreduction. Further, in this report of unselected patients the median survival for both groups was approximately 24 months, much lower than what has been reported from tertiary centers in the US [35].

Ultimately, better screening tests are needed for ovarian cancer to help reduce the burden of advanced-stage disease. For those women with advanced-stage tumors, newer therapeutic strategies may help prolong survival and increase the chance of cure. Further prospective clinical trials as well as novel methods of analyzing population-based data will help to shed light on how best to individualized the treatment of women with newly diagnosed, advanced stage tumors.

3 The Role of Lymphadenectomy in Endometrial Cancer

3.1 Background

Endometrial cancer is the most common gynecologic cancer in the United States. In 2014, it is estimated that 52,630 women will be diagnosed with the disease and 8,590 women will die from uterine cancer [36]. For the vast majority of women primary treatment entails surgery. Surgical management of endometrial cancer consists of hysterectomy and usually bilateral salpingo-oophorectomy [37]. Lymphadenectomy, or removal of the regional lymphatics, may be a part of the primary surgical effort as well. Hysterectomy for endometrial cancer can be performed via laparotomy, or, more recently using minimally invasive surgery with either laparoscopy or robotic assistance [38].

The surgical treatment of endometrial cancer has evolved over the last four decades. Historically, treatment for all women with endometrial cancer was initiated with intracavitary radiation [39]. Intracavitary radiation was most frequently administered using capsules loaded directly into the uterine cavity. Radiation was followed by hysterectomy. In the 1980s, treatment paradigms began to shift. In lieu of primary radiation, hysterectomy was often employed as initial therapy and followed by tailored, adjuvant radiotherapy. Lymphadenectomy was performed in some women to help guide adjuvant radiotherapy [39]. This treatment shift and the recognition of the role of lymphadenectomy in endometrial cancer was recognized in 1988 when a revised surgical staging system for endometrial cancer was introduced by the International Federation of Obstetrics and Gynecology [40].

A series of surgical pathology studies have demonstrated that women with high-risk uterine features including higher tumor grade, greater depth of myometrial invasion, and lymphvascular space invasion were at higher risk for nodal metastasis [41]. Further, these studies suggested that the presence of nodal metastases was among the strongest adverse predictors of survival in women with endometrial cancer [42]. The primary goal of lymphadenectomy is to identify occult metastatic disease to help guide adjuvant therapy. Women identified with metastatic disease could thus be triaged to adjuvant therapy in the form of chemotherapy and radiation and those women without nodal disease could forego additional therapy and its associated toxicity [43]. In addition to treatment planning, some studies have suggested that lymphadenectomy has a therapeutic role [44, 45]. The therapeutic role of lymphadenectomy may be the result of resection of microscopic nodal disease.

The potential benefits of lymphadenectomy are weighed against the increased operative time and morbidity associated with performance of the procedure. Currently, debate around lymphadenectomy centers on whether lymphadenectomy should be performed universally in all patients, or, whether the procedure should be performed selectively in high-risk patients or omitted entirely [46]. More recently, sentinel lymph node biopsy has been described for endometrial cancer [47].

3.2 Evidence

Observational studies have defined a strong rationale for performance of lymphadenectomy in women with apparent uterine-confined endometrial cancer. First, it is well accepted that the presence of nodal metastasis is highly prognostic for endometrial cancer. International data as well as studies from the National Cancer Database have suggested that survival for stage I–II endometrial cancer is >80 % but decreases to approximately 40–50 % in women with nodal disease [48–50]. Identification of occult nodal metastasis therefore provides important prognostic information for patients, and ideally would identify a subset of patients who could receive adjuvant therapy.

The argument for universal lymphadenectomy for endometrial cancer is further bolstered by the difficulty in accurately identifying women with nodal disease without pathologic assessment. The premise of selective lymphadenectomy relies on classification of patients based on preoperative and intraoperative factors into a high-risk group that would undergo lymphadenectomy and similarly, a population at low-risk for lymph node metastases that could safely forego lymphadenectomy [50]. Risk stratification relies on utilization of pathologic factors, most commonly tumor grade, depth of myometrial invasion, and size. Investigators from the Mayo Clinic have identified a subgroup of patients at very low-risk for lymph node metastasis. In a series of 328 patients with grade 1 or 2 endometrioid tumors, ≤2 cm in diameter and <50 % myometrial invasion, the rate of nodal metastasis was 5 % and 5-year survival was 97 % [51]. These criteria were further examined prospectively as well as through a multi-institutional evaluation that noted a negative predictive value of 98.2 % [52, 53].

Despite the high negative predictive value of utilizing preoperative and intraoperative assessment to stratify patients, concern has been raised that data available to surgeons at the time of decision making frequently changes after complete pathologic evaluation of the surgical specimens. For example, in the GOGs surgicopathology study, 20 % of tumors classified as grade 1 preoperatively were upgraded and frequently myoinvasive [41]. A prospective, blinded study of the accuracy of frozen section in women with endometrial cancer found an overall poor correlation between frozen section findings in the operating room and final pathology. These investigators noted that tumor grade at frozen section correlated with final pathology in only 58 % of cases while depth of invasion correlated in 67 % of patients. Overall, 28 % of patients were upstaged from the intraoperative assessment to final pathology [54]. Similarly, a report of 181 women with a diagnosis of grade 1 endometrial cancer who underwent staging lymphadenectomy found that 19 % of the neoplasms were upgraded, 18 % upstaged while adjuvant therapy was affected by the results of lymphadenectomy in 26 % of women [55]. Lastly, intraoperative gross inspection and palpation of the lymph nodes has very poor sensitivity in identifying nodal metastases [41]. Proponents of lymphadenectomy have argued that universal lymphadenectomy saves women from re-exploration when unexpected pathologic findings are noted postoperatively.

The theoretic benefit of lymphadenectomy is to identify women with positive nodes who can undergo adjuvant therapy and increase the chance of cure as well as to spare lower risk women potentially toxic therapy. This argument depends on two factors. First, there must be an effective treatment that improves survival for women with nodal metastasis. Second, a large portion of women without nodal metastases should be at low enough risk to be able to forego adjuvant therapy, or, alternatively, undergo a less toxic intervention than patients with nodal disease. Historically, pelvic radiotherapy was the treatment of choice for women with nodal disease from endometrial cancer. More recently, the GOG has demonstrated that combination chemotherapy is superior to radiation therapy [56]. In practice, multimodal therapy employing both chemotherapy and radiation is often utilized for women with node positive endometrial cancer [57].

Several observational reports have suggested that the results of lymphadenectomy are associated with decision making for adjuvant therapy [55, 58, 59]. An analysis of over 58,000 patients with stage I-II endometrioid adenocarcinomas in the Surveillance, Epidemiology, and End Results database noted that lymphadenectomy was performed in approximately 44 % of patients. Among low-risk women with tumors confined to the endometrium, performance of lymphadenectomy was not associated with patterns of adjuvant therapy. Among women with myoinvasive tumors, lymphadenectomy was associated with treatment with women who underwent lymphadenectomy being more likely to receive brachytherapy and those women who did not undergo lymphadenectomy more frequently receiving pelvic radiation. For example, among women <60 years of age with grade 2 tumors invading >50 % of the myometrium, whole pelvic radiation was used in 40 % of women who underwent lymphadenectomy versus 61 % of those who did not, while vaginal brachytherapy was used in 11 and 2 %, respectively [59]. Similarly, a single institution study of 95 patients found that 13 % of patients received extended field radiation due to para-aortic nodal disease while 52 % of patients had negative nodes and avoided treatment [58].

A fourth argument for the performance of universal lymphadenectomy stems from the potential therapeutic benefit of the procedure [44, 45, 60, 61]. The potential therapeutic benefit of lymphadenectomy for women with negative lymph nodes was first described by Kilgore and colleagues in 1995. In this report of 649 patients, there was a trend toward increased survival in women who underwent multi-site sampling [45]. A single institution analysis of 509 patients with endometrial cancer noted that removal of >11 nodes was associated with improved survival in women with grade 3 tumors, but node count had no impact on survival in those with grade 1 and 2 neoplasms [44]. Data on over 12,000 patients registered in the Surveillance, Epidemiology, and End Results database suggested that more extensive lymphadenectomy improved survival for intermediate and high-risk patients (<50 % myoinvasion and grade 3, > 50 % myoinvasionn, and stages II–IV). Lymph node count remained significant after adjustment for clinical and demographic variables as well as receipt of adjuvant radiotherapy [60]. In contrast, several retrospective reports have shown no association with lymphadenectomy and survival, particularly among low-risk patients [51, 62, 63].

Despite potential benefits in prognostication and treatment planning, the most important question is whether lymphadenectomy ultimately improves survival in women with apparent early-stage endometrial cancer. Two randomized controlled trials have now directly addressed this issue [64, 65] (Table 2). The first study examined 514 women with endometrial cancer apparently confined to the uterus. Patients were randomizedto either systematic pelvic lymphadenectomy or no lymphadenectomy. Removal of bulky lymph nodes was permitted in the no lymphadenectomy arm. Adjuvant therapy was based on the discretion of the treating clinician. The study was powered to detect an 8 % difference in 5-year survival. The median number of pelvic lymph nodes removed in the lymphadenectomy arm was 26, while 22 % of patients in the no lymphadenectomy arm had enlarged nodes and underwent resection. Only 14 % of the 56 patients with enlarged nodes in the no lymphadenectomy arm had metasatic disease. Choice of adjuvant therapy did not differ statistically between the two arms ($P = 0.07$). Early and late postoperative complications were more common in the lymphadenectomy arm. After a median follow-up of 49 months, the recurrence rate was 12.9 % in the lymphadenectomy arm versus 13.2 % in the no lymphadenectomy arm. Similarly, there was no difference in survival; 5-year overall survival was 86 % in the lymphadenectomy arm versus 90 % in the no lymphadenectomy arm ($P = 0.50$) [64].

A second RCT examining the role of lymphadenectomy, A Study in the Treatment of Endometrial Cancer (ASTEC), analyzed 1,408 women treated in 85 centers across 4 countries. ASTEC randomized women with apparent uterine confined disease to either lymphadenectomy or standard surgery without lymphadenectomy. Patients underwent a second randomization after surgery for adjuvant therapy. The study was powered to detect a 10 % improvement in 5-year survival. The median number of nodes removed in the standard surgery group was 12 while 5 % of women in the no lymphadenectomy arm had some nodal tissue removed. Operative time and complications were longer in the lymphadenectomy arm. 5-year recurrence-free survival was 79 % in the no lymphadenectomy arm versus 73 % in the lymphadenectomy arm while 5-year overall survival was 81 % in the no lymphadenectomy compared to 81 % in the no lymphadenectomy arm and 80 % in the lymphadenectomy cohort. The authors concluded that pelvic lymphadenectomy had no benefit on survival and should not be recommended outside of clinical trials [65].

3.3 Areas of Uncertainty and Future Study

Despite the publication of 2 randomized trials, the role of lymphadenectomy for early-stage endometrial cancer remains actively debated [43, 46, 66]. A number of methodologic concerns have been raised regarding the design of the two clinical trials. While both trials included quality control, neither trial required para-aortic

Table 2 Outcomes of randomized controlled trials of lymphadenectomy for endometrial cancer

Study	Arms	Subjects	Lymphadenectomy (median nodes removed)	Operating room time (median) (min)	Radiation received (%)	Recurrence (%)	5-year recurrence free survival (%)	5-year overall survival (%)
Benedetti Panici (2008)								
	No pelvic lymphadenectomy	264	22 %	120	25	13.2	82	90
	Pelvic lymphadenectomy	273	100 % (30)	180	17	12.9	81	86
ASTEC (2009)								
	No pelvic lymphadenectomy	704	5 %	60	33	Not reported	79	81
	Pelvic lymphadenectomy	704	92 % (12)	90	33	Not reported	73	80

lymphadenectomy and the node counts, particularly in ASTEC, were relatively low overall [43, 66]. There is growing recognition that isolated para-aortic node metastases are not infrequent among women with endometrial cancer [52]. Similarly, both trials included a relatively low-risk population in which the overall rates of lymph node metastases were low. While actively debated, it has been argued that any benefit of lymphadenectomy is more likely to be detected in a higher risk patient population. A decision analysis that reviewed many of the statistical assumptions of the 2 RCTs suggested that a survival difference of 10 % was only detectable if the rate of isolated pelvic nodal metastasis rose to 15 %. This analysis concluded that the populations studied in these trials rendered both studies underpowered to detect a difference in survival [43, 46].

Finally, neither trial had a standard protocol for adjuvant therapy and, as such, differences in outcome may be due not only to lymphadenectomy, but also to differences in postoperative treatment. This concern focuses not just on lymphadenectomy, but also on endometrial cancer in general where recommendations for adjuvant therapy are highly variable. Most women with advanced stage disease (including nodal metastasis) are treated with chemotherapy often combined with radiation [57]. However, there is now greater recognition that uterine factors may be nearly as important in prognosis as nodal disease [67, 68]. This awareness has led to increased use of chemotherapy, often combined with vaginal brachytherapy, for early-stage tumors [69]. If adjuvant therapy is similar for patients whether or not they undergo lymphadenectomy then any survival benefit for the procedure would require a benefit to the resection of microscopic metastatic disease. The changing patterns of adjuvant therapy may thus further confound trials of lymphadenectomy.

There is much debate about how to proceed to further study the role of lymph node dissection in apparent early-stage endometrial cancer. To achieve adequate power, it appears that analysis of a higher-risk patient population enriched for nodal metastasis will be required to achieve statistical significance [43, 46]. Future prospective trials will likely also need to include sentinel lymph node dissection, translational science endpoints and quality of life evaluations [43]. However, as has been pointed, using various treatment appropriations to endometrial cancer, 3-year survival rates range from 88 to 93 %. The overall favorable prognosis of the disease raises question as to the value of large scale, randomized trials in this scenario as these trials, even if designed optimally, would result in very small differences in survival [43, 46].

Given the difficulties in conducting large-scale randomized trials there is also clearly room for alternative study designs. Previous observational studies of endometrial cancer and lymphadenectomy are strongly influenced by selection bias and likely unmeasured confounding. Particularly as endometrial cancer patients are elderly and often have substantial comorbidity, a number of measured and unmeasured factors undoubtedly influence decision making and influence outcomes. Statistical analysis with newer methodology such as instrumental variable analysis may help mitigate some of these confounding factors. Large, population-based studies can not only analyze survival in real world populations but also assess the impact of lymphadenectomy on downstream decision making. Ultimately further work is needed to develop novel imaging strategies and biomarkers that can perhaps identify high-risk patients without the need for a surgical intervention such as lymphadenectomy [43].

4 Adjuvant Therapy for Ovarian Cancer

4.1 Background

At the time of diagnosis nearly three quarters of women with ovarian cancer present with advanced stage disease (stage III or IV). For these women, standard treatment entails either primary surgery or neoadjuvant chemotherapy. Surgery is typically followed by adjuvant chemotherapy.

The last three decades have seen significant improvement in the chemotherapeutic treatment options for women with ovarian cancer [10, 70–72]. In the 1970s and 1980s treatment often employed agents such as doxorubicin and cyclophosphomadie. In the 1980s platinum-analogue showed efficacy for ovarian cancer and are still considered the most active agents for the disease. A series of studies completed by the GOG in the United States and by cooperative groups throughout the world have explored the incorporation of a number of chemotherapeutic drugs, examined alternative strategies to administer these agents, and tested how novel biologic agents can be used for the treatment of ovarian cancer.

Despite the advances in the chemotherapeutic armamentarium for ovarian cancer, how to choose the best therapy for individual patients often remains elusive. Increased efficacy of chemotherapy is often accompanied by increased toxicity. A major challenges for oncologists is how to balance efficacy, toxicity, and quality of life in decision making.

4.2 Evidence

The standard of care for the adjuvant therapy of advanced stage ovarian cancer changed rapidly in the mid-1990s with presentation of data examining taxanes in the treatment of ovarian cancer. GOG protocol 111 randomized 386 women who underwent suboptimal tumor cytoreduction (>1 cm residual tumor) to 6 cycles of chemotherapy with either cyclophosphamide and cisplatin or cisplatin and paclitaxel (Table 3). The overall response rate was 60 % in the cisplatin/cyclophosphamide group compared to 73 % in the cisplatin/paclitaxel arm. With a median follow-up of 37 months, the median progression free survival in was 13 months in cisplatin/cyclophosphamide arm compared to 18 months in the cispltain/paclitaxel arm ($P < 0.0001$). Median overall survival was 24 versus 38 months, respectively [72]. A similar, confirmatory trial (OV10) was conducted by investigators in Europe and Canada to compare cisplatin/cyclophosphamide to cisplatin/paclitaxel.

In this analysis of 680 patients the response rate as well as progression-free and overall survival were superior in the paclitaxel-treated patients [73].

Subsequent work by the GOG was focused on reducing the toxicity and enhancing convenience of platinum and taxane based therapy. GOG protocol 158 randomized 792 patients to treatment with either cisplatin and paclitaxel or carboplatin and paclitaxel. The study followed a non-inferiority design and found that the carboplatin/paclitaxel combination was less toxic, easier to administer, and not inferior to the cisplatin-containing doublet. With these findings the combination of carboplatin and paclitaxel has remained the most frequently used regimen for ovarian cancer [30]. Subsequent modifications of the carboplatin/paclitaxel backbone for ovarian cancer focused on adding additional cytotoxic agents to upfront therapy. An international trial of over 4,300 women led by the GOG (protocol 182) randomized patients to carboplatin and paclitaxel with some combination of gemcitabine, liposomal doxorubicin, or topotecan given either as triplets or sequential doublets. The final analysis revealed no difference in survival for any of the combinations [74].

While the addition of additional cytotoxic agents to initial therapy appears to be of little value, there has been great interest in alternate ways to deliver cytotoxic chemotherapy. Intraperitoneal chemotherapy allows the administration of chemotherapy directly into the abdominal cavity. Given that ovarian cancer predominately spreads within the peritoneal cavity, there is a strong rationale for this method of delivery. Numerous preclinical studies have demonstrated that intraperitoneal administration of chemotherapy results in a higher cellular concentration of a number of agents. Similarly, the feasibility of intraperitoneal chemotherapy has been shown in a number of phase II and phase III trials [10, 75, 76].

One of the first large randomized trials of intraperitoneal chemotherapy was reported by the Southwest Oncology Group (SWOG) in 1996. In this randomized controlled trial, 654 patients with optimally cytoreduced ovarian cancer were randomized to intravenous cyclophosphamide and cisplatin or an experimental regimen of intravenous cyclophosphamide with intraperitoneal cisplatin. The intraperitoneal chemotherapy arm was associated with an 8 month improvement in overall survival (49 vs. 41 months) [75]. Despite the survival benefit demonstrated with intraperitoneal chemotherapy, there was little attention to this method of treatment delivery until the publication of GOG protocol 172 in 2006. In this protocol, 429 women with optimally cytoreduced ovarian cancer were randomized to intravenous cisplatin and paclitaxel or an experimental arm of intravenous paclitaxel on day 1, intraperitoneal cisplatin on day 2 and intraperitioneal paclitaxel on day 8 (intraperitoneal arm). Intraperitoneal chemotherapy was associated with an improvement in both progression-free (24 vs. 18 months) and overall (66 vs. 50 months) survival. The improved survival was however, accompanied by greater toxicity. Within the cohort of women who received intraperitoneal chemotherapy, only 42 % were able to complete all 6 intraperitoneal cycles. Grade 3–4 myosuppression, renal, neurologic, infectious, metabolic and hepatic toxicity as well as fatigue and metabolic events were all more frequent in the intraperitoneal chemotherapy arm. While quality of life was worse during treatment for those women in

Table 3 Sentinel studies of adjuvant therapy for advanced stage ovarian cancer

Study	Arms	Subjects	Completed all scheduled therapy (%)	Response rate (%)	Median progression-free survival (months)	Median overall survival (months)
GOG 111 (1996)						
	Cisplatin and cyclophosphamide	202	78	60	13	24
	Cisplatin and paclitaxel	184	87	73	18	38
OV10 (2000)						
	Cisplatin and cyclophosphamide	338	–	45	12	26
	Cisplatin and paclitaxel	342	–	58	16	36
GOG 158 (2003)						
	Cisplatin and paclitaxel	400	85	–	19	49
	Carboplatin and paclitaxel	392	87	–	22	57
GOG 172 (2006)						
	Intravenous cisplatin and paclitaxel	210	90	–	18	50
	Intraperitoneal cisplatin and paclitaxel	205	42 (intraperitoneal)	–	24	66
GOG 218 (2011)						
	Carboplatin and paclitaxel	625	16	–	10	39
	Carboplatin and paclitaxel and bevacizumab	625	17	–	11	39
	Carboplatin and paclitaxel and prolonged bevacizumab	623	24	–	14	40
JGOG 3016 (2009)						
	Carboplatin and paclitaxel every 3 weeks	320	73	–	18	62
	Carboplatin and dose dense paclitaxel	317	62	–	28	101

the intraperitoneal therapy arm, there was no difference in quality of life 1 year after treatment [10].

There has also been interest in incorporating novel, molecularly targeted agents into the upfront treatment of ovarian cancer. To date, the greatest interest has focused on bevacizumab, a humanized anti-vascular endothelial growth factor [71]. GOG protocol 218 randomized 1,873 women with incompletely resected stage III and IV ovarian cancer to chemotherapy with carboplatin and paclitaxel to three arms: placebo, bevacizumab for 6 cycles or bevacizumab during chemotherapy and as consolidation therapy for a total of 22 cycles. The median progression-free survival was 10.3 months in the control grouop, 11.2 in the bevacizumab during chemotherapy arm and 14.1 in the prolonged bevacizumab arm. PFS was statistically significantly longer in the prolonged bevacizumab arm compared to the control arm. Median overall survival was 39.3, 38.7, and 39.7 months respectively [71]. A second study of bevacizumab reported similar results; bevacizumab was associated with improved progression-free survival [70]. The benefits were greatest in patients at highest risk for recurrence.

Lastly, as an alternative to delivery of the maximum tolerated dose of intravenous chemotherapy, recently studies have explored combinations using more frequent, lower doses of these agents (dose dense chemotherapy). The Japanese Gynecologic Oncology reported long-term results of a dose dense chemotherapy regimen for adjuvant therapy (JGOG protocol 3016). In this study, 631 women with stage II-IV ovarian cancer were randomly assigned to carboplatin and paclitaxel every weeks or to carboplatin on day 1 and paclitaxel on days 1, 8 and 15 of a 3 week cycle. With a median follow-up of 77 months, the investigators found an improvement in both progression free (28 months vs. 17 months) and overall (101 months vs. 62 months) survival for women who received dose dense treatment. The improvement in survival was most pronounced in those women with suboptimally cytoreduced tumors. Grade 3–4 anemia was more common in the dose dense group, but both regimens were relatively well tolerated [77, 78].

4.3 Areas of Uncertainty and Future Study

Data from a variety of sources and using a number of study designs can help inform the debate regarding the best adjuvant therapy for advanced stage ovarian cancer. Currently, standard therapy remains carboplatin and paclitaxel administered every 3 weeks. Intraperitoneal chemotherapy has been consistently associated with improved overall survival but also accompanied by substantial toxicity [10]. The addition of bevacizumab appears to improve progression-free survival, particularly if administered for a prolonged course, but this therapy has not resulted in improved overall survival, is associated with added toxicity and substantial cost [70, 71]. Finally, dose dense paclitaxel resulted in impressive survival improvements but this data is based on one study outside of the United States [77, 78].

To help tailor a number of prospective, phase III trials are currently underway. Many of these studies are cooperative group trials and are comparing strategies of standard intravenous chemotherapy, dose dense chemotherapy, intraperitoneal chemotherapy and bevacizumab in various combinations. Many of these trials are also focused on developing less toxic regimens to enhance the therapeutic profile and minimize impact on quality of life.

While randomized controlled trials are optimal for minimizing bias, a major concern is that these trials often lack generalizability to "real world" populations. Particularly in the cooperative group setting, trial inclusion criteria are often extensive with exclusion of elderly patients and those with comorbid medical conditions. While RCTs maximize precision, the results may not be directly applicable to the daily practice of oncology. A recent analysis compared eligibility and outcomes of patients treated on 21 SWOG trials to non-trial participants from throughout the United States captured through analysis of SEER. The analysis noted that trial participants were significantly younger than non-trial participants with similar tumors. Among 11 good-prognosis studies trial participation was not associated with survival. However, among 10 poor-prognosis studies survival was better in trial participants. The impact of trial participation was predominately noted in the first year after treatment likely due to the exclusion of patients with comorbidity [79].

To help design treatment strategies for real world populations, observational data and comparative effectiveness studies are of great utility [80]. Unlike randomized trials, these studies can show actual treatment trends in community practice and examine risks and benefits in specific patient populations or groups of subjects with particular characteristics. A major limitation of observational data is confounding, both measured and unmeasured. Newer methodology to help limit this bias is now more commonly employed for oncology studies [81–83].

In oncology there is now a greater focus on quality of life. One aspect of measuring quality of life is specifically examining outcomes that matter to patients. While patient-reported outcomes (PROs) are now being more frequently described, many oncology trials are still designed with insufficient focus on PROs. A recent systematic review examined PROs in randomized trials of brain tumors. Among 14 RCTs including over 3,000 patients, only 2 studies incorporated PROs that sufficiently satisfied methodologic criteria to provide high-quality PROs [84]. Use of PROs in gynecologic oncology remains in its infancy and clearly this will be a focus of study over the next decade.

Finally, there is growing concern about the cost of incorporating new therapeutic agents into the treatment regimens. In particular, controversy has surrounded use of bevacizumab for solid tumors [85, 86]. In a cost-effectiveness analysis of treatment strategies using bevacizumab for ovarian cancer based on the results of GOG 218, the costs of treatment for patients on each arm were approximately $2.5 million for carboplatin/paclitaxel, $21.4 million for carboplatin/paclitaxel and initial bevacizumab and $78.3 million for carboplatin, paclitaxel and extended bevacizumab. This translated into an incremental cost-effectiveness ratio of $479,712 per progression-free life-year saved for initial bevacizumab and $401,088 per progression-free life-year saved for prolonged bevacizumab [85]. These studies highlight the difficulty in utilizing costly new drugs of uncertain value. Clearly moving forward with cost constraints on oncology, decision analyses and cost effectiveness studies will play an important role in helping to shape public policy for the treatment of gynecologic malignancies (Tables 1, 2 and 3).

References

1. Bristow RE, Tomacruz RS, Armstrong DK, Trimble EL, Montz FJ (2002) Survival effect of maximal cytoreductive surgery for advanced ovarian carcinoma during the platinum era: a meta-analysis. J Clin Oncol 20:1248–1259
2. Hoskins WJ, McGuire WP, Brady MF et al (1994) The effect of diameter of largest residual disease on survival after primary cytoreductive surgery in patients with suboptimal residual epithelial ovarian carcinoma. Am J Obstet Gynecol 170:974–980; discussion 9-80
3. Wright JD, Lewin SN, Deutsch I et al (2011) Defining the limits of radical cytoreductive surgery for ovarian cancer. Gynecol Oncol 123:467–473
4. Gerestein CG, Damhuis RA, Burger CW, Kooi GS (2009) Postoperative mortality after primary cytoreductive surgery for advanced stage epithelial ovarian cancer: a systematic review. Gynecol Oncol 114:523–527
5. Wright JD, Herzog TJ, Neugut AI et al (2012) Effect of radical cytoreductive surgery on omission and delay of chemotherapy for advanced-stage ovarian cancer. Obstet Gynecol 120:871–881
6. Wright J, Doan T, McBride R, Jacobson J, Hershman D (2008) Variability in chemotherapy delivery for elderly women with advanced stage ovarian cancer and its impact on survival. Br J Cancer 98:1197–1203
7. Everett EN, French AE, Stone RL et al (2006) Initial chemotherapy followed by surgical cytoreduction for the treatment of stage III/IV epithelial ovarian cancer. Am J Obstet Gynecol 195:568–574; discussion 74-6
8. Hou JY, Kelly MG, Yu H et al (2007) Neoadjuvant chemotherapy lessens surgical morbidity in advanced ovarian cancer and leads to improved survival in stage IV disease. Gynecol Oncol 105:211–217
9. Chi DS, Musa F, Dao F et al (2012) An analysis of patients with bulky advanced stage ovarian, tubal, and peritoneal carcinoma treated with primary debulking surgery (PDS) during an identical time period as the randomized EORTC-NCIC trial of PDS versus neoadjuvant chemotherapy (NACT). Gynecol Oncol 124:10–14
10. Armstrong DK, Bundy B, Wenzel L et al (2006) Intraperitoneal cisplatin and paclitaxel in ovarian cancer. N Engl J Med 354:34–43
11. Griffiths CT (1975) Surgical resection of tumor bulk in the primary treatment of ovarian carcinoma. Natl Cancer Inst Monogr 42:101–104
12. Hoskins WJ (1994) Epithelial ovarian carcinoma: principles of primary surgery. Gynecol Oncol 55:S91–S96
13. Aletti GD, Dowdy SC, Gostout BS et al (2006) Aggressive surgical effort and improved survival in advanced-stage ovarian cancer. Obstet Gynecol 107:77–85
14. Chi DS, Eisenhauer EL, Lang J et al (2006) What is the optimal goal of primary cytoreductive surgery for bulky stage IIIC epithelial ovarian carcinoma (EOC)? Gynecol Oncol 103:559–564
15. Chi DS, Eisenhauer EL, Zivanovic O et al (2009) Improved progression-free and overall survival in advanced ovarian cancer as a result of a change in surgical paradigm. Gynecol Oncol 114:26–31
16. Chi DS, Franklin CC, Levine DA et al (2004) Improved optimal cytoreduction rates for stages IIIC and IV epithelial ovarian, fallopian tube, and primary peritoneal cancer: a change in surgical approach. Gynecol Oncol 94:650–654

17. Chi DS, Liao JB, Leon LF et al (2001) Identification of prognostic factors in advanced epithelial ovarian carcinoma. Gynecol Oncol 82:532–537
18. Eisenkop SM, Friedman RL, Wang HJ (1998) Complete cytoreductive surgery is feasible and maximizes survival in patients with advanced epithelial ovarian cancer: a prospective study. Gynecol Oncol 69:103–108
19. Aletti GD, Eisenhauer EL, Santillan A et al (2011) Identification of patient groups at highest risk from traditional approach to ovarian cancer treatment. Gynecol Oncol 120:23–28
20. Gerestein CG (2010) Nieuwenhuyzen-de Boer GM, Eijkemans MJ, Kooi GS, Burger CW. Prediction of 30-day morbidity after primary cytoreductive surgery for advanced stage ovarian cancer. Eur J Cancer 46:102–109
21. Inciura A, Simavicius A, Juozaityte E et al (2006) Comparison of adjuvant and neoadjuvant chemotherapy in the management of advanced ovarian cancer: a retrospective study of 574 patients. BMC Cancer 6:153
22. Kang S, Nam BH (2009) Does neoadjuvant chemotherapy increase optimal cytoreduction rate in advanced ovarian cancer? Meta-analysis of 21 studies. Ann Surg Oncol 16:2315–2320
23. Morice P, Dubernard G, Rey A et al (2003) Results of interval debulking surgery compared with primary debulking surgery in advanced stage ovarian cancer. J Am Coll Surg 197:955–963
24. Morrison J, Haldar K, Kehoe S, Lawrie TA (2012) Chemotherapy versus surgery for initial treatment in advanced ovarian epithelial cancer. Cochrane Database Syst Rev 8:CD005343
25. Schwartz PE, Rutherford TJ, Chambers JT, Kohorn EI, Thiel RP (1999) Neoadjuvant chemotherapy for advanced ovarian cancer: long-term survival. Gynecol Oncol 72:93–99
26. Vergote I, Leunen K, Amant F (2012) Primary surgery or neoadjuvant chemotherapy in ovarian cancer: what is the value of comparing apples with oranges? Gynecol Oncol 124:1–2
27. Dewdney SB, Rimel BJ, Reinhart AJ et al (2010) The role of neoadjuvant chemotherapy in the management of patients with advanced stage ovarian cancer: survey results from members of the society of gynecologic oncologists. Gynecol Oncol 119:18–21
28. Vergote I, Amant F, Leunen K (2010) Neoadjuvant chemotherapy in advanced ovarian cancer: what kind of evidence is needed to convince US gynaecological oncologists? Gynecol Oncol 119:1–2
29. Chi DS, Bristow RE, Armstrong DK, Karlan BY (2011) Is the easier way ever the better way? J Clin Oncol 29:4073–4075
30. Ozols RF, Bundy BN, Greer BE et al (2003) Phase III trial of carboplatin and paclitaxel compared with cisplatin and paclitaxel in patients with optimally resected stage III ovarian cancer: a gynecologic oncology group study. J Clin Oncol 21:3194–3200
31. Vergote I, Trope CG, Amant F et al (2010) Neoadjuvant chemotherapy or primary surgery in stage IIIC or IV ovarian cancer. N Engl J Med 363:943–953
32. Bristow RE, Eisenhauer EL, Santillan A, Chi DS (2007) Delaying the primary surgical effort for advanced ovarian cancer: a systematic review of neoadjuvant chemotherapy and interval cytoreduction. Gynecol Oncol 104:480–490
33. Vergote I, Trope CG, Amant F, Ehlen T, Reed NS, Casado A (2011) Neoadjuvant chemotherapy is the better treatment option in some patients with stage IIIc–IV ovarian cancer. J Clin Oncol 29:4076–4078
34. Herzog TJ, Armstrong DK, Brady MF et al (2014) Ovarian cancer clinical trial endpoints: society of gynecologic oncology white paper. Gynecol Oncol 132:8–17
35. Wright JD, Ananth CV, Tsui J et al (2014) Comparative effectiveness of upfront treatment strategies in elderly women with ovarian cancer. Cancer 120:1246–1254
36. Siegel R, Ma J, Zou Z, Jemal A (2014) Cancer statistics, 2014. CA Cancer J Clin 64:9–29
37. Wright JD, Buck AM, Shah M, Burke WM, Schiff PB, Herzog TJ (2009) Safety of ovarian preservation in premenopausal women with endometrial cancer. J Clin Oncol 27:1214–1219
38. Wright JD, Burke WM, Wilde ET et al (2012) Comparative effectiveness of robotic versus laparoscopic hysterectomy for endometrial cancer. J Clin Oncol 30:783–791

39. Wright JD, Medel NIB, Sehouli J, Fujiwara K, Herzog TJ (2012) Contemporary management of endometrial cancer. Lancet 379:1352–1360
40. Creasman W (2009) Revised FIGO staging for carcinoma of the endometrium. Int J Gynaecol Obstet 105:109
41. Creasman WT, Morrow CP, Bundy BN, Homesley HD, Graham JE, Heller PB (1987) Surgical pathologic spread patterns of endometrial cancer: a gynecologic oncology group study. Cancer 60:2035–2041
42. Morrow CP, Bundy BN, Kurman RJ et al (1991) Relationship between surgical-pathological risk factors and outcome in clinical stage I and II carcinoma of the endometrium: a Gynecologic Oncology Group study. Gynecol Oncol 40:55–65
43. McMeekin DS (2012) Designing the next lymphadenectomy trial: what should we learn for our prior experiences. Gynecol Oncol 126:1–2
44. Cragun JM, Havrilesky LJ, Calingaert B et al (2005) Retrospective analysis of selective lymphadenectomy in apparent early-stage endometrial cancer. J Clin Oncol 23:3668–3675
45. Kilgore LC, Partridge EE, Alvarez RD et al (1995) Adenocarcinoma of the endometrium: survival comparisons of patients with and without pelvic node sampling. Gynecol Oncol 56:29–33
46. Naumann RW (2012) The role of lymphadenectomy in endometrial cancer: was the ASTEC trial doomed by design and are we destined to repeat that mistake? Gynecol Oncol 126:5–11
47. Khoury-Collado F, Murray MP, Hensley ML et al (2011) Sentinel lymph node mapping for endometrial cancer improves the detection of metastatic disease to regional lymph nodes. Gynecol Oncol 122:251–254
48. Creasman WT, Odicino F, Maisonneuve P et al (2003) Carcinoma of the corpus uteri. Int J Gynaecol Obstet 83(Suppl 1):79–118
49. Partridge EE, Shingleton HM, Menck HR (1996) The national cancer data base report on endometrial cancer. J Surg Oncol 61:111–123
50. Chan JK, Kapp DS (2007) Role of complete lymphadenectomy in endometrioid uterine cancer. Lancet Oncol 8:831–841
51. Mariani A, Webb MJ, Keeney GL, Haddock MG, Calori G, Podratz KC (2000) Low-risk corpus cancer: is lymphadenectomy or radiotherapy necessary? Am J Obstet Gynecol 182:1506–1519
52. Mariani A, Dowdy SC, Cliby WA et al (2008) Prospective assessment of lymphatic dissemination in endometrial cancer: a paradigm shift in surgical staging. Gynecol Oncol 109:11–18
53. Convery PA, Cantrell LA, Di Santo N et al (2011) Retrospective review of an intraoperative algorithm to predict lymph node metastasis in low-grade endometrial adenocarcinoma. Gynecol Oncol 123:65–70
54. Case AS, Rocconi RP, Straughn JM Jr et al (2006) A prospective blinded evaluation of the accuracy of frozen section for the surgical management of endometrial cancer. Obstet Gynecol 108:1375–1379
55. Ben-Shachar I, Pavelka J, Cohn DE et al (2005) Surgical staging for patients presenting with grade 1 endometrial carcinoma. Obstet Gynecol 105:487–493
56. Randall ME, Filiaci VL, Muss H et al (2006) Randomized phase III trial of whole-abdominal irradiation versus doxorubicin and cisplatin chemotherapy in advanced endometrial carcinoma: a gynecologic oncology group study. J Clin Oncol 24:36–44
57. Secord AA, Havrilesky LJ, O'Malley DM et al (2009) A multicenter evaluation of sequential multimodality therapy and clinical outcome for the treatment of advanced endometrial cancer. Gynecol Oncol 114:442–447
58. Lo KW, Cheung TH, Yu MY, Yim SF, Chung TK (2003) The value of pelvic and para-aortic lymphadenectomy in endometrial cancer to avoid unnecessary radiotherapy. Int J Gynecol Cancer 13:863–869
59. Sharma C, Deutsch I, Lewin SN et al (2011) Lymphadenectomy influences the utilization of adjuvant radiation treatment for endometrial cancer. Am J Obstet Gynecol 205(562):e1–e9

60. Chan JK, Cheung MK, Huh WK et al (2006) Therapeutic role of lymph node resection in endometrioid corpus cancer: a study of 12,333 patients. Cancer 107:1823–1830
61. Mohan DS, Samuels MA, Selim MA et al (1998) Long-term outcomes of therapeutic pelvic lymphadenectomy for stage I endometrial adenocarcinoma. Gynecol Oncol 70:165–171
62. Carey MS, O'Connell GJ, Johanson CR et al (1995) Good outcome associated with a standardized treatment protocol using selective postoperative radiation in patients with clinical stage I adenocarcinoma of the endometrium. Gynecol Oncol 57:138–144
63. Eltabbakh GH, Piver MS, Hempling RE, Shin KH (1997) Excellent long-term survival and absence of vaginal recurrences in 332 patients with low-risk stage I endometrial adenocarcinoma treated with hysterectomy and vaginal brachytherapy without formal staging lymph node sampling: report of a prospective trial. Int J Radiat Oncol Biol Phys 38:373–380
64. Panici PB, Basile S, Maneschi F et al (2008) Systematic pelvic lymphadenectomy vs. no lymphadenectomy in early-stage endometrial carcinoma: randomized clinical trial. J Natl Cancer Inst 100:1707–1716
65. Kitchener H, Swart AM, Qian Q, Amos C, Parmar MK (2009) Efficacy of systematic pelvic lymphadenectomy in endometrial cancer (MRC ASTEC trial): a randomised study. Lancet 373:125–136
66. Creasman WT, Mutch DE, Herzog TJ (2010) ASTEC lymphadenectomy and radiation therapy studies: are conclusions valid? Gynecol Oncol 116:293–294
67. Kwon JS, Qiu F, Saskin R, Carey MS (2009) Are uterine risk factors more important than nodal status in predicting survival in endometrial cancer? Obstet Gynecol 114:736–743
68. Medel NIB, Herzog TJ, Deutsch I et al (2011) Comparison of the prognostic significance of uterine factors and nodal status for endometrial cancer. Am J Obstet Gynecol 204:248 e1–e7
69. Susumu N, Sagae S, Udagawa Y et al (2008) Randomized phase III trial of pelvic radiotherapy versus cisplatin-based combined chemotherapy in patients with intermediate- and high-risk endometrial cancer: a Japanese gynecologic oncology group study. Gynecol Oncol 108:226–233
70. Perren TJ, Swart AM, Pfisterer J et al (2011) A phase 3 trial of bevacizumab in ovarian cancer. N Engl J Med 365:2484–2496
71. Burger RA, Brady MF, Bookman MA et al (2011) Incorporation of bevacizumab in the primary treatment of ovarian cancer. N Engl J Med 365:2473–2483
72. McGuire WP, Hoskins WJ, Brady MF et al (1996) Cyclophosphamide and cisplatin compared with paclitaxel and cisplatin in patients with stage III and stage IV ovarian cancer. N Engl J Med 334:1–6
73. Piccart MJ, Bertelsen K, James K et al (2000) Randomized intergroup trial of cisplatin-paclitaxel versus cisplatin-cyclophosphamide in women with advanced epithelial ovarian cancer: three-year results. J Natl Cancer Inst 92:699–708
74. Bookman MA, Brady MF, McGuire WP et al (2009) Evaluation of new platinum-based treatment regimens in advanced-stage ovarian cancer: a phase III trial of the gynecologic cancer intergroup. J Clin Oncol 27:1419–1425
75. Alberts DS, Liu PY, Hannigan EV et al (1996) Intraperitoneal cisplatin plus intravenous cyclophosphamide versus intravenous cisplatin plus intravenous cyclophosphamide for stage III ovarian cancer. N Engl J Med 335:1950–1955
76. Markman M, Bundy BN, Alberts DS et al (2001) Phase III trial of standard-dose intravenous cisplatin plus paclitaxel versus moderately high-dose carboplatin followed by intravenous paclitaxel and intraperitoneal cisplatin in small-volume stage III ovarian carcinoma: an intergroup study of the Gynecologic Oncology Group, Southwestern Oncology Group, and Eastern Cooperative Oncology Group. J Clin Oncol 19:1001–1007
77. Katsumata N, Yasuda M, Isonishi S et al (2013) Long-term results of dose-dense paclitaxel and carboplatin versus conventional paclitaxel and carboplatin for treatment of advanced epithelial ovarian, fallopian tube, or primary peritoneal cancer (JGOG 3016): a randomised, controlled, open-label trial. Lancet Oncol 14:1020–1026

78. Katsumata N, Yasuda M, Takahashi F et al (2009) Dose-dense paclitaxel once a week in combination with carboplatin every 3 weeks for advanced ovarian cancer: a phase 3, open-label, randomised controlled trial. Lancet 374:1331–1338
79. Unger JM, Barlow WE, Martin DP et al (2014) Comparison of survival outcomes among cancer patients treated in and out of clinical trials. J Natl Cancer Inst 106:dju002
80. Hershman DL, Wright JD (2012) Comparative effectiveness research in oncology methodology: observational data. J Clin Oncol 30:4215–4222
81. Stukel TA, Fisher ES, Wennberg DE, Alter DA, Gottlieb DJ, Vermeulen MJ (2007) Analysis of observational studies in the presence of treatment selection bias: effects of invasive cardiac management on AMI survival using propensity score and instrumental variable methods. JAMA 297:278–285
82. Earle CC, Tsai JS, Gelber RD, Weinstein MC, Neumann PJ, Weeks JC (2001) Effectiveness of chemotherapy for advanced lung cancer in the elderly: instrumental variable and propensity analysis. J Clin Oncol 19:1064–1070
83. Hadley J, Yabroff KR, Barrett MJ, Penson DF, Saigal CS, Potosky AL (2010) Comparative effectiveness of prostate cancer treatments: evaluating statistical adjustments for confounding in observational data. J Natl Cancer Inst 102:1780–1793
84. Dirven L, Taphoorn MJ, Reijneveld JC et al (2014) The level of patient-reported outcome reporting in randomised controlled trials of brain tumour patients: a systematic review. Eur J Cancer 50(14):2432–2448
85. Cohn DE, Kim KH, Resnick KE, O'Malley DM, Straughn JM Jr (2011) At what cost does a potential survival advantage of bevacizumab make sense for the primary treatment of ovarian cancer? A cost-effectiveness analysis. J Clin Oncol 29:1247–1251
86. Dawood S, Shaikh AJ, Buchholz TA et al (2012) The use of bevacizumab among women with metastatic breast cancer: a survey on clinical practice and the ongoing controversy. Cancer 118:2780–2786

MIX
Papier aus verantwortungsvollen Quellen
Paper from responsible sources
FSC® C105338

If you have any concerns about our products,
you can contact us on
ProductSafety@springernature.com

In case Publisher is established outside the EU,
the EU authorized representative is:
Springer Nature Customer Service Center GmbH
Europaplatz 3, 69115 Heidelberg, Germany

Printed by Libri Plureos GmbH
in Hamburg, Germany